Endorsements by Health Equity Leaders

As we like to say at the Satcher Health Leadership Institute, many Black women have risen to positions of leadership because they cared enough, they knew enough, they had the courage to do enough, and they persevered until the job was done.

To those Black women, we owe a sincere debt of gratitude.

—David Satcher, MD, PhD, Four-Star Admiral for the US Public Health Service, 16th US Surgeon General

A remarkable journey that transports us from the consequential realities of health disparities to the optimism of seeking and finding healing health—collectively and individually. Black women who read this book will find themselves powerfully represented within. The beauty of this narrative is its potential to inspire, captivate, and motivate all.

—Joan Y. Reede, MD, MPH, MBA, Professor and Dean for Diversity and Community Partnership, Harvard University

Black Women and Resilience is a powerful exposé on the health and well-being of Black women by Black women scholars. It is a solid contribution to the field of women's health and important reading for all interested in understanding and improving the health status of Black women.

—Georges Benjamin, MD, Executive Director, American Public Health Association

Black Women and Resilience provides a glimpse of the magnetic richness of Black women striving for ideal health. I applaud Drs. Holden and Jones for delineating an examination of complex systemic issues, demarcating some of the contributors to political determinants of health, and identifying approaches to help strengthen community health.

—Daniel Dawes, JD, Executive Director, Satcher Health Leadership Institute, Morehouse School of Medicine

This exceptional book is a rich compilation of thought leadership that offers the reader intersectional angles about Black women in the pursuit of optimal health and wellness. It weaves together a tapestry of cultural experiences that engender resilience and addresses significant issues that are relevant to public health within diverse communities.

—Beverly Daniel Tatum, PhD, President Emerita, Spelman College

Praise is warranted for this amazing volume of narrative which chronicles the multifaceted intricacies of Black women's health. It is imperative that diverse leaders in our nation prioritize use of a lifespan developmental approach to understanding aspects of women's health. Support of efforts for innovative interventions and prevention strategies are essential for improving population health.

—Vivian Pinn, MD, Senior Scientist Emerita, Fogarty International Center, Founder and Inaugural Director, Office of Research on Women's Health, National Institutes of Health

Black Women and Resilience

SUNY Series in Black Women's Wellness
Stephanie Y. Evans, editor

Black Women and Resilience
Power, Perseverance, and Public Health

Edited by
Kisha Braithwaite Holden
and Camara Phyllis Jones

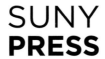

Cover Art: "Memories Like Mountains," Brandie Adams-Piphus.

© 2024 State University of New York

All rights reserved

Printed in the United States of America

No part of this book may be used or reproduced in any manner whatsoever without written permission. No part of this book may be stored in a retrieval system or transmitted in any form or by any means including electronic, electrostatic, magnetic tape, mechanical, photocopying, recording, or otherwise without the prior permission in writing of the publisher.

For information, contact State University of New York Press, Albany, NY www.sunypress.edu

Library of Congress Cataloging-in-Publication Data

Names: Holden, Kisha Braithwaite, editor. | Jones, Camara Phyllis, editor.
Title: Black women and resilience : power, perseverance, and public health / [edited by] Kisha Braithwaite Holden and Camara Phyllis Jones.
Description: Albany, NY : State University of New York Press, [2024] | Series: SUNY series in black women's wellness | Includes bibliographical references and index.
Identifiers: LCCN 2022053659 | ISBN 9781438494234 (hardcover : alk. paper) | ISBN 9781438494241 (ebook) | ISBN 9781438494227 (pbk. : alk. paper)
Subjects: LCSH: African American women—Social conditions. | Women, Black—United States—Social conditions. | Resilience (Personality trait)—United States. | Perseverance (Ethics) | Health services accessibility—United States. | Public health—United States.
Classification: LCC HQ1163 .B56 2023 | DDC 305.48/896073—dc23/eng/20230126
LC record available at https://lccn.loc.gov/2022053659

10 9 8 7 6 5 4 3 2 1

About the Cover Art

The cover art, the description, and the poem below, "Memories Like Mountains," were conceptualized by Brandie Adams-Piphus, a remarkable Black woman artist. The artistic expression is about

> transcending past negative memories and traumas. You must confront them again and again until you have risen above them. This piece is a figurative exploration of this process. The subject is one with the mountains (her memories) because often our past memories are interwoven with our identity. We may partly choose to define ourselves by our past hurts and pain. The mountains are shown as inside the subject's head to symbolize memories, which often are like mountainous terrain with many different layers and inclines. The color is returning to her as she reaches the top of the mountain to illustrate her transformation and ascension over her past.

Memories, like mountains,
With their winding paths and steep inclines,
Must be scaled
Again, and again.
Until you reach the top.

Kisha Braithwaite Holden

In memoriam of my beloved mother, guardian angel, and queen, Mrs. Judy Moore Braithwaite, and my exquisite grandmother Mrs. Mittie Elizabeth Kellum Moore. They both inspired me and gingerly taught me to truly trust and believe in myself through being intuitive, inquisitive, insightful, inventive, imaginative; and demonstrating integrity.

To my extraordinary bonus/stepdaughter Michele and impeccable bonus daughter-niece Myla for cultivating indelible footprints of excellence as burgeoning young scholars.

Camara Phyllis Jones

To the amazing Black women in my life:

My late mother, Camille Greta Patterson Jones, whose boundless love, commitment to excellence, and insistence that the world recognize her royal humanity shaped me and continue to guide me.

My sisters, Dr. Camille Arnel Jones and Dr. Clara Yvonne Jones, who surrounded me with their brilliance and creativity and fearlessness growing up, and who continue to demonstrate what unconditional love and support look like.

My daughter, Calah Camara Mzee Singleton, an amazing writer, artist, and visionary who is brilliant, creative, and strong; healthy, happy, and delightful; kind, and wise, and loving, with a beautiful spirit!

Contents

LIST OF ILLUSTRATIONS	xv
ACKNOWLEDGMENTS	xvii
LOVE LETTER TO THE MOSAIC BEAUTY, RADIANCE, AND HUMANITY OF BLACK WOMEN *Kisha Braithwaite Holden and Camara Phyllis Jones*	xix
FOREWORD *Valerie Montgomery Rice*	xxi
INTRODUCTION *Kisha Braithwaite Holden and Camara Phyllis Jones*	1

Part One
Cultural Narratives about Black Womanhood

POEM 1 Jubilation *Calah Singleton*	13
CHAPTER 1 Black Motherhood: Deeply Rooted *Malika B. Gooden and Raquel Brown*	15

CHAPTER 2
Dispelling Negative Stereotypes and Images: Black Girl Magic,
Black Girls Rock! 31
  Regina Davis Moss

CHAPTER 3
The Superwoman (Sojourner) Syndrome and African American/
Black Women 47
  Tabia Henry Akintobi, Adrienne Chevelle Glymph Foster,
  Bridg'ette Israel, and Taylor A. Wimbly

CHAPTER 4
The Making of a Black American Quilt: Discussing the Threads
of the Strong Black Woman Image through Family Narratives
and Media Storytelling 65
  Asha S. Winfield

COMMENTARY: NOTHING CAN BREAK YOU UNLESS YOU GIVE
IT PERMISSION TO! 77
  Tonyka McKinney

CONVERSATIONS WITH THOUGHT LEADERS: BEACONS OF LIGHT 81
  Annelle B. Primm, Linda Goler Blount, and Cedrice Davis

Part Two
Toward an Optimal Health Agenda:
The Importance of Our Survival

POEM 2
Face Your Pace 87
  Adele Browne

CHAPTER 5
The Black Women's Health Study: An Epidemiologic Snapshot
of Black Women's Health 89
  Lynn Rosenberg, Yvette C. Cozier, and Julie R. Palmer

CHAPTER 6
Obesity, Heart Disease, and the Influence of Dietary Guidelines
among Black Women 101
   Jennifer Rooke

CHAPTER 7
When Resilience Hits Its Ceiling: The Burden of the
COVID-19 Pandemic 117
   *Rhonda Reid, Kristian T. Jones, Chidi Wamuo,
and Christopher Villongco*

CHAPTER 8
Black Women and HIV: From Surviving to Thriving 129
   *Rhonda C. Holliday, Kimberly A. Parker, and
Alyssa G. Robillard*

CHAPTER 9
The Nexus of Chronic Stress, Autoimmune Disorders, and
Black Women 143
   Lesley Green-Rennis, Lisa Grace-Leitch, and Anika Thrower

CHAPTER 10
Mindfulness Matters: Mental Health Risks and Protective
Factors for Black Women 157
   *Kisha Braithwaite Holden, Sharon A. Rachel,
Ricardo D. LaGrange, Glenda Wrenn Gordon, and
Cynthia Major Lewis*

CHAPTER 11
Reckoning with Resilience: Black Breastfeeding 171
   Kimarie Bugg, Ifeyinwa V. Asiodu, and Andrea Serano

CHAPTER 12
The Color Line of Infertility: Reproductive Disparities in
Black Women 185
   *Yoann Sophie Antoine, Blessing Chidiuto Lawrence,
Shubhecchha Dhaurali, Beverly Udegbe, Lauren Cohen,
Paige E. Feyock, Mildred Watson-Baylor, and
Ndidiamaka Amutah-Onukaga*

COMMENTARY: ABORTION IS A REPRODUCTIVE JUSTICE ISSUE
FOR BLACK FAMILIES AND COMMUNITIES   199
   Joia Crear-Perry, Nia Mitchell, Donna L. Brazile, and Rachel Villanueva

CONVERSATIONS WITH THOUGHT LEADERS: BEACONS OF LIGHT   209
   Henrie M. Treadwell, Helene D. Gayle, and Gail E. Wyatt

Part Three
Journey to Wellness and Community Healing

POEM 3
Corona Reflections   215
   Tamia A. McEwen

CHAPTER 13
On the Frontlines: Stressors of Black Women Caring for
Children of Incarcerated Parents   217
   Shenique Thomas-Davis, Vivian C. Smith, and Bahiyyah M. Muhammad

CHAPTER 14
Resilience, Recovery, and Resistance: Black Women Overcoming
Intersectional Complex Trauma   231
   Brenda Ingram and Amorie Robinson

CHAPTER 15
"I Feel Some Type of Way": Experiences of Relationship
Violence, Resilience, and Resistance among Urban Black Girls   247
   LeConté J. Dill, Bianca D. Rivera, Shavaun S. Sutton, and Elizabeth O. Ige

CHAPTER 16
Womanist Theological Bioethics: A Healing and
Culturally Responsive Approach to Death and Dying in
Black Communities   265
   Nicole Taylor Morris

CHAPTER 17
Blissful Balance: Spirituality, Healing, and Restoration 279
Imani Ma'at and Cheryl Taylor

COMMENTARY: ORGANIZED RESISTANCE IS NECESSARY 297
Linda Rae Murray

CONVERSATIONS WITH THOUGHT LEADERS: BEACONS OF LIGHT 303
Jennifer F. Kelly, Jemea Dorsey, and Addie Briggs

Part Four
Advocacy and Activism for Social Justice

POEM 4
Sandra Bland 309
Imani Ma'at

CHAPTER 18
#SayHerName: Honoring Black Women Victims of Violence 311
Maisha Standifer and Sydney Love

CHAPTER 19
Black Women, Public Health, and Resilience: Political Power 317
Brian McGregor and Anana Johari Harris Parris

CHAPTER 20
Standing on the Shoulders of Those Before Us 333
Allyson S. Belton, Ashley Kennedy Mitchell, and Katrina M. Brantley

CHAPTER 21
Multimedia: Changing the Narrative 345
Crystal R. Emery and Carmen Clarkin

CHAPTER 22
Anti-Racism Primer: Naming Racism and Moving to Action 365
Camara Phyllis Jones, Clara Y. Jones, and Camille A. Jones

Commentary: Looking Back to Move Forward 389
  Camara Phyllis Jones, Byllye Y. Avery, Linda Rae Murray,
  and Kisha Braithwaite Holden

Conversations with Thought Leaders: Beacons of Light 409
  Melissa Harris-Perry, Christine Beatty, and Sandra Harris-Hooker

List of Contributors 413

About the Coeditors 427

Index 429

Illustrations

Figures

1.1	Black motherhood: work-life balance.	23
6.1	Food consumption by ethnicity.	104
6.2	US meat consumption by ethnicity.	105
6.3	Factors underlying obesity in Black women.	106
12.1	Resiliency in action.	191
15.1	Spaces of Black girl resilience and resistance enactment.	255
17.1	Spiritual dimensions of Black women's resilience.	291
22.1	States with jurisdictions declaring "Racism is a public health crisis."	370
22.2	Levels of health and social intervention: A Cliff Analogy.	373
22.3	Allegories communicating four key messages about racism.	374
22.4	Summary image from the Gardener's Tale allegory "Levels of Racism: A Theoretic Framework and a Gardener's Tale."	378
C.1	Maternal health fact sheet.	205
C.2a–b	Cancer fact sheet.	206–207

Tables

1.1	Foundations that honor legacies.	27

9.1	Common autoimmune disorders. *Source*: Author.	145
10.1	Selected stressful anxiety-provoking issues. *Source*: Author.	159
13.1	Reported health outcomes/conditions.	224
17.1	Black women's resilience: spirituality research review of literature.	281

Acknowledgments

The coeditors would like to thank Brandie Adams-Piphus for the book cover art and poem entitled "Memories like Mountains." It captures the kaleidoscope essence and fluidity of womanhood—movement forward, resilience.

Kisha Braithwaite Holden would like to thank coeditor Dr. Camara Phyllis Jones, who embodies remarkable talents; and for weaving together a powerful narrative that contextualizes the experiences of Black women. I offer a special thanks to the chapter authors, poets, and thought leaders who demonstrated brilliance in delineating the multiple layers of excellence of Black women. Immense gratitude is given to my illustrious mentors Dr. Veronica G. Thomas (Howard University), Dr. Henrie M. Treadwell (Morehouse School of Medicine), Dr. Nadine Kaslow (Emory University), Dr. Brenda Hayes (Morehouse School of Medicine), and Dr. David Satcher (16th US Surgeon General) who helped me to elucidate and "use my voice" through the critical study of Black women, families, and communities. Immense appreciation is extended to Daniel Dawes, JD (Executive Director, Satcher Health Leadership Institute at Morehouse School of Medicine) for his unwavering support and guidance for the book development. Recognition is well deserved for one of my mentees Dr. Jammie Hopkins for his steadfast commitment and gentility in establishing various book elements. Loving gratitude is given to my linesisters of Delta Sigma Theta, Inc., a public service sorority. A plethora of grace, honor, and gratefulness is offered to my big sister and best friend Dr. Malika B. Gooden for paving the way for me to flourish as a Black woman. Gratitude is given to my father, Dr. Ronald Braithwaite for teaching me about the complexities of navigating through academia.

Camara Phyllis Jones acknowledges with immense gratitude Dr. Kisha Braithwaite Holden, the lead editor of this volume, for her vision, energy, and dedication to getting these words and agendas of Black women onto the national stage. Kisha, you demonstrate sisterhood, resilience, and collectivity for all the world to see! I would also like to acknowledge the amazing Black men in my life: My late father, Dr. Arnold Melvin Jones, whose gentle strength, twinkly humor, and work as a surgeon in service of his community modeled masculinity as deep humanity. My husband, Dr. Herbert Alfred Singleton, who is not only a wonderful pediatrician but whose nurturing spirit and boundless energy have kept our household going on so many levels for so long to support me in my work. Thank you for teaching me how to show love through action and for loving me so! And my son, Malcolm Herbert Arnold Mzee Singleton, a masterful listener, healer, and bridge builder who is brilliant, creative, and happy; majestic, magical, strong, and free; kind, and wise, and loving, with a beautiful spirit!

Love Letter to the Mosaic Beauty, Radiance, and Humanity of Black Women

Dear Grandmother, Mother, Daughter, Niece, Sister, Aunt, Friend:

Black women are divine anchors of community and the souls of our families. Rooted in a fierce independence of mind, wisdom, and creativity—Black women epitomize excellence. Your demonstration of intelligence, actualization of resilience, and endurance of misogynoir is extraordinary. A wealth of gratitude and reverence must be given to Black women for the numerous groundbreaking inventions and innovative discoveries, for stellar leadership in a myriad of multidisciplinary professional fields, and for paving a robust foundation for brilliance to flourish. Despite an intricate matrix of barriers and challenges that have been encountered, Black women rise above it all; and in some cases, "make a way, out of no way." The unique experiences and winding path of a journey through intersectionality of identities, systemic biases, atypical socialization, marginalization, internalization of convoluted emotions, and perceptions of invisibility create a montage of an incomparable framework that has been ascended by many Black women. Through kinship networks, sisterhood circles, mentoring, allyships, and adaptable relationships the nexus of bonds give birth to a formidable grid of distinction. Black women are at the center of nature and nurture. We stand with you against the Black maternal health crisis; social injustices against Black, Indigenous, People of Color (BIPOC) communities; systemic racism, sexism, and classism; and the many complex issues that contribute to health inequities. We understand the need to balance strength and vulnerability.

Even in all your glory, synchronicity, and rhythm with life, self-care is essential. Compassion to yourself must be prioritized in order to maintain a strong armor of protection for you to continue serving as warriors of cultural preservation, health, and wellness. And, despite negative notions about you, you continue to engender an ethos of brilliance and offer the many special ways that you teach and support individuals, families, and communities. Remarkably, countless undertakings are seamlessly accomplished while you simultaneously balance personal life expectations. Yet, strategies for prevention of chronic diseases (e.g., diabetes, heart disease, auto-immune diseases), stress management, preclusion of workplace, home, and school burn-out as well as bolstering your mental health are all critical priorities that must be endorsed by you. Yes, you are gorgeous, impeccable, luminous, and influential. And discussions, action, and engaging in comprehensive quality healthcare specific to your personal health and well-being must become embedded in your lifestyle. The success of your health is under your control. You are enough—worthy of everything that your heart desires.

Relish your regal beauty, grace, and genuine love of life. Challenge the diverse sociocultural, economic, political, and ecological stressors that you experience. This will further allow you to cultivate fertile ground for planting seeds of hope, confidence, and optimism for future generations. This is your time to shine brightly! Thank you for being phenomenal women of enchanting elegance, courageous spirit, regal dignity, and unyielding humanity.

Patently, the distance between where we began and where we are today is the measure of the strength of Black women. The hopes for a better future are contingent upon our willingness to safeguard our most vital human resource. Let's relish the exquisite ingenuity and courage of Black women. It is in that spirit that this collection is offered.

Love,
Kisha and Camara

Foreword

Valerie Montgomery Rice

Take an enchanted journey traveling through pathways of the minds and hearts of many Black women, and at the intersection of these two key entities, at the core, is resilience cultivated by Grace, Fortitude, Tenacity, and Perseverance. Drs. Holden and Jones brilliantly curate this collection as a vehicle that takes the reader on an exploratory wave of (1) shaping cultural narratives that numerous Black women engender, (2) identifying significant health priorities for Black women, (3) promoting wellness and community healing, and (4) signifying the importance of advocacy and activism to achieve social justice.

Health equity aims to give individuals, families, and communities what they need, when they need it, and in the amount that they need it to reach their optimal levels of health. Black women are central gatekeepers to reifying this notion. Within the US, numerous Black people, Indigenous people, and other people of color experience health disparities at alarming rates. In fact, the quest to tackle and eliminate health disparities has no historical model to help guide national and global efforts. It requires a transformational change in the way that we are currently addressing the issue. It also requires commitment at the local, state, regional, and federal levels. The Minority Health and Health Disparities Research and Education Act of 2000 established the National Center on Minority Health and Health Disparities (NCMHD) at the National Institutes of Health (NIH), providing a clear mandate of leading and coordinating biomedical research on minority health and health disparities. The congressional act charged the NCMHD with conducting and supporting research, training, and dissemination of information related to health disparities. The legislation also charged the NCMHD with leading the development of an NIH-wide Strategic Plan for eliminating health disparities. Later, the National Institute on Minority Health and Health Disparities (NIMHD) was established to lead scientific research to improve minority health and eliminate health disparities.

The NIMHD envisions "an America in which all populations will have an equal opportunity to live long, healthy and productive lives; and to accomplish this, NIMHD raises national awareness about the prevalence and impact of health disparities and disseminates effective interventions to reduce and encourage elimination of health disparities." This is critically important, because at the bedrock of survival for communities of color lies health and wellness. It is imperative that we confront any moral conundrums, navigate ambiguity, focus on diverse perspectives, eradicate critical points of inflection, and dissolve platitudes of disdain by accepting the simple reality that health is a human right. Collectively, the current time and climate are ripe for community members, policy makers, educators, clinicians, and researchers to maximize opportunities to advance health equity.

Historic Black women "firsts" masterfully plant seeds of hope and prosperity for young Black girls. Selected individuals include: Kamala Harris (Vice President of the United States), Michelle Obama (Former First Lady of the United States), Stacey Abrams (first Black woman to run for Governor in Georgia), Madame C. J. Walker (first Black woman millionaire), Oprah Winfrey (billionaire philanthropist), Misty Copeland (principal ballerina of the American Ballet Theatre), Vernice Armour (America's first Black female combat pilot), Henrietta Lacks (Black woman whose cancer cells were immortalized for medical research), Venus Williams (first Black woman to be ranked number one in the world for the sport of tennis) and her sister Serena Williams, who has earned the most tennis accolades of all time, Mae Jemison (physician, engineer, NASA astronaut) that became the first Black woman to travel into space, Justice Ketanji Brown Jackson (first Black woman to serve on the US Supreme Court), and me—the first Black woman President and CEO named to lead a freestanding medical school.

We use our intellectual flexibility, creativity, curiosity, and boldness to retract curtains of vulnerability. We recognize that vulnerability is a strength. In times of great joy and great unrest, Black women remarkably thrive and shower others with a tapestry of abundance of courage to execute and demonstrate excellence. Through thoughtful leadership, boundless internal beauty, and resilience, let's visualize majestic and imperial crowns bestowed upon Black women; and in the words of poet laureate Maya Angelou, "Still I Rise."

Introduction

KISHA BRAITHWAITE HOLDEN AND
CAMARA PHYLLIS JONES

Purpose

The aim of *Black Women and Resilience: Power, Perseverance, and Public Health* is to help nurture community exchange of ideas between scholars by providing an infusion of qualitative and quantitative approaches examining resilience at the nexus of Black women and public health. We use a health equity lens, understanding that achieving health equity requires valuing all individuals and populations equally, recognizing and rectifying historical injustices, and providing resources according to need (Jones, 2014). This edited volume provides a critical examination of the unique experiences and contributions of Black women as thought leaders and catalysts for transformation in the United States. *Black Women and Resilience: Power, Perseverance, and Public Health*, part of the SUNY Press Black Women's Wellness Series, is divided into four interconnected parts: part 1, "Cultural Narratives about Black Womanhood"; part 2, "Toward an Optimal Health Agenda: The Importance of Our Survival"; part 3, "Journey to Wellness and Community Healing"; and part 4, "Advocacy and Activism for Social Justice." Each of these sections elucidates core constructs and strategies for empowerment from academic experts and community leaders. There is recognition that intersectional identities exist; and this collection does not cover all aspects or specific diseases/disorders encountered by all Black women. Nevertheless, this volume highlights practical approaches for promoting self-care, emotional intelligence, and balance in responding to daily life demands. Throughout the book, the signifiers Black and African-American are used interchangeably.

Organization of the Book: A Communal Approach to Black Women's Health and Well-being

The organization of this book reflects our deep understanding that the health and well-being of Black women are communal processes rooted in history, in culture, and in recognizing, celebrating, and sharing our gifts with one another. Our authors include those who responded to an open call for contributions as well as those who were specifically invited, and represent a broad range of ages, expertise, and perspectives. Each of the four sections of the book opens with depictions and explanations of four adinkra symbols and with a poem. Each section includes a "Commentary" in addition to more academic chapters, and each section ends with a "Conversation with Thought Leaders," where we present the collective wisdom gleaned in a group conversation around structured questions. We close the volume with a dialogue in which we look back to move forward, recognizing the importance of sustaining our work across generations. This book is very much a community endeavor and reflects our recognition that assuring the conditions for Black women's health will require collective action.

Cultural Narratives about Black Womanhood

Part 1 delineates cultural realities illustrated within the experiences of many Black women. It offers a depiction of selected aspects of Black womanhood. It includes four chapters—"Black Motherhood: Deeply Rooted," "Dispelling Negative Stereotypes and Images: Black Girl Magic, Black Girls Rock!," "The Superwoman (Sojourner) Syndrome and African American/Black Women," "The Making of a Black American Quilt: Discussing the Threads of the Strong Black Woman Image through Family Narratives and Media Storytelling"—and one commentary entitled "Nothing Can Break You Unless You Give It Permission To!" This section aims to illuminate some of the core issues that are germane to understanding of Black womanist ideology.

Toward an Optimal Health Agenda: The Importance of Our Survival

Part 2 discerns a canopy of information about significant health issues that impact Black women. It includes eight chapters—"The Black Women's Health Study: An Epidemiologic Snapshot of Black Women's Health," "Obesity, Heart Disease, and the Influence of Dietary Guidelines among Black Women," "When Resilience Hits Its Ceiling: The Burden of the COVID-19 Pandemic," "Black Women and HIV: From Surviving to Thriving," "The Nexus of Chronic Stress, Autoimmune Disorders, and Black Women," "Mindfulness Matters: Mental Health Risks and Protective Factors for Black Women," "Reckoning with Resilience: Black Breastfeeding," "The Color Line of Infertility: Reproductive Disparities in Black Women"—and one commentary entitled "Abortion Is a Reproductive Justice Issue for Black Families and Communities." Also, two Centers for Disease Control and Prevention fact sheets concerning Maternal Health and Cancer are offered. This section aims to explicate selected health topics of significance to Black women utilizing a health equity lens. It is recognized that a vast array of diseases/disorders/illnesses are not represented. Nevertheless, the selected health conditions provide a foundation for fostering a health agenda that may be rooted in particular challenges encountered by some Black women.

Journey to Wellness and Community Healing

Part 3 offers a compilation of topics to encourage well-being and growth among Black women in five chapters—"On the Frontlines: Stressors of Black Women Caring for Children of Incarcerated Parents," "Resilience, Recovery, and Resistance: Black Women Overcoming Intersectional Complex Trauma," "'I Feel Some Type of Way': Experiences of Relationship Violence, Resilience, and Resistance among Urban Black Girls," "Womanist Theological Bioethics: A Healing and Culturally Responsive Approach to Death and Dying in Black Communities," "Blissful Balance: Spirituality, Healing, and Restoration"—and one commentary entitled "Organized Resistance Is Necessary." This part seeks to illustrate selected relevant issues that are central to the plethora of ways to promote robust living, wellness, and healing within communities.

ADVOCACY AND ACTIVISM FOR SOCIAL JUSTICE

Part 4 illustrates the importance of disentangling significant concepts related to justice and empowerment for Black women in the United States. Five chapters—"#SayHerName: Honoring Black Women Victims of Violence," "Black Women, Public Health, and Resilience: Political Power," "Standing on the Shoulders of Those before Us," "Multimedia: Changing the Narrative," "Anti-Racism Primer: Naming Racism and Moving to Action"—and a dialogue of significance entitled "Looking Back to Move Forward" are offered. This section gives a glimpse into the veracity of lived experiences for many Black women and gives approaches that may be used for integrity-centered servant leadership. It also highlights the need for collective action, because collective action propels us, informs us, inspires us, and protects us.

Black Women Trailblazers and Thought Leaders

There are many Black women thought leaders who have shattered the "glass ceiling" and laid a stellar foundation of brilliance for achievement of excellence by future generations. Separate key informant interviews and related analyses were conducted by medical anthropologist Maisha Standifer, PhD, and psychologist Kisha Braithwaite Holden, PhD, MSCR, with twelve innovative Black women. These phenomenal women represent diverse fields in public health, medicine, psychology, women's health, health equity, Black women's wellness, pediatrics, psychiatry, political science, and academia. They share perspectives relative to their conceptualizations of how resilience is actualized among Black women. Excerpts and quotes from these amazing interviews are laced throughout the volume as concluding conversations in each of the four sections of the book.

Conceptualization of Community Resilience

Resilience is important for optimal physical and mental health functioning across a variety of populations and settings, and across the human life span (Tsai & Freedland, 2022). The American Psychological Association defines individual resilience as "the process of adapting well in the face of adversity, trauma, tragedy, threats, or significant sources of stress—such as family and relationship problems, serious health problems, or workplace and financial stressors." As much as resilience involves "bouncing back" from these difficult experiences, it can also involve profound personal growth (APA, 2020). Psychological resilience has been recognized for centuries by civilizations around the world as a core element of human development and growth (Masten & Wright, 2010; Nicoll & Zerboni, 2020). This notion is further reinforced by research studies that suggest that resilience involves behaviors, thoughts, and actions that are invoked in response to challenging situations (Holden et al., 2016–2017; Connor-Davidson, 2003; Siebert, 2005). Moreover, studies have identified developmental, neurobiological, health, and psychosocial factors that are associated with resilience among children and adults (Iflaifel et al., 2020; Tsai et al., 2017); and the field of resilience research is ripe with opportunities to utilize new conceptual frameworks, extend investigations to understudied populations, and develop more effective interventions (Elliott et al., 2019; Meyer et al., 2019; Robertson et al., 2015; Rutter, 2013; Tsai et al., 2018).

The concept of community resilience has been addressed across multiple disciplines, including environmental sciences, engineering, sociology, psychology, and economics (Koliou et al., 2020), and comprehensive community resilience models typically encompass the performance of individuals within a community, and environmental and socioeconomic infrastructure systems that are largely interdependent (Matarrita-Cascante et al., 2017). Magis (2010) suggests that community resilience is "the existence, development, and engagement of community resources by community members to thrive in an environment characterized by change, uncertainty, unpredictability, and surprise."

The notion of community resilience provides an optimal framework for building healthier communities (Holden et al., 2016). Moreover, this concept is particularly salient with an awareness that equity in health implies that ideally everyone should have a fair opportunity to attain their full health potential. We purport that collectively community members, public health professionals, practitioners, researchers, policymakers, and other stakeholders should elevate strategies to cultivate community resilience, even as they also work to decrease the stresses and assaults on individuals and communities.

On Public Health

Public health is the science and practice of caring for the health and well-being of whole communities. Public health is more than the sum of the health status of individuals. Public health is about the health of communities, which includes both individuals and the ties that bind individuals; individuals and the contexts in which those individuals thrive or are wasted; individuals and the power structures that either celebrate or deny their full humanity.

As opposed to medical care, which is concerned about the health and well-being of individuals one by one, public health acknowledges that each of us is part of a greater collective, that we are inextricably interconnected, that we are all in this together. Public health concerns itself with distributions of measures across populations, and with contexts that aid in interpretation of the measures. The measure of community health is not the level of health enjoyed by only the healthiest member in a community; public health is judged by how widely distributed the enjoyment of good health is in that community. And the pathway to good community health is through assurance of the conditions for optimal health for all people. And that requires recognizing that health is not created within the health sector. Public health requires the bridging of health sectors to nonhealth sectors, including education, housing, justice, transportation, environment, immigration, agriculture, business, and other sectors that shape our contexts and our interactions. Because the distribution of goods and services in communities is not random, public health must address the root causes of the uneven distribution of exposures and opportunities, thus concerning itself with all of the structures, policies, practices, norms, and values that shape group differences in contexts. This means addressing racism, sexism, heterosexism, capitalism, and other systems of structured inequity. This means that public health should also concern itself with social/societal issues. No person lives in a vacuum, even those being punished with solitary confinement. We are all impacted by the choices of others in our society, whether we acknowledge that or not. Yet we differ in our ability to access power and to practice self-determination, which is based on the power to decide, the power to act, and control of resources.

We live in community with one another, whether we want to acknowledge that truth or not. What I do impacts you and what you do impacts me. Your breath affects my ability to breathe. Your greed affects my ability to eat. Your fear affects my ability to live. Our individual health and the health of our communities are shaped by power-sharing and valuing of one another. On the other hand, selfishness undermines our health and the health of our communities.

This volume weaves together the wisdom of Black women for and about Black women for the betterment of the whole of society. We understand that the health and well-being of the public are a community-level concern. And we also understand that they are an individual concern because in truth, we *are* all in this together. The planet on which we live. The air we breathe. The water we drink. The brilliance in which we invest or that we instead squander. The humanity that we recognize or that we instead dehumanize to our great loss. The creativity that we nurture or that we instead constrain with our soul-crushing disinvestment in communities that we "other." Our very limited conceptions of "my children" versus "your children" that keep us from recognizing that all children are our children.

Black women have held these truths through the ages and continue to be living beacons of collective consciousness, collective caring, collective action. When we lose fear, we gain health. When we share our material resources, we gain health. When we share our talents, we gain health. When we acknowledge the full humanity of all of us, we gain health. And wealth. And joy. And strength as a community.

References

American Psychological Association. (2020). *Building your resilience.* http://www.apa.org/topics/resilience/building-your-resilience.

Connor, K., & Davidson, J. (2003). Development of a new resilience scale: The Connor-Davidson Resilience Scale (CD-RISC). *Depression and Anxiety, 18*(2), 76–82. https://doi.org/10.1002/da.10113

Elliott, T. R., Hsiao, Y.-Y., Kimbrel, N. A., DeBeer, B. B., Gulliver, S. B., Kwok, O.-M., Morissette, S. B., & Meyer, E. C. (2019). Resilience facilitates adjustment through greater psychological flexibility among Iraq/Afghanistan war veterans with and without mild traumatic brain injury. *Rehabilitation Psychology, 64*(4), 383–397. https://doi.org/10.1037/rep0000282

Holden, K., Akintobi, T., Hopkins, J., Belton, A., McGregor, B., Blanks, S., & Wrenn, G. (2016). Community engaged leadership to advance health equity and build healthier communities. *Social Sciences, 5*(1), 2. https://doi.org/10.3390/socsci5010002

Holden, K. B., Hernandez, N. D., Wrenn, G. L., & Belton, A. S. (2016–2017). Resilience: Protective factor for depression and post-traumatic stress disorder among African Americans. *Health, Culture, and Society, 9/10*, 12–29. https://doi.org/10.5195/hcs.2017.222

Iflaifel, M., Lim, R. H., Ryan, K., & Crowley, C. (2020). Resilient health care: A systematic review of conceptualisations, study methods and factors that develop resilience. *BMC Health Services Research, 20*(1), article 324. https://doi.org/10.1186/s12913-020-05208-3

Jones, C. P. (2014). Systems of power, axes of inequity: Parallels, intersections, braiding the strands. *Medical Care, 52*(10, suppl. 3), S71–S75.

Koliou, M., Lindt, J. W. van de, McAllister, T. P., Ellingwood, B. R., Dillard, M., & Cutler, H. (2020). State of the research in community resilience: Progress and challenges, *Sustainable and Resilient Infrastructure, 5*(3), 131–151. https://doi.org/10.1080/23789689.2017.1418547

Meyer, E. C., Kotte, A., Kimbrel, N. A., DeBeer, B. B., Elliott, T. R., Gulliver, S. B., & Morissette, S. B. (2019). Predictors of lower-than-expected posttraumatic symptom severity in war veterans: The influence of personality, self-reported trait resilience, and psychological flexibility. *Behaviour Research and Therapy, 113*, 1–8. https://doi.org/10.1016/j.brat.2018.12.005

Nicoll, K., & Zerboni, A. (2020). Is the past key to the present? Observations of cultural continuity and resilience reconstructed from geoarchaeological records. *Quaternary International, 545*, 119–127. https://doi.org/10.1016/j.quaint.2019.02.012

Magis, K. (2010). Community Resilience: An indicator of social sustainability. *Society and Natural Resources, 23*(5), 401–416. https://doi.org/10.1080/08941920903305674

Masten, A. S., & Wright, M. O. (2010). Resilience over the lifespan: Developmental perspectives on resistance, recovery, and transformation. In J. W. Reich, A. J. Zautra, & J. S. Hall (Eds.), *Handbook of adult resilience* (pp. 213–237). Guilford Press.

Matarrita-Cascante, D., Trejos, B., Qin, H., Joo, D., & Debne, S. (2017). Conceptualizing community resilience: Revisiting conceptual distinctions. *Community Development, 48*(1), 105–123. https://doi.org/10.1080/15575330.2016.1248458

Robertson, I. T., Cooper, C. L., Sarkar, M., & Curran, T. (2015). Resilience training in the workplace from 2003 to 2014: A systematic review. *Journal of Occupational and Organizational Psychology, 88*(3), 533–562. https://doi.org/10.1111/joop.12120

Rutter, M. (2013). Annual research review: Resilience—clinical implications. *Journal of Child Psychology and Psychiatry, 54*(4), 474–487. https://doi.org/10.1111/j.1469-7610.2012.02615.x

Siebert, A. (2005). *The resiliency advantage: Master change, thrive under pressure, and bounce back from setbacks.* Berrett-Kohler.

Tsai, J., & Freedland, K. E. (2022). Introduction to the special section: Resilience for physical and behavioral health. *Health Psychology, 41*(4), 243–245. http://dx.doi.org/10.1037/hea0001179

Tsai, J., Harpaz-Rotem, I., Pietrzak, R. H., & Southwick, S. M. (2017). Trauma resiliency and posttraumatic growth. In S. Gold, C. Dalenberg, & J. Cook (Eds.), *APA handbook of trauma psychology: Vol. 2. Trauma practice* (pp. 89–113). American Psychological Association. https://doi.org/10.1037/0000020-005

Tsai, J., Jones, N., Pietrzak, R. H., Harpaz-Rotem, I., & Southwick, S. M. (2018). Susceptibility, resilience, and trajectories. In F. J. Stoddard, D. M. Benedek, M. R. Milad, & R. J. Ursano (Eds.), *Trauma- and stressor-related disorders* (pp. 223–238). Oxford University Press.

Part One

Cultural Narratives about Black Womanhood

Adinkra symbols are from Ghana, West Africa, and represent concepts or aphorisms that are used extensively in fabrics, logos, pottery, and architectural features. The symbols have a decorative function but also represent objects that encapsulate evocative messages conveying traditional wisdom, aspects of life, or the environment. There are many symbols with distinct meanings, often linked with proverbs. Selected Adinkra symbols have been chosen to support introduction of the various parts of the book to reflect close alignment with the chapter content elucidated; and for empowerment related to cultural nuances relative to experiences of African American/Black individuals, families, and communities across the diaspora.

Grace/grās/
Elegance or beauty of form, manner, motion, or action.

Ananse Ntontan
West African Adinkra Symbol for Wisdom, Creativity, and the Complexities of Life

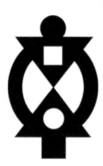

Boa Me Na Me Mmoa Wo
West African Adinkra Symbol for Cooperation and Interdependence

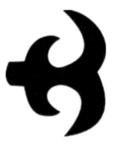

Akoko Nan
West African Adinkra Symbol for Nurturing and Discipline

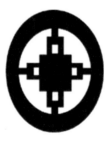

Dame-Dame
West African Adinkra Symbol for Intelligence and Ingenuity

Jubilation

Calah Singleton

on the island we stayed underground
sweaty shoulders touching
the air so close my breath was yours
four walls and us
standing in the blackberry darkness
so deep so they could not hear us

to every thing there is a season
or rather
this is a way of saying
we have lived in black squares
and died in even darker places

and yet.

i want flowers
for each time i have stumbled across a video
i could not watch
again
a petal for each deep breath taken
in memory of those who could
not

each clicked heart reviving one that was stolen

i want all of us weaving lives together
not rending garments
i want our phones cracked on the ground
soaking minerals back into homelands
i want all of us together
our hands clasped
faces to the widening sky
finding, each day, a new reason for
jubilation

Chapter 1

Black Motherhood
Deeply Rooted

MALIKA B. GOODEN AND RAQUEL BROWN

"The most disrespected person in America is the Black woman. The most unprotected person in America is the Black woman. The most neglected person in America is the Black woman"—sentiments of the late visionary Malcolm X that still ring true today—although it's been more than fifty years since he first uttered those powerful words. And yet, for some individuals on the opposite end of that spectrum, what also rings true is the most resilient woman in America is the Black woman. And not just the Black woman, an exclusive tribe, the "Black Mother." From paleoarchaeologic findings to intraracial and intraethnic generational stories, Black mothers are deeply rooted like the genus Adansonia, made in variations of the deciduous Baobab.[1]

Before there was ever a Malcolm or other known human life, there was Lucy—the three-million-year-old hominin radiometric dated fossil, the original "Black Mother," who has rewritten the story of humanity. And anchored in African ancestry is the Cradle of Civilization—approximately 50 km northwest of Johannesburg, South Africa, in the Gauteng Province is Fossil Hominid Sites of South Africa, and in Hadar in the Awash Valley of the Afar Triangle lies the birthplace of humankind. Lucy or by her African given name Dinknesh, meaning "you are marvelous," has become the cultural ambassador for Africa (Jethro, 2016) and is the cultural ancestor of humankind and humanity. The significance of the Dinknesh fossil finding underscores the depth and breadth of the Black Mother and her distinctive contribution to the evolution of mankind and humanity.

Mother, motherly, mothering—whether a noun, adjective, or verb, mindfulness matters in the sacred sisterhood of being Black Mothers—an archipelago of cultures and experiences but one tribe with a clear understanding of issues common only to them. Functioning within a society of multigenerational, ethno-sociopolitical trauma, triggers, and stressors as the problem and no easy answers, resilience continues to be the potent elixir guiding the internal paths of Black Mothers as they journey through life with pride, purpose, and patience.

Black Motherhood: Mother-Child Bond

Whether subscribed to as a biological, social, or functional construct, being a mother is multifaceted and connotes various meanings depending on your ideology. As well, becoming a mother considers a diversity of contexts and circumstances (Farrell, 2013). That aside, the Black Mother–child bond is a unique and dynamic relationship. Entering the world disadvantaged from the womb, there is a baseline understanding of differences that will occur in nurturing, protecting, and raising a Black child. Yet, within those differences are the very factors that begin the building blocks of an internal resiliency matrix that Black children carry within themselves throughout the duration of their lives.

Mother—"traditionally" a woman or female parent of a child who performs the role of bearing the child(ren) who may or may not be their biological offspring. Yet, Black Mother expounds and extends beyond "mother" including both nuclear and extended family; from biologic mother and grandmothers to adopted-mothers, surrogate-mothers, godmothers, stepmothers, "bonus-mothers," "auntie-mothers," "cousin-mothers," to any colloquial named mother figure or combination thereof that more accurately defines and distinguishes the Black Mother village. And without distinguishing between a "good" or "bad" mother nor taking into account factors such as socioeconomic status, age, religion, and parenting style, there are some truths within Black motherhood held to be self-evident, which is an ability to withstand the impact of intentional circumstances placed upon them.

Like the African Baobab "tree of life," the Black Mother plays a key role within the mother-child ecosystem. And while some Black mothers can become paralyzed with insecurity and doubt about their abilities to overcome systems of racism, prejudice, and conscious and unconscious biases at the root of many issues, it is the symbiotic relationship between the Black Mother and her child(ren) that keeps her grounded, connected through trials and tribulations, and empowers her to overcome adversities. Yet, the systemic challenges Black Mothers face also correlate with health issues and related concerns encountered.

Black Motherhood: Matriarchal Stories of Resilience

Black Mothers across centuries have faced challenges on every front, often investing all of their time and energy into everyone and everything at the expense of their own health and self-care. And, it is the matriarchs of many families that have long "held it down," kept things together, and passed customs on to continue the legacies, understandings, and traditions relative to withstanding adversity and overcoming societal challenges.

Beautiful, brilliant, Black matriarchal mothers like *Harriett Tubman*, who was a political abolitionist and born a slave. She risked her life to free others. *Rebecca Lee Crumpler*, the first Black woman medical doctor in the US. And Congresswoman *Yvonne Braithwaite Burke*, the first Black Woman to serve Congress while pregnant. She was an advocate for women to receive maternity leave, and spoke out against racism. Other notable Black mothers who had a significant impact in history are *Katherine Johnson*, a NASA mathematician, whose orbital calculations and trajectories were critical in the launch of space shuttles to the moon; *Mary Jackson*, a mathematician and NASA's first Black woman aerospace engineer; *Dorothy Vaughn*, a "human computer," mathematician, and expert FORTRAN programmer at NASA and its first Black supervisor and manager; *Maya Angelou*, a decorated African American orator, author, and poet; *Michelle Obama*, first African American First Lady of the United States, attorney, author, and wife of the first African American President of the United States, Barack Obama; *Kamala Harris*, first woman and African American Vice President of the United States, currently the highest ranking female official in US history; and *Hester Ford*, a supercentenarian and native to the Carolinas who was the oldest living African American mother that passed in April 2021 at 115 years old. These esteemed matriarchs, thought leaders, and teachers, and many unnamed sheroes, have not only paved the way but each have a story steeped in Black Motherhood. Their stories, like those of many Black mothers, are the roots, the trunk, the branches, and the leaves forever leading the tribe. Hear their whispers and feel their roars:

> Resilience is not simply fighting to overcome whatever challenge that is in front of you (health issues with your children, endless racist death threats, government-supported attempts against your husband's life, finding the money to pay every mortgage and tuition bill) but it is doing so knowing that when that specific battle is won, another far greater challenge is waiting around the corner, and yet pushing forward anyway. (Lillian E. Gregory, mama, freedom fighter, civil rights activist, humanitarian honoree, mother of eleven children [one who was lost to SIDS], 83 years old, and wife of the late human rights icon and comedian Dick Gregory)

> After losing my mom at the tender age of 12, due to complications while giving birth to my younger brother, me and my five siblings practically lived with my grandparents who had 12 children of their own. Growing up in the south in Pompeytown included picking cotton among other things and I can authentically say I hated it. Since I proved to be bad at cotton-picking, my grandmother kept me close by her side in the kitchen, where I learned to be an excellent cook. After marriage, I had two beautiful daughters and several "like-a-daughters." When my children were babies, I made a conscious decision to stay home, raise them, and take care of my family. I'm proud to say my girls have inherited my cooking skills and cook with love, knowing how to add a little bit of this and a dash of that without a recipe, just as I learned from my grandmother. To this day, my mac 'n' cheese is expected at every family gathering. Family is everything! I'm a resilient Black Mother. (mama Lila Benjamin, 90 years old)

> My resilience as a Black Mother means that I did those things because I knew I had to. I lost one child and raised four beautiful children (including twin boys). I had *no* fear going through cancer and heart surgeries. I had to do what I needed

for my family and I survived. I did *not* go out here and do big things, but I did what needed to be done. (mama Dorothy Stokes, 82 years old)

As a Black Mother, resiliency means weathering the storms of widowhood as a young mother with a baby son, raising three successful children while completing a master's degree, challenging myself to leave the legacy of love and faith left to me by my Mother, to make the impossible, possible. (mama Esther Brinson, 78 years old)

Oldest of 12 children, I was responsible for helping my siblings at a very young age and I even had to miss school every Friday to do so. And, despite the strong desire, I wasn't able to attend college. However, I had the loving support of a grandmother who encouraged me to be independent and I went on to put my two daughters through college, own a successful full-service salon business, and survive cancer all by the grace of God. That is my resilience as a Black Mother and woman. (mama Mimi Martin, 77 years old)

"I am who I am, I cannot change my ethnicity or my innate abilities, you are who you are; why not work together to effect change in the things we can." My mantra as a strong, gifted, and vibrant African woman perpetrates resilience through uplifting others to reach their God-given destiny. A mother of two adultren who are the center of my being, are achieving their goals instilled through my love, their relentless determination, and my nurturing from birth. My resilience is framed in witnessing the fruits of my labor realized when I pour positive energy into humankind. (mama Lydia Patton, 75 years old)

For me, Black motherhood resilience begins and ends with faith: a divinely inspired conviction and determination that says you can raise a young Black man alone, while building a home and career; that you can somehow put yourself through graduate school, all the while helping him with his undergraduate education; that you can have enough love and faith in his ability to make good decisions for himself, even when they are contrary to your worldview of success; that you can be patient and respectful enough to acknowledge that his life belongs to him and not you; and when death comes to him all too early in your view, that you can look back on his short life and be proud of the wonderful, loving, caring, and generous person you had the honor and privilege of helping through life and accept that his time on earth has passed; that you can remain confident that God is in the midst of everything, that he is okay and so are you. (mama Linda Brown, 75 years old)

As the middle child of nine children, with an alcoholic, dominating father, and an abused mother, I became filled with the stress of my environment and desired to always "do the right thing" to stay under the parental radar. I missed much of my childhood. Books became my escape. Thus began my journey to serve people who cannot speak up for themselves as a lifelong counselor, community activist, motivational speaker, and published author. While working full-time and achieving my master's degree, I raised two children using a totally wholistic approach. Resilience for me has been not allowing my birth circumstances to deter God's purpose for my life. I am satisfied. (mama Adele Browne, 73 years old)

Black Mother stories are deep rooted stories of the past, present, and future; and they are vast. Dinknesh stories, slavery stories, strange fruit stories, freedom stories, war stories, civil rights stories, love stories, higher education stories, college stories, spades stories, family gathering stories, soul food stories, sister and brother stories, "good hair" and "bad hair" stories, salon stories, melanin stories, girls trip stories, black men and women we love stories, sexuality stories, marriage stories, pregnancy stories, baby stories, miscarriage stories, vilomah stories, menopause, hot-flash stories, in-law stories, infidelity stories, abuse stories, divorce stories, single mother stories, good girlfriend stories, prayer circle stories, first Black president and First Family stories, racial injustice stories, cultural appropriation stories, Karen stories, mental and physical health stories, medical mistreatment stories, gun violence stories, police brutality stories, black lives don't matter stories, survival stories, resiliency stories, sacred sisterhood stories, Black Mother tribe stories.

These stories are the stories of generations, legacies, and ancestral transformation that have shaped the Black Mother collective.

Black Motherhood: Mindfulness Matters

Within the "Black community," it is widely accepted and understood that Black Mothers are resourceful, "can make something out of nothing," and quite simply get the job done no matter what, especially when it comes to their children and families—long standing facts that transcend professional and personal ideologies of life—reinforced by the "Black Girl Magic" phenomenon and movement established by CaShawn Thompson in 2013 to celebrate the beauty, influence, and resilience of Black women. Yet, the expectation to consistently be strong and exhibit "Black Girl Magic" often requires expansive, unhealthy commitments, leaving no time to balance or to recharge mentally, emotionally, spiritually, physically, and financially. And, as CNN commentator Abby Phillips indicated, "Black mothers teach their daughters how to walk through fire"; in response to how Justice Ketanji Brown Jackson handled the intense confirmation hearings convened by the US Congress for her to serve on the US Supreme Court. An early 2006 study published in the *American Journal of Public Health* established that Black women may face greater exposure in varying social classes and have higher rates of stress-induced "wear and tear" on their bodies than their white female or male peers, leading to early health issues (Geronimus et al., 2006). Unfortunately, this exposure persists today.

Black motherhood mindfulness is an intentional practice of Black mothers allowing themselves time to reflect, balance, adapt, and refuel within the commitments of motherhood, familial responsibilities, and professional ambitions.

Black Motherhood: Balancing Act

There is a common notion that women must choose between becoming a mother and having a professional career or working. Yet, the legacy of Black motherhood has debunked this secular ideology of having to choose, but rather taking on both, either as a personal choice or out of necessity. Clemetson (2006) documented, "for generations Black women have viewed work as a means for elevating not only their own status as women, but also as a crucial force in elevating their family, extended family and their entire race."

Many Black Mothers strive to achieve work-life balance amidst the challenges of inequities and racism that they may face in the professional realm and within society. It is important to expound the notion of a linear view of motherhood work-life balance as Black mothers build on ancestral strength while evolving within modern society to create foundations of resilience and success for themselves and their progeny. Just as being black is not monolithic and shades of melanin vary, so are the needs, priorities, and structures within black families. From the bellows of poverty to the upper crust of the Black elite, there remains a common thread of survival nurturing for biological children and nonbiological children within the collective village among Black Mothers and families.

There is untapped power in the legacy of Black Motherhood. And, it is essential for Black Mothers to validate their place of importance within society, personally within their homes, and professionally at the workplace. Understanding how Black mothers define themselves individually and within the context of various cultural groups helps them to better achieve work-life balance and overall health and wellness. Paramount to achieving this balance are "Black Mother Mindfulness Exercises." Through a series of self-reflective questions—for example, What are my daily/weekly priorities? What priorities can I rotate? What is important to my professional life? What is important to my personal family life? What is important to me for self-care?—these mindfulness exercises allow a space of grace for mentally prioritizing and mindful planning.

Mindful planning and the identification of top personal and professional obligations, and the ability to rotate priorities, becomes attainable; keeping in mind the tasks that can never be neglected and those that can be combined or suspended without compromising the desired outcome(s). Keeping a log or journal in a consistent manner, whether daily, weekly, or monthly, and rotating top priorities by manner of time constraints, overall impact (e.g., on health, education, finances), and crisis management will create a healthier more focused internal mental environment and diminish guilt or anxiety as Black motherhood mindfulness, work-life balance, and positive health outcomes increase. Likewise, reevaluating personal bandwidths at appropriate, predetermined intervals helps to better understand strengths, shortcomings, and limitations, which supports effective life management.

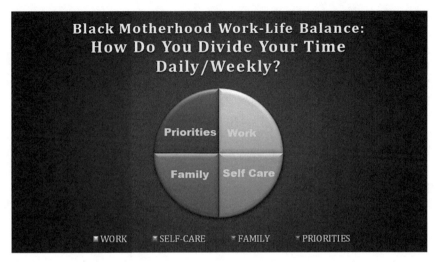

Figure 1.1. Black motherhood: work-life balance. *Source*: Author.

Black Motherhood: Adaptability

"If you don't bend, you break"—a subtle chastising yet endearing generational phrase often uttered from Black mothers and grandmothers to their children when the child stubbornly stands their ground on a matter—oblivious to the lessons of adaptability and compromise in the moment. "Black women bear much of the responsibility for the social and economic survival of Black families, kinship networks, and communities" (Geronimus, 2006). Symbolic is a Black Mother doing it all, against all odds, and yet Black Mothers are often marginalized, compromised, and depleted with maintaining their own mental and physical health and well-being. Black women have long established trends of resilience as evident in "what was known as the notorious matriarchy in Blacks is now regarded as female-centered families in the white community" (Johnson & Staples, 2004).

Managing and accomplishing much with little time to spare creates high-capacity resourcefulness; and it can also create mental and physical health deficiencies within the individual mother and the tribe. As a result, some Black Mothers acquire tunnel vision on how to better manage as mothers while juggling multiple responsibilities. As public health researcher Arline Geronimus documented in 2006, Black Motherhood exudes resilience in the troughs of "weathering" through life with racism and other disparities that exist. This resilience persists along with stigmas of vulnerability, shame, and incompetence some Black mothers carry. Jackson and Kiehl (2017) found that recent resilience-oriented models suggest high levels of social support and positive appraisal associated with traumatic loss. Bailey et al. (2013), indicated that positive adjustment processes and successful adaptation were critical to Black Mothers dealing with adversity. It is imperative not only that Black mothers adopt adaptability principles but that they are more self-aware and mindful of their priorities, work-life balance, and support needs. Subscribing to principles that foster healthy life choices and promote balance in the most important facets of life encourages mindful Black mothers and women to "bend and not break." As indicated, Black motherhood adaptability principles are necessary for balance and overall health and wellness.

Black Motherhood Adaptability Principles

Express Your Feelings

"If you are feeling it, it is real," says Alexandra Sacks in describing how Black mothers are invisible to medical professionals (Braithwaite, 2019). Some Black mothers suffer in silence, afraid, or find it difficult to express vulnerabilities. But it is important for Black mothers to express their feelings and fears to better determine their wants and needs and proactively address health issues and concerns for better outcomes.

Discover and Appreciate Your Worth

Self-worth is associated with self-esteem. Determine the people, places, activities, routines, rituals, and environments that help boost self-esteem and also provide healthy, safe, positive landing places (Everet alt et al., 2016). Refrain from allowing anything or anyone to devalue your self-worth. Be kind to yourself and love yourself!

Embrace and Promote Black Consciousness

Being comfortable in one's own skin is critical. Black Mothers must cultivate their value and share this consciousness with their children (Dow, 2019).

Promoting Black is beautiful, Black is positive, Black is intelligence, Black is love, and the "flattery" (like you, not you) aspect of cultural appropriation, so Black children understand their value and worth and believe in themselves and their abilities anywhere in the world.

SEEK AND ACCEPT HELP

Qualities of self-coping, internalizing angst, and becoming emotionally and physically depleted are common among Black Mothers. And seeking and accepting professional help to proactively address health issues like depression or mental illness is often a last resort for Black Mothers and their children (Atkins, 2016), in part due to stigmas within the black community and personal choices. It is important that stigmas are neutralized and Black women seek the care they need.

INCORPORATE COMPLEMENTARY AND ALTERNATIVE MEDICINE (CAM)

Along with mainstream allopathic medicine, incorporate integrative approaches to address health issues and concerns. Include natural complementary and alternative medicine (CAM) for whole-body health and wellness, including but not limited to naturopathy, chiropractic, and acupuncture, as well as safe, tried and true remedies handed down generations. According to a 2017 national report by the NIH National Center for Complementary and Integrative Medicine, there was an increase in the use of yoga, meditation, and chiropractors, which were identified as commonly used approaches to health and wellness, between 2012 and 2017 (Clark et al., 2018).

ENGAGE IN PHYSICAL ACTIVITY

Engaging in regular physical activity is not only beneficial to physical health, but also mental and emotional health. Benefits include, but are not limited to, sleep enhancement, inspired physical intimacy, weight control, joint health, increased strength, decreased blood pressure, pain management, and increased endorphins and dopamine production, which triggers a pleasure effect and decreased stress and feelings of pain, while boosting energy and improving mood.

ACKNOWLEDGE AND CELEBRATE "WINS"

Slow down and "take time to smell the roses." Give yourself permission to celebrate the "wins"—the positive achievements, changes, and resolutions.

EVOLVE

The resilience of Black Motherhood is the capability to stand on the strength of the ancestors before them but also evolve as mothers. And with evolving and adapting comes balance, enhanced quality of life, and a more consistent, sustainable feeling of wholeness.

Black Mother, Queen, Prophetess, Earth Angel, Warrior Goddess, Child Bearer, Dinknesh—there is no earthly being above you—you are the "Matriarch of Mankind—the Resilient One." Keep your head held high, face to the sun, and allow yourself to be uplifted and ascend. After all, Black Motherhood is a blessing of resilience and ancestral birthright. A mother's love is "endless, all encompassing, and a force of nature that is unrivaled."

Recommendations and Call for Action

Black Mothers, women, and organizations across the globe need to continue to support, focus efforts, organize, and mobilize locally, regionally, nationally, and internationally. Efforts must persist to advance Black Mothers and women in the areas of health, finance, business, leadership, human rights and justice, science, technology, engineering, the arts, innovation, and beyond, despite the cacophony of societal challenges.

Organizations and foundations like Black Mamas Matter Alliance (BMMA), which is focused on research and policy change to advance Black maternal healthcare; the National Black Women's Justice Institute (NBWJI), which is focused on reducing racial and gender disparities in justice systems; and the Judy M. Braithwaite Family Foundation, Inc. (JMBF Foundation), which is focused on providing merit-based scholarships to college-bound students, are a few of many vested organizations committed to the progress of Black women, mothers, and families.

Supporting the efforts of organizations, foundations, and small businesses through research, funding, donations, and patronage significantly and positively impacts the lives of Black Mothers, children, and families.

Table 1.1. Foundations that honor legacies

AyannaGregory.com	Focus is therapeutic healing and empowerment through music and creative arts.
Black Career Women's Network	Focus is career advancement and networking.
Black Mamas Matter Alliance	Focus is research and policy change to advance black maternal health care.
Black Women's Blueprint	Focus is forefronting issues like health care, education, and economy.
Mocha Moms	Focus is support through all phases of motherhood and national advocation.
Moms Rising	Focus is nonpartisan cultural and legislative change.
Premier Spine Center, M. B. Gooden	Focus is patient-centered, integrative chiropractic care for whole body health and wellness.
SisterLove	Focus is HIV/AIDS education, prevention, and self-help.
The Black Maternal Health Caucus	Focus is improving health outcomes during pregnancy and postpartum.
The Black Women's Agenda	Focus is data-based policy changes and economic, social, and civil liberties education.
The Black Women's Health Imperative	Focus is evidence-based programs to improve health and wellness.
The Black Women's Playwright Group	Focus is supporting playwrights through networking with actors, directors, and producers.
The Foundation for Black Women's Wellness	Focus is eliminating health disparities.
The Judy M. Braithwaite Family Foundation	Focus is providing merit-based scholarships to college-bound students.

continued on next page

Table 1.1. Continued.

The Loveland Foundation	Focus is providing financial support to Black women and girls seeking mental health support.
The National Association of Colored Women's Clubs	Focus is advancing economic and social welfare.
The National Black Women's Justice Institute	Focus is reducing racial and gender disparities in justice systems.
The National Coalition of 100 Black Women	Focus is health, education, and economic empowerment.
The National Congress of Black Women	Focus is educational, political, and cultural development.
The National Council of Negro Women	Focus is small business initiatives and programs that address national obesity.

Source: Author.

And, although the resiliency of Black Mothers knows no bounds, the importance of protecting, respecting, and cherishing the Black Mother and woman is paramount. It matters.

Note

1. The approach to writing this chapter was based on a collection of direct and indirect experiences and stories of Black Mothers across generations, accepted generalities with the "Black community," and philosophical contributions. The chapter does not analyze, distinguish, or expound on Black Mothers born in the U.S. versus Africa, the Caribbean, or any other related geographical areas/countries/continents globally nor distinguish "good" vs "bad" Black Mothers, mothering, motherhood, or issues like parenting style to address such issues. Black and African-American are used interchangeably and often capitalized (as is Black Mother) for emphasis as a distinguishable group.

References

Atkins, R. (2016). Coping with depression in single black mothers. *Issues in Mental Health Nursing, 37*(3), 172–181. https://doi.org/10.3109/01612840.2015.1098760

Bailey, A., Sharma, M., & Jubin, M. (2013). The mediating role of social support, cognitive appraisal, and quality health care in black mothers' stress-resilience process following loss to gun violence. *Violence and Victims, 28*(2). https://doi.org/10.1891/0886-6708.11-00151

Braithwaite, P. (2019, September 30). Mental health in Black moms is largely ignored—5 ways we can improve it. *Self.*

Clark, T., Barnes, P., Black L., Stussman, B., & Nahin, R. (2018). *Use of yoga, meditation, and chiropractors among US adults aged 18 and older* (National Center for Health Statistics, Data Brief no. 325).

Clemetson, L. (2006, February 9). Work vs. family, complicated by race. *The New York Times*, G1.

Dow, D. M. (2019). Introduction: Not part of that White motherhood society. *Mothering while Black: Boundaries and burdens of middle-class parenthood.* University of California Press.

Everet alt, J. E., Marks, L. D., & Clarke-Mitchell, J. F. (2016). A qualitative study of the Black mother-daughter relationship: Lessons learned about self-esteem, coping, and resilience. *Journal of Black Studies, 47*(4). https://doi.org/10.1177/0021934716629339

Farrell, C. (2013). Motherhood and medical ethics: Looking beyond conception and pregnancy. *AMA Journal of Ethics, 15*(9), 743–745. https://doi.org/10.1001/virtualmentor.2013.15.9.fred1-1309

Geronimus, A. T., Hicken, M., Keene, D., & Bound, J. (2006). "Weathering" and age pattern of allostatic load scores among Blacks and Whites in the United States. *American Journal of Public Health, 96*(5), 826–833. https://doi.org/10.2105/AJPH.2004.060749

Jackson, B., & Kiehl, E. M. (2017). Adaptation and resilience in African American mothers. *SAGE Open Nursing, 3.* https://doi.org/10.1177/2377960817701137

Jethro, D. (2016, June 21). Meet 3-million-year-old Lucy—She'll tell you a lot about modern African heritage. *The Conversation.* https://theconversation.com/meet-3-million-year-old-lucy

Johnson, L. B., & Staples, R. (2004). *Black families at the crossroads: Challenges and prospects* (rev. ed.). Jossey-Bass.

Chapter 2

Dispelling Negative Stereotypes and Images
Black Girl Magic, Black Girls Rock!

Regina Davis Moss

Throughout history to the present day, Black women have been unfairly subjected to myths and stereotypes about their lives. Black women have been ascribed negative and inferior images as the result of a long-lived legacy of racism, sexism, and oppression. The distorted representation of the Black woman was extremely important for the creation and maintenance of the political, economic, and social structure of America, particularly during slavery. When the Slave Trade Act of 1807 ended, enslaved Black women were repeatedly coerced, raped, and forced to breed enslaved children for their owners' financial gain (Sublette & Sublette, 2016; Bridgewater, 2000). To justify their dehumanization, the conceptualization of images that continuously discredit and "other" Black women became the foundation for framing Black women's identities. Prevailing stereotypes of Black womanhood include the Jezebel, Mammy, Tragic Mulatto, Sapphire, Matriarch, Welfare Mother, and Strong Black Woman archetypes.

Jezebel

The Jezebel is an attractive seductress who is governed by her libido and matters of the flesh (White, 1999). She is deemed a hypersexual woman with insatiable, animalistic passions, and therefore morally undisciplined. The historical portrayal of the Jezebel's sexual greed was diametrically opposed to the idolized passionlessness of the "true woman," who was chaste, delicate, pure, and white. The stereotype of sexually promiscuous also defined Black women as bad mothers who procreate with abandon (Roberts, 2017).

It is important to note the construct of the licentious temptress served to justify the sexual abuse of slave women by their owners, and thus the jealousy and resentment of White women (Hill Collins, 2000; Villarosa, 1994). American society widely believed Black women drew on their sexual relationships with their White masters to not only satisfy their own desires, but to gain freedom and other privileges (Stephens & Phillips, 2003). This reinforced the myth that Black women are responsible for their own rape and sexual coercion. Indeed, from the moment they set foot in America, Black women have been vulnerable to rationalized sexual exploitation.

The image of the lascivious and devious Black woman was systematical, perpetuated long after the ending of slavery (Roberts, 2017). Modern-day portrayals are seen in music videos and often reinforced in mass media, including television shows, movies, and magazines that feature images of Black women.

Mammy

In direct contradiction to the Jezebel, the obsequious and matronly Mammy represented the embodiment of the ideal Black woman. Generally, pictured as dark-skinned, thick-lipped, rotund, and handkerchiefed, the Mammy portrayed the content servant, skilled cook, most devoted housekeeper, and capable nurturer of the master's children (Roberts, 2017). She was also depicted as asexual and nonthreatening to her mistress's femininity due to her old age, physical strength, and obesity.

The Mammy archetype highlighted the social prestige of Southern White families, the South's romanticization of the Black-White relationship, and a historical legitimation for slavery and segregation (Morton, 1991). The image preserved the convenient script of the happy, docile, Black female servant during a period when Black women were transitioning from unpaid house slaves to paid domestic workers (Stephens & Phillips, 2003).

Despite evidence affirming Mammy was a largely mythical figure with little basis in the lived experiences of Black women (Walker-Barnes, 2014), the caricature became a cult figure during the Jim Crow era. Mammy was embodied in Aunt Jemima for the Chicago Columbia Exposition in

1893 and appeared on pancake boxes for decades (Roberts, 2017). In June 2020, Quaker Oats announced it would retire the name and characters, acknowledging one of its major brand's origins were based on a racial stereotype. The Mammy image, however, continues to proliferate, whether partly disguised or totally unchanged, today.

Tragic Mulatto

As slaves or as free domestic servants, Black females' proximity to their White masters made them more likely to be sexually harassed or raped. One result of interracial rape was miscegenation and the emergence of mulattos (Mgadmi, 2009). The mulatto is the offspring of a White slaveholder and his Black female slave. Despite her mixed Black and White ancestry the mulatto was considered Black in the light of the pervasive "one-drop rule," which held that "a single drop of 'Black blood'" made a person a Black (Davis, 1991).

Being "whitish" and regarded thus as more beautiful than fullblooded Black women, many mulattas were also during slavery sold for the exclusive purpose of prostitution and concubinage. The mulatta's imagery was conspicuously dichotomized between "good" and "bad," between the elevated "whitish" and degraded "Blackness," and capable of progress (Mgadmi, 2009).

Most strikingly, the mulatto was perceived as the product of an unnatural relationship committed by either Blacks or Whites and miscegenation was considered the greatest sin of all (Fredrickson, 1987). She was loathed by White society for being living proof that the color line had been crossed and stigmatized in the Black community for being born of a mother who had not exhibited standards of sexual purity. All these factors were contributory to the emergence of the image of "the tragic mulatto," who figured as an unstable, dangerous person who despised her descent, her family, and herself (Morton, 1991).

Sapphire

The Sapphire image is a loud, bitter, and domineering female who controls men and usurps their role. She is characterized as angry, disagreeable, hypersensitive, and emasculating, and her berating is directed at her partners and children (Stephens & Phillips, 2003). The Sapphire caricature is a harsh label used to punish Black women who violate the societal norms that encourage them to be passive, servile, nonthreatening, and unseen. This image became the prelude to the Matriarch and *Angry Black Women*.

Matriarch

The Matriarch is the unwed mother whose overbearing attitude is insinuated to be the cause of family instability. The stereotype holds that Black women's independence damages their families in two ways: they demoralized Black men and they transmitted a pathological lifestyle to their children, perpetuating generational poverty and antisocial behavior (Roberts, 2017). Assistant Secretary of Labor Daniel Patrick Moynihan popularized this myth when he commissioned a 1965 report, *The Negro Family: The Case for National Action*, that stated the African American experience was problematized by a family structure that was under the sexual controls of its women (Moynihan, 1967). Through his use of the term "matriarch," Moynihan presented African American women as emasculating and contemptuous females who did not need a man beyond using his seed for childbearing (Stephens & Phillips, 2003).

Welfare Mother

The Welfare Mother archetype is one that is lazy, uneducated, and purposefully breeding children to take advantage of public assistance programs (Hill Collins, 2000; Stephens & Phillips, 2003). Black mothers are portrayed as calculating, unable to adequately care for their children, a burden on taxpayers, and deserving of harsh discipline (Roberts, 2017).

Despite White and working people always having comprised the majority of those receiving government assistance, this stigmatizing stereotype was attributed to the Black female. This shift in narrative has enabled those in power to continue to monitor and control Black and female bodies under the guise of assistance.

Strong Black Woman

In an attempt to project an image of strength and, in part, push back against negative stereotypes such as Jezebel, Mammy, or Welfare Mother,

Black women created the narrative of the Strong Black Woman (SBW). The SBW role, also often referred to as the Superwoman, obligates Black women to present an image of strength, suppress emotions, resist dependence on others, succeed despite limited resources, and prioritize caregiving over self-care (Woods-Giscombé, 2010).

In her book *Too Heavy a Yoke: Black Women and the Burden of Strength*, Walker-Barnes (2014) contends, "The myth of Black women's strength is dangerously seductive in that it imbues Black women with a certain moral and emotional superiority, providing a psychic balm against the daily insults incurred from social injustice." Accordingly, Black women consider emotional strength a birthright, and moments of deviation cultural flaws or failure.

The stereotype of the SBW may be an emblem of a Black woman'ss value to her community; but it can also compromise her well-being. The obligation to perform as though she is superhuman conceals her vulnerabilities, isolation, and dissociation from any suffering (Bryant, 2018).

Texturism

Black women also experience texturism during which we are discriminated against based on how our hair naturally grows out of our heads. The length and texture of a Black woman's hair can have an impact on access to education, religious institutions, relationships, and employment opportunities (Mbilishaka, 2018; Johnson and Bankhead, 2014). Hair is often an overwhelming force in the negotiation of self-image for Black women (Capodilupo, 2015; Lewis, 1999). Black women make a personal and psychological decision to style their hair using heat, chemical, or nonchemical methods, such as twists, braids, locs, weaves, wigs, and straightened styles (Ellis-Hervey et al., 2016). Eurocentric beauty standards of long, flowing hair place pressure on Black women to focus on length retention and straightening procedures to permanently, or semipermanently alter the texture of their hair (Hargro, 2011). The adoption of these practices in the Black community is rooted in institutionalized ideas of racial hierarchy, acceptance, and advancement as a race in post-slavery America.

For many Black women, wearing a natural or unprocessed hair style is an identity that affirms ethnicity, in solidarity with others doing the same, and often a statement of direct opposition to mainstream ideals of beauty (Berry-McCrea, 2018; Barner, 2017). While we are currently witnessing a shift in the cultural understanding of natural hairstyles, the texture and style of Black women's hair continue to play a role in how they are viewed and appraised by others in society and the workplace. Studies have found Black women may be denied jobs based on stereotypes that natural hairstyles are unprofessional, unclean, unkempt, or intimidating (Dove, 2019; Constantinides et al., 2019). Such grooming and appearance policies exacerbate anti-Black bias and transcend across employment, school, athletics, and other areas of daily living. On January 1, 2020, California became the first state to implement the CROWN Act (2019), which updates the definition of "race" in the California Fair Employment and Housing Act and the California Education Code to be "inclusive of traits historically associated with race, including, but not limited to, hair texture and protective hairstyles." CROWN stands for Create a Respectful and Open World for Natural Hair and is a law that prohibits discrimination based on hair style and hair texture. While there is a strong movement to enact the CROWN Act in other states and localities, Black women are currently only afforded legal protections from discrimination against natural Black hairstyles in three states: California, New York, and New Jersey. When Black women are able to fully express their love for their natural hair, it helps to undo generations of teaching that Black hair in its natural state is not beautiful, or something to be hidden or covered up. Until then, many will be forced to choose between embracing their identities and individuality and professional advancement (Griffin, 2019; Dove, 2019).

The Politics of Respectability

Although the demeaning stereotypical perception of Black women was conditioned by White patriarchal ideals, Black women's efforts to counter these negative images were paradoxically based on the very values that condemned, enslaved, and degraded them. The debate and discourse about respectability within the Black community that pervaded the Progressive Era was at the heart of a strategy to "uplift" the race (Mgadmi, 2009). As biological and social reproducers, it is natural that Black women would be a key focus of the respectability discourse. Racial advancement placed an exaggerated importance on Black females abiding by the canons of respectability that rested on bourgeois values of thrift, sexual restraint, cleanliness, and hard work (Wolcott, 2001). Many Black women participated in domestic training courses and were instructed to wear modest and subdued clothing. Black intellectuals, activists, and institutions for racial reform such as the Urban League, the National Association for the Advancement of Colored People, and the National Association of Colored Women were actively instrumental in these reform tactics (Mgadmi, 2009). Black scholars of the period such as Booker T. Washington, Du Bois, and members of "The Talented Tenth," often perpetuated negative stereotypes about Black women by emphasizing domesticity, monogamy, sexual restraint, passionlessness, and other White patriarchal values of true womanhood. In their view, it reframed the "bad" image of Black women into a "good" feminine picture capable of rise in status. However, it also reflected an acceptance and internalization of such representations, a yielding to cultural inferiority, and narrow identity for Black women.

The Politics of Silence

Despite, the passionlessness and "sexually pure" identity projected upon them, which contradicted that of the Jezebel, Black women of all classes were distinctly left to contend with its actualization. The aim was to instill dignity and self-respect while also challenging negative, stereotypical images, which was not without costs. Working-class Black women may have been able to use this approach as a shield against sexual harassment, exploitation, and rape in private homes, while aspiring or middle-class Black women may have had to endure to appeal to Whites and gain status. In both cases, Black women were ushered into a cult of secrecy and silence even when sexually abused and harassed (Hine, 1994). In addition to dissemblance defining much of their public life, Black women's silence was a denial and repression of their own sexuality and emotions. There is a clear dichotomization between the privileges of femininity and protection from violence for Black women. How the law currently deals with a Black woman's rape reinscribes the historical notion that for Black women, sex is never against their will (Dagbovie-Mullins, 2013).

Dictated by a social and political purpose, the responsibility of the Black woman toward justice and equality for the Black community was made coterminous with her desire as a woman—a desire that was expressed as a dedication to elevating the race through respectability, reform, and a new gendered racial identity.

Impact on Health and Sexuality

It is important to explore the effects of stereotypes on health outcomes. There is evidence that stereotypes can be harmful to the well-being of Black women through at least two mechanisms: (1) stereotype threat and (2) stereotyping leading to discrimination (Rosenthal & Lobel, 2016). Stereotype threat is when an individual is worried or anxious about the possibility of confirming or being judged according to stereotypes about their group (Steele & Aronson, 1995). Patients who feel judged by healthcare workers are more likely to mistrust their health providers and delay treatment of health problems. They are also less likely to access available preventive care and follow medical instructions (Jones et al., 2013). Stereotype threat related to unique stereotypes about African American women have led Black women to experience greater distress throughout their lifetime and specifically during pregnancy (Rosenthal & Lobel, 2016). A large body of research indicates that chronic stress predicts greater risk of adverse birth outcomes for Black women, including maternal mortality, preterm birth, and low birth weight (Geronimus, 1992; Giscombé & Lobel, 2005; Parker Dominguez et al., 2008).

Stereotypes of Black women held by health care providers may also lead to conscious or unconscious discrimination and biases that can affect provision of care (Rosenthal & Lobel, 2016). A landmark study found many White medical students wrongly believe Black people have a higher pain tolerance than White people, impacting the accuracy of treatment recommendations. Of all participants, 73% held at least one false belief about the biological differences between races. Examples of these beliefs include Black people having thicker skin, less sensitive nerve endings, or stronger immune systems (Hoffman et al., 2016). In ample quantitative and qualitative studies, Black women report receiving lower quality of care including poor or disrespectful communication, rushed care, dismissed concerns, denial of treatment, and invasive procedures without consent, regardless of socioeconomic status.

Some healthcare stereotyping may be an unintended consequence of health awareness campaigns that often communicate and reinforce negative stereotypes about certain groups of people. Examples include those aimed at educating Black women about contraception, sexual risk-taking, and prevention of sexually transmitted infections. This does not contend certain health concerns should not be addressed in specific communities. However, messaging and interventions tend to focus on adverse sexual and reproductive outcomes and seldom include sex-positive data about experiences, rendering Black women's sexuality invisible. Black women are inundated with messages of how to have sex, with whom to have sex, and where to have sex. Few have heard sex and emotional pleasure discussed in the same breath (Stephens & Phillips, 2003).

Many Black researchers and feminists (Wyatt, 1997; Hill Collins, 2000; hooks, 1992) have long noted that Black female sexuality is stereotypically represented as inherently "abnormal," "excessive," and "disproportionate." Black women and girls are unable to escape the ways in which culture has used their gender and race to shape a monolithic image of deviant sexuality. Sarah (Saartjie) Bartmann, so-called Hottentot Venus, is known to be the original portrait of Black female sexuality. Persuaded to leave Cape Town, South Africa, she was forcibly put on display throughout Europe to illustrate the ways the exotic, animalistic bodies of African women—specifically the skin color, buttocks, and genitalia—broadcasted a presumed hypersexuality of Black women not associated with White standards of beauty and female sexuality (Flowers, 2018). During her performances, she was displayed partially nude, with a skin-colored loincloth as her only coverage (Gould, 1985).

The field of gynecology was born when Dr. J. Marion Sims explored vesico-vaginal fistulas using enslaved Black women as research subjects. These women—Anarcha, Lucy, and nine others—were forced to endure repeated exploratory, experimental, painful, and life-threatening vaginal surgeries without anesthesia or their consent (Flowers, 2018).

Black women are simultaneously fetishized and desexualized. On one hand they experience others as being attracted and drawn to them because of their physical appearance, while at the same time, our society's cultural ideals and social norms offer few sexual scripts. The everyday reinforcement of limited scripts has a direct impact on Black women's sexual self-concept, behaviors, and decision-making processes (Morton, 1991).

How Black women's health concerns, physical appearance, intellectual prowess, sexuality, and bodily autonomy are affirmed may influence their health experiences and outcomes (Wyatt, 1997). Healthcare providers and staff training focused on the multiple social and institutional factors that contribute to ongoing health disparities as well as how to provide patient-centered, culturally congruent care can break down stereotypes and ensure Black women feel understood and welcomed in the healthcare environment.

Influence of Media

Although there are more representations of African American women available for consumption in the mass media than ever before, the substance of these images has changed little over the past century (Wyatt, 1997; Stephens & Phillips, 2003). The exoticizing of African American women as wild, sexually promiscuous, and amoral continues to be normalized by descriptors that are widely circulated, accepted, and used to frame ideas about this population (hooks, 1992; Stephens & Phillip, 2003).

Media impacts our environments by influencing our beliefs, value systems, public ideology, and relation to one another other. What information the media presents to the general public regarding a particular group of people becomes how the public learns to understand the behaviors, expectations, and image of others. When audiences do not possess direct knowledge or experiences with such a group, they become particularly reliant upon the media to inform them.

Throughout history, the mass media, in various forms, have tended to support the power of the dominant group by presenting highly negative, emotion-evoking images of minority groups (Luther et al., 2011). This includes the news, network television series, reality TV, advertisements, music videos, and social media that portray Black women in ways that reify stereotypical gendered schemas. With these considerations in mind, it is important to understand the consequences that present themselves as a result of biased content. For example, media portrayals of economically disadvantaged Black women during the welfare debate and society's response to such portrayals play an important role in creating and sustaining the trope of the Welfare Queen. The picture is made all the more frightening by always depicting crack babies as Black children on welfare. The media sets up an assumption that all Black American girls grow up in the projects or city streets and all Black women, often regardless of their socioeconomic status, get placed in the same societal categorization. This stereotype is not a real person but a unidimensional stick figure who lives in the public imagination (Lamb, 2001).

Of note, not all media portrayals of Black women are negative or disempowering. However, it is particularly troubling that the images available for emulation exceedingly portray women in such limited, inferior, and frequently offensive ways. The content not only activates and reinforces existing stereotypical beliefs of consumers who have little contact with members of other racial or ethnic groups, but persistent exposure may also shape how African American females come to feel about themselves. Research has shown that television, particularly entertainment programming, is the most important source of information and socialization for African American adolescents. It has also been found that, when comparing by race and gender, African Americans and women spend the greatest amount of time watching television (Stephens & Phillips, 2003). As consumers of media, it is important we challenge the dominant discourse and hold the creators of content that promotes stereotypical images accountable.

In 2006, celebrity DJ Beverly Bond founded Black Girls Rock! (BGR!) to challenge stereotypical social constructs of Black women. The multifaceted media, entertainment, philanthropic, education, and empowerment platform showcases empowering images of women of color and promotes positive role models for girls. BGR! is a leading force in highlighting the spectrum of brilliance among Black women and a cultural paradigm shift where Black women's narratives, presence in society, and prominence in mainstream media are being elevated like never before.

Recommendations and Call for Action

This critical examination of adverse stereotypical images has practical implications for public health practitioners as well as individuals in any field who work and interact with Black women. It is important to increase awareness of how unique stereotypes about Black women, due to the intersection of race and gender, explicitly or implicitly affect perceptions, judgments, and their treatment. Further, it is valuable for policymakers to understand their application to persistent inequities in access to socioeconomic opportunities and the potential for broader public policy.

Given current interest in diversity, equity, and inclusion approaches that foster positive intergroup relations in diverse settings, the issues outlined above lend critical vocabulary and can be used to facilitate constructive dialogue about how beliefs, assumptions, and biases become institutionalized, and ultimately impact organizational priorities. This includes creating safe spaces for the important work of consciousness-raising, acknowledgment, and cultural appreciation.

Theoretical underpinnings for research and interventions serving Black women and girls should be informed by scholars of color whose work forms the basis of the field's knowledge. Loretta J. Ross, Kimberlé Williams Crenshaw, Patricia Hill Collins, and many others have provided foundations for sociocultural learning and understanding that prioritize Black women's lives (Ross et al., 2017; Crenshaw, 1991; Hill Collins, 2000; Flowers, 2018). In addition to looking back, we should also encourage more scholarship. This can be accomplished through support from philanthropic grants, private donors, and faculty-supported student-led research, as well as through the development of culturally congruent graduate courses and curricula (Flowers, 2018).

What's missing from the care of Black women is their centered voice, validation of experience, and freedom to choose and be informed. Black women need respectful care that is free of implicit and explicit bias (Black Mamas Matter Alliance, 2018). Expanding training and education in clinical settings is critical to promoting awareness of how bias affects care and places Black women's lives at risk.

Current findings, along with past evidence of the damaging effects of societal stereotypes, underscore the importance of diversifying images of Black women in media and including more positive, complex, and dynamic portrayals (Mastro, 2015). The extent to which audiences perceive negative, and often uncontested, portrayals as realistic are associated with endorsement of social scripts and decreased agency. How media content is formed, selected, and presented is heavily subjected to the opinions of those involved in the industry. Educators must be intentional about designing media literacy curricula that help young people think critically about the ways they internalize and embody stereotypes, interact with one another, and navigate imbalances of power in gender, race, and socioeconomics (Flowers, 2018). Closer study is also needed of the type of programming and genres in young people's media diets, as some may be more stereotypical than others (Ward, 2003).

Moving this paradigm-shifting work forward in the United States will only be accomplished by identifying and confronting the fallacies on which stereotypical images are constructed. It also requires critically exploring why they have persisted for centuries and what social and institutional structures are connected to their maintenance.

As part of a celebratory address delivered during the 1982 Malcolm X weekend at Harvard University, influential feminist scholar Audre Lorde stated, "[That is how I learned that if] I didn't define myself for myself I would be crunched into other people's fantasies for me and be eaten alive." In the face of repressive stereotypes, Black women's resilience prevails and continues the long struggle to write our own narrative filled with self-love and admiration. Hill Collins (2000) contends that, within

African American communities, Black women fashion an independent standpoint about the meaning of Black womanhood. As always, Black women use innate gifts and magic to organize and respond, center our voices, and determine our own destiny.

Resources

Black Girls Rock! https://www.blackgirlsrock.com

Morton, P. *Disfigured images: The historical assault on Afro-American women.* Greenwood, 1991.

Wyatt, G. *Stolen women: Reclaiming our sexuality, taking back our lives.* Wiley, 1997.

References

Barner, B. (2017, July 6). The personal is digital: Exploring race, beauty and hair online. *Flow Journal.* https://www.flowjournal.org/2017/07/the-personal-is-digital

Berry-McCrea, E. L. (2018). "To My Girls in Therapy, See Imma Tell You This fo Free . . .": Black Millennial Women Speaking Truth to Power in and across the Digital Landscape. *Meridians, 16*(2), 363–372.

Black Mamas Matter Alliance. (2018). *Setting the standard for holistic care of and for Black women.* https://blackmamasmatter.org/wp-content/uploads/2018/04/BMMA_BlackPaper_April-2018.pdf.

Bridgewater, P. D. (2000). Reproductive freedom as civil freedom: The Thirteenth Amendment's role in the struggle for reproductive rights. *Journal of Gender, Race and Justice, 3*(2), 401–425.

Bryant, C. (2018). Re-membering ourselves: Confession as a pathway to conscientization. *Meridians, 16*(2), 351–362.

California Government Code § 12926. California Fair Employment and Housing Act.

California Government Code Id. § 212.1. California Education Code.

Capodilupo, C. M. (2015). One size does not fit all: Using variables other than the thin ideal to understand Black women's body image. *Cultural Diversity and Ethnic Minority Psychology, 21*(2), 268–278.

Constantinides, D., Sennott, S., Davis, C. (2019). *Sex therapy with erotically marginalized clients: Nine principles of clinical support.* Routledge.

Crenshaw, K. (1991). Mapping the margins: Intersectionality, identity politics, and violence against women of color. *Stanford Law Review, 43*(6), 1241–1299.

CROWN Act (Create a Respectful and Open Workplace for Natural Hair), Senate Bill 188 (CA, 2019). https://leginfo.legislature.ca.gov/faces/billTextClient.xhtml?bill_id=201920200SB188

Dagbovie-Mullins, S. (2013). Pigtails, ponytails, and getting tail: The infantilization and hyper-sexualization of African American females in popular culture. *Journal of Popular Culture, 46*(4), 745–774.

Davis, F. (1991). *Who is Black? One nation's definition.* Pennsylvania State University Press.

Dove. (2019). *The CROWN research study.* https://static1.squarespace.com/static/5edc69fd622c36173f56651f/t/5edeaa2fe5ddef345e087361/1591650865168/Dove_research_brochure2020_FINAL3.pdf

Ellis-Hervey, N., Doss, A., Davis, D., Nicks, R. &Araiza, P. (2016). African American personal presentation: Psychology of hair and self-perception. *Journal of Black Studies, 47*(8), 869–882.

Flowers, S. C. (2018). Enacting our multidimensional power: Black women sex educators demonstrate the value of an intersectional sexuality education framework. *Meridians, 16*(2), 308–325.

Fredrickson, G. (1987). *The Black image in the White mind: The debate on Afro-American character and destiny, 1817–1914* (with new introd.). Wesleyan University Press.

Geronimus, A. T. (1992). The weathering hypothesis and the health of African-American women and infants: evidence and speculations. *Ethnicity and Disease, 2*(3):207–221.

Giscombé, C. L., & Lobel, M. (2005). Explaining disproportionately high rates of adverse birth outcomes among African Americans: The impact of stress, racism, and related factors in pregnancy. *Psychological Bulletin, 131*(5), 662–683.

Griffin, C. (2019, July 3). How natural Black hair at work became a civil rights issue. *JSTOR Daily.* https://daily.jstor.org/how-natural-black-hair-at-work-became-a-civil-rights-issue/

Gould, S. J. (1985). The Hottentot Venus. In *The Flamingo's smile: Reflections in natural history* (pp. 291–305). Norton.

Hargro, B. (2011). *Hair matters: African American women and the natural hair aesthetic* [master's thesis, Georgia State University]. https://scholarworks.gsu.edu/art_design_theses/95

Hill Collins, P. (2000). *Black feminist thought: Knowledge, consciousness, and the politics of empowerment* (2nd ed.). Routledge.

Hine, D. (1994). Rape and the inner lives of Black women in the Middle West: Preliminary thoughts on the culture of dissemblance. In V. L. Ruiz & E. C. DuBois(eds.), *Unequal sisters: A multicultural reader in U.S. women's history* (2nd ed.). Routledge.

Hoffman, K., Trawalter, S., Axt, J., Oliver, M. (2016). Racial bias in pain assessment and treatment recommendations, and false beliefs about biological differences between blacks and whites. *Proceedings of the National Academy of Sciences, 113*(16) 4296–4301.

hooks, b. (1992). *Black looks: Race and representations.* Between the Lines Press.

Johnson, T. A., & Bankhead, T. (2014). Hair it is: Examining the experiences of Black women with natural hair. *Open Journal of Social Sciences, 2*(1), 86–100.

Jones, P. R., Taylor, D. M., Dampeer-Moore J., Van Allen, K. L., Saunders, D. R., Snowden, C. B., & Johnson, M. B. (2013). Health-related stereotype threat predicts health services delays among Blacks. *Race and Social Problems, 5*, 121–136.

Lamb, S. (2001). *The secret lives of girls: What good girls really do—Sex play, aggression, and their guilt.* Free Press.

Lewis, M. L. (1999). Hair combing interactions: A new paradigm for research with African American mothers. *American Journal of Orthopsychiatry, 69*(4), 504–514.

Lorde, Audre. (1984). *Sister outsider: Essays and speeches.* Crossing Press.

Luther, C., Ringer Lepre, C., Clark, N. (2011). *Diversity in U.S. mass media.* Wiley.

Mastro, D. (2015). Why the media's role in issues of race and ethnicity should be in the spotlight. *Journal of Social Issues, 71*(1), 1–16.

Mbilishaka, A. (2018). PsychoHairapy: Using hair as an entry point into Black women's spiritual and mental health. *Meridians, 16*(2), 382–392.

Mgadmi, M. (2009). Black women's identity: Stereotypes, respectability and passionlessness (1890–1930). *Revue LISA, 7*(1), 40–55.

Morton, P. (1991). *Disfigured images: The historical assault on Afro-American women.* Greenwood.

Moynihan, D. P. (1967). The Negro family: A case for national action. In L. Rainwater & W. L. Yancey (Eds.), *The Moynihan report and the politics of controversy* (pp. 41–124). MIT Press.

Parker Dominguez, T., Dunkel-Schetter, C., Glynn, L., Hobel, C., & Sandman, C. (2008). Racial differences in birth outcomes: The role of general, pregnancy, and racism stress. *Health Psychology, 27*(2), 194–203.

Roberts, D. (2017). *Killing the black body: Race, reproduction, and the meaning of liberty.* Vintage.

Rosenthal, L., & Lobel, M. (2016). Stereotypes of Black American women related to sexuality and motherhood. *Psychology of Women Quarterly, 40*(3), 414–427.

Ross, L., Roberts. L., Derkas, E., Peoples, W., & Bridgewater Toure, P. (2017). *Radical reproductive justice: Foundations, theory, practice, critique.* Feminist Press.

Steele, C. M., & Aronson, J. (1995). Stereotype threat and the intellectual test performance of African Americans. *Journal of Personality and Social Psychology, 69*(5), 797–811.

Stephens, D. P., & Phillips, L. D. (2003). Freaks, gold diggers, divas, and dykes: The sociohistorical development of adolescent African American women's sexual scripts. *Sexuality and Culture, 7*(1), 3–49.

Sublette, N., & Sublette, C. (2016). *The American slave coast: A history of the slave-breeding industry*. Lawrence Hill Books.

Thompson, C. (2009). Black women, beauty, and hair as a Matter of being. *Women's Studies, 38*(8), 831–856.

Villarosa, L. (1994). *Body and soul: The African American women's guide to physical health and emotional well-being*. Harper Perennial.

Walker-Barnes, C. (2014). *Too heavy a yoke: Black women and the burden of strength*. Cascade Books.

Ward, L. M. (2003). Understanding the role of entertainment media in the sexual socialization of American youth: A review of empirical research. *Developmental Review, 23*(3), 347–388.

White, D. G. (1999). *Ar'n't I a woman: Female slaves in the plantation South*. Norton.

Wolcott, V. (2001). *Remaking respectability: African American women in interwar Detroit*. University of North Carolina Press.

Woods-Giscombé, C. L. (2010). Superwoman schema: African American women's views on stress, strength, and health. *Qualitative Health Research, 20*(5), 668–683.

Wyatt, G. (1997). *Stolen women: Reclaiming our sexuality, taking back our lives*. Wiley.

Chapter 3

The Superwoman (Sojourner) Syndrome and African American/Black Women

TABIA HENRY AKINTOBI,
ADRIENNE CHEVELLE GLYMPH FOSTER,
BRIDG'ETTE ISRAEL, AND TAYLOR A. WIMBLY

> That man over there says that women need to be helped into carriages, and lifted over ditches, and to have the best place everywhere. Nobody ever helps me into carriages, or over mud-puddles, or gives me any best place! And ain't I a woman? Look at me! Look at my arm! I have ploughed and planted, and gathered into barns, and no man could head me! And ain't I a woman?
>
> —Sojourner Truth (Ain't I a Woman, 1851)

African American/Black women's resilience is rooted in individual or collective historical experiences from which recovery is required. Recovery may be from personal trauma or the social injustices inherent with the dual identities of membership in a systemically less powerful race/ethnicity and gender. It is also associated with the bruises and bumps related to the personal and public drive to be excellent. African American/Black (AA/B) women often hold a subconscious intent to *prove* worthiness and competence to some who expect less and others who know that they will get the job done at all costs. There are also stressors associated with the attempt to juggle a perpetually changing set of balls—some chosen (e.g., mother, boss, partner), and some required. The "bounce back" associated with resilience may be to a happier existence or one reflecting the perfect proverbial "balance" that does not exist. Whatever the reason, the weight, crown, and magic associated with being strong, AA/B, and female creates both welcome and unexpected stress. In this chapter we will unpack its root, consequences, and a path forward.

Sojourner Truth, born Isabella Baumfree, was sold into slavery at the young age of nine. For nearly 30 years she was enslaved and experienced physical, mental, and sexual abuse at the hands of her slave owners. Upon receiving emancipation, Sojourner became an avid women's rights activist and abolitionist. Sojourner embodied strength, independence, and resilience. She is well-known for her speech *Ain't I a Woman*, given at the 1851 Women's Convention in Akron, Ohio (Truth, 1851). In this speech she discusses the differences in how she was treated as an AA/B woman compared to White women, citing how she was never "helped into carriages" and "lifted over ditches." She goes on to discuss how she has "ploughed and planted and gathered into barns," tasks that are manual labor and typically done by men. Her speech spoke to the societal lack of regard for AA/B women's womanhood and showcases the strength to persevere in times of hardship. During this time in history, AA/B women were utilized for hard manual labor, while White women were seen as more fragile and unable to handle such tasks (Lekan, 2009).

Researchers have coined Sojourner as one of the first "strong Black women" alongside others like Harriet Tubman. In 1997, Leith Mullings first conceptualized the Sojourner Syndrome (SS) framework. This framework provided a culturally relevant way to explain the inequalities in race, class, and gender experienced by AA/B women (Mullings, 2002). The SS represents the survival skills displayed by AA/B women that held the community together to survive 400 years of slavery, segregation, and discrimination (Lekan, 2009, p. 35). Many researchers have noted that the SS can be compared to the John Henryism (JH) framework (Lekan, 2009; Warren-Findlow, 2006). John Henry was an AA folk hero known for his strength in driving railroad spikes. He proved he was better, faster, and stronger than a machine in saving jobs for AA men and ultimately died from exhaustion (Lekan, 2009). JH framework describes the act of being vigilant to confront barriers (Warren-Findlow, 2006). Similarly, in the SS framework AA/B women are seen as strong, hardworking, head of the household, and resilient in the face of obstacles. The characteristics of strength and striving to and attaining success are all commendable attributes, but, altogether, are hard to navigate without self-awareness and attention to self-care.

SS is defined as a condition when the intersection of race, gender, and class combine to potentially cause mental and physical health issues. It has been determined that AA/B women are the subgroup that identifies with this condition most, and therefore the name of the abolitionist and women's rights activist was chosen. The name represents resilience and a need for a strategic approach to undo the damage of this silent assassin.

The propaganda that has repeatedly played out in movies, novels, and songs has taught society to question *all* women's capabilities, relevance, and values. Then to be an AA/B woman is second strike. For years, AA/B women have dealt with being labeled as a Jezebel (promiscuous and overly sexualized), Mammy (older AA woman caretaker), and Welfare Queen (reference to misuse of welfare funds) (Woods-Giscombe, 2010). The Superwoman Schema (SWS) can be imagined as a modernized version of the SS recently emerging as a coping strategy for racism and oppression in AA/B women as result of the negative stereotypes. Cheryl Woods-Giscombe (2010) conducted a qualitative study with AA/B women from various socioeconomic backgrounds between the ages of 19 and 72. Findings from the focus groups led her to the five characterizations that make up the SWS. Those characteristics are (1) obligation to manifest strength, (2) obligation to suppress emotions, (3) resistance to being vulnerable or dependent, (4) determination to succeed despite limited resources, and (5) obligation to help others (Woods-Giscombe, 2010).

Since SS framework's conception, AA/B women have continued to fight for equality and respect in society. AA/B women are constantly seeking to change the narrative and move away from the stereotypes placed among them through the media. Vines et al. (2006) detailed their survey of AA/B, with 93% who identified with being a victim of racism and/or discrimination. Discriminatory acts and the fear of these actions cause daily and unnecessary stress. Malcolm X stated in one of his iconic speeches that "the most disrespected person in America is the black woman" (X, 1962).

Since history recorded the initial presence of the AA/B women as naked on the auction block, one can understand why they are desired, but not respected. This tale of uninvited vulnerability and servitude, along with being seen as property, solely for the pleasure of others, has been inherited by each generation, despite civil and gender rights progress. Today, the sting is still just as deadly. The Sojourner woman strives to survive while serving as an example of strength, determination, and excellence.

The Unique Leadership Position of African American/Black Women

The Personal and Professional Juggling Act

The Forbes Fortune 500 list only included four Black CEOs in 2020 after Jide Zeitlin resigned. Rosalind Brewer will lead Walgreens as CEO starting March 2021 and become the only Black female CEO of a Fortune 500 company (Kowitt & Zillman, 2021). The number of AA/B leaders are disproportionate when compared to their Caucasian counterparts. United States president, Catholic clergy member, head coach of a major sport, and secretary of defense are just a short list of leadership positions that have never been filled by women (Gillett, 2018). These data would suggest women are not qualified for leadership positions, but that couldn't be further from the truth.

Stacey Abrams became the first Black female governor nominee of a major party when she won the democratic vote in 2018 (Martin & Burns, 2018). Though Brian Kemp defeated her in that election by a narrow margin, she continued to do great work for her constituents in Georgia. This was a minor defeat, which placed her in the perfect position to oversee the voting process in Georgia during the 2020 presidential election. Abrams and her team maintained an accurate count, resulting in the Biden-Harris win in Georgia. Turning Georgia blue in 2020 helped the democratic ticket earn enough Electoral College votes to win the election, making Kamala Harris the first woman vice-president of the United States and first person of color to hold this office.

Black Excellence comes at a price and AA/B women pay with their mental and physical health. Finding balance between home and work is an uphill battle for women. Many women have responsibilities within their families, careers, and social circles, making it all look so easy because the more we have to do the more we get done. The will to survive changes the focus of countless AA/B women from thriving in social settings to career success. Relationships with family and friends once served as a healthy way of venting and releasing stress but now has gotten lost in the life of a busy Sojourner woman.

Some refer to it as a juggling act, while others seek balance. Nonetheless the outcome is the same. There is a need for a deliberate approach to identify the unique characteristics that gives this resilient group their edge. Sharpening the tools the world gave them in order to provide this world with what it so desperately needs. Sojourner women are determined, ambitious, and insightful leaders who need to take care of themselves so they can better serve humanity (Mullings, 2005). Against all odds, these women thrive in work environments that were not designed with them in mind.

The road AA/B women travel to secure leadership positions is narrow, not well-paved or well-traveled. Translated differently, AA/B women may have wonderful male or female mentors who don't look like them and provide sound advice, but they may not represent the same lived experience central to the AA/B and female experiences. This, in turn, does not adequately prepare them for how the SS and SWS can negatively manifest. There are lots of meetings you may not receive an invitation to. As we make strides to higher heights and breaking glass ceilings, we must also put forth an effort to help other AA/B women. This will protect and strengthen all of humanity, because a diverse workplace is a place that could foster novel ideas. Everyone can benefit in such an environment through exposure to diversity, being stretched toward valuing the importance of inclusion and integration of those with different lenses and perspectives toward more comprehensive programs, interventions, and solutions. There are still so many firsts for Black women to achieve, so our dedication to helping the next generation prepare for the future will provide perpetuity of all women in the spaces we desire to occupy.

The Weight and Responsibility of the Pursuit of Wealth

The SS and SWS is correlated with the attainment of wealth for AA/B women. Wealth—what is owned minus what is owed—is a buffer between unexpected setbacks and economic catastrophe. Without savings or wealth, resilience from unplanned disruptions like job loss or health emergencies can domino into negative mental and physical consequences from which recovery can be potentially insurmountable. For most women, the dream is for the next generation—whether one's children or community—to do better than they have. Zaw et al. (2017) posit that "wealth is associated with the well-being of the next generation, as it provides parents with the ability to help pay for their children's college education and can also be passed down from generation to generation." More often, African American families and the women within are experiencing first- or second-generation wealth with welcomed cultural responsibility that compounds the negative effects of the SS, if not attended to.

At the intersection of race and gender, AA/B women reflect the least realization of wealth when compared to other groups. According to the Panel Study of Income Dynamics (PSID), AA/B women who are not married typically fare the worst. Single White women without a college degree have $3,000 more in median wealth than single AA/B with a college degree. Marriage does not reap wealth dividends for AA/B women. White women have more than five times the wealth of their black counterparts. While single White mothers have a median wealth of $3,000, AA/B single mothers experience the largest wealth disadvantage with a median wealth of zero (Zaw et al., 2017).

Millennials (those born between 1981 and 1996) are one of the first generations to rapidly reflect portfolios closing the wealth gap (Dorsainvil, 2019). AA/B women in this group experience great success as they strive. They are the demographic with the highest growth rate of college enrollment when compared to other groups, and are increasingly working in management, professional, and related jobs. They are, however, frequently the financial backbones of not only their families but of others whom they seek to bring along toward similar success.

The realities of race and wealth attainment, particularly for AA/B women, represent important considerations amid their Sojourner identity because not only are they to be strong and achieve, but also bring their village with them. They do, however, experience concurrent guilt, pressure, and responsibilities as their wealth grows. Moreover, African Americans are significantly more likely to become a family caregiver over the course of their lifetime, often while maintaining part- or full-time employment (Flynn, 2018). This reality reflects a financial responsibility that can take a negative toll, not only on their wealth trajectory, but on their health.

Sojourner Syndrome, Superwoman Schema, and Health Disparities among African American/Black Women

Living up to the SS and SWS ideals can in turn cause AA/B women to be more susceptible to disease and illness. The SS is constantly paired with the theoretical hypothesis, weathering (Lekan, 2009; Mullings, 2002; Warren-Findlow, 2006; Mullings, 2005). Weathering conceptualizes the impact of consistent stress, due to institutional inequalities, across the life span that contributes to excessive morbidity and mortality in AA women (Lekan, 2009; Warren-Findlow, 2006). Weathering can begin early in life and worsen with age. Stressors experienced from maintaining resilience through hardships (i.e., SS) contribute to weathering. Qualitative research has found that chronic stress is related to the continued discrimination of race, gender, class, and age in AA/B women. Studies show that AA/B women are in alignment with SS, seeking to manifest strength in the face of adversity, being the center of the family, taking on the role as the primary caretaker, maintaining a job, and making life better for all those around them (Lekan, 2009). This level of stress taken on by AA/B women has led to health disparities in chronic illnesses such as heart disease (Lekan, 2009; Mullings, 2002; Warren-Findlow, 2006; Mullings, 2005).

The SS framework helps to clarify the intersection between race, class, and gender. Not only are there inequities associated with simply being a woman but also being AA can inherently affect class status. The SS provides a broad explanation for the burden of poorer health. AA/B women experience utilizing Sojourner Truth at the center as the "strong Black woman." Woods-Giscombe (2010) describes the role of Superwoman as a "double-edged sword" for health in AA/B women (p. 669). The SWS has proven to have both positive and negative effects. On the one hand it serves to empower women to have fortitude and support others, thinking of the women that came before them. On the other hand, it can be detrimental to the health of AA/B women by giving the idea that there's no room for weakness or vulnerability and can negatively enforce shame in asking for help.

AA/B women make up roughly 7% of the total US population and 52% of the AA population (CDC Wonder, 2020). However, they exceed all races in mortality for heart disease, cancer, and stroke (Adkins-Jackson et al., 2019). The SS and SWS are both considered helpful for black women's survival and self-preservation. They can, however, be harmful to self-care behaviors due to greater prioritization of others' needs when compared to their own (Stanton et al., 2017). SWS characteristics are associated with perceived stress, depressive symptoms, emotional eating, sleep disturbance, and sedentary behavior in African American women (Woods-Giscombe et al., 2016; Allen et al., 2019). In a recent study looking at the effect of SWS on mental health in AA women, researchers found that several of the participants described SWS characteristics as reasons for not seeking mental health care. For example, participants stated they did not want to be "perceived as weak," which aligns with SWS characteristic "obligation to present an image of strength." Participants also discussed the "obligation to suppress emotions," naming their mothers, grandmothers, and other caregivers that came before them and held things in because they were the backbones of the family (Allen et al., 2019). AA/B women in this study also discussed the role faith played in their desire to pursue mental health services. Many agreed on the phrases "God wouldn't put more on me than I can bear," "What doesn't kill you makes you stronger," and "Give the situation to God" (Allen et al., 2019). These comments align with SWS "resistance to being vulnerable about depending on others." Findings from the study suggest that cultural expectations around faith influence women's decisions about using mental health services and the appearance of strength is a proxy for degree of faith in God (Allen et al., 2019). In a second study with a group of prediabetic AA/B women, participants mentioned feelings of guilt related to delaying their own self-care but still believed their family's needs superseded their own (Sheffield-Abdullah & Woods-Giscombe, 2021). They also recognized how this can have negative impacts on their personal health. "Even though you know something wrong with you, it's like you put it on the back burner and say 'Aw, I can do it later.' And then you get obesity when—you don't really do it, but you start eating the good stuff because everybody has stressed you out and this is how you cope with it," said one participant (Sheffield-Abdullah & Woods-Giscombe, 2021).

Implications for Psychological, Spiritual, and Emotional Well-Being

As AA/B women continue to embrace the SWS, this narrative is greatly impacting their overall health and general well-being from a psychological and physiological perspective and subsequently the genetic level. This stress (distress and eustress) impacts all aspects of the human body and affects all organs. This issue includes head—emotional/psychological, concentration problems, lack of energy, mood swings, panic attacks, anxiety; and from the largest organ, skin—acne, eczema, dermatitis, skin rashes, and random breakouts; heart—increased blood pressure, high cholesterol, fast heartbeat, increased risk of heart attack, stroke, and increased high cholesterol; stomach—irritable bowel syndrome (IBS), inflammatory bowel disease (IBD), food allergies, stomach cramps, nausea, and weight fluctuation; intestines—lowered nutrient absorption, reduced metabolism, decreased enzymatic output, increased risk of IBD, and diabetes; pancreas—elevated secretion of insulin, damaged arteries, and obesity; reproductive system—decreased estrogen production leading to reduced fertility and loss of sexual drive; immune system—suppressed immune system to fight and recover from illness, high levels of inflammation in the body, thus increased potential for chronic health conditions (Conway-Phillips et al., 2020; Adkins-Jackson et al., 2019; Kang et al., 2018; Woods-Giscombe et al., 2016).

This effect is an ongoing fight or flight response with little time for relaxation, recovery, and recharge. The Superwoman Schema identifies neglect of self-care as one of the stress related health behaviors that can be perceived as a liability in the SWS (Woods-Giscombe et al., 2016). This belief is a form of kryptonite for the Superwoman Syndrome. In addition to the psychological and physiological affect, there is an impact on a genetic level. Exposure to stress can modify DNA methylation, which has the potential to alter gene expression and thus contribute to disease phenotypes.

The AA/B Superwoman has forsaken her own needs and self-care over generations to assist and support others. The occasional visit to the beauty shop was the extent of self-care for many. The idea of leisure or down-time was unheard of and not embraced. The belief was more often centered on utilizing religiosity as an approach for self-care. In recent years with groups like Girl Trek and Outdoor Afros, there has been a wanting to get out and exercise and explore, moving from helping and supporting everyone else to giving themselves permission to be a priority, moving the care of the AA woman higher up on the necessary priority list.

Our Sisters' Sentiments

As we examined the relevance of the SS and SWS on the historical and current lives of AA/B women we invited their engagement to make our inquiry more formal and expand on the secondary literature. A Qualtrics survey was disseminated and completed by 125 AA/B women. The survey contained Likert scale questions through which participants selected a value from 0 to 5 representing their level of stress and how well they handled stress. They also indicated their age range, any health or medical conditions, and their highest level of education completed. Group 1 was comprised of women at the beginning of their careers (18–34 years of age) and made up 37.1% of those surveyed. Group 2 consisted of women with work experience (age 35–54), representing 50.8%. Women who were nearing retirement or retired made up Group 3 (≥ 55), composing 12.1% of the total. Nine women (three per group) agreed to participate in follow-up key informant interviews. There was no significant difference in the stress levels based on education or age. Most women (84%) identified with having a stressful life that they managed well. Though these women perceive they are handling their stress well, they suffer from various health issues that stem from stress. High blood pressure was most frequently reported (31.7%) when compared to the other heath conditions that included high cholesterol (15%), diabetes (8.7%). and chronic migraine headaches (8.7%), respectively. Women could choose more than one health issue. Women who participated in key informant interviews were asked to share the inherent balls that seemed immovable as well as those that they have chosen. Both were part of the psychological, social, or emotional realities in the "balance" and "juggle" of the demands of their excellence, time, and intentions to last. A few reflections are noted in the sections that follow.

Superwoman (Sojourner) Syndrome: Factors Outside of Her Control

Tarita B. (Group 2), executive director of a community-based organization, indicated that she cannot control the determinants of "employee motivation, performance and professionalism" of those that make up her organization. This is challenging because she sometimes wants to employ the social work skills central to her passion and training to get to the root of the matter but knows this is not her role. She must refrain from the SWS that tempts her to want to fix this. It is an "inner struggle" that creates stress for those she knows are simply seeking a paycheck versus following a passion. She must still expect a certain level of professionalism that does not always manifest.

Nachae' J. (Group 1), entrepreneur, artist, and therapist, discussed that family turmoil or challenges are among the issues that are well outside of her locus of control. "As the newer kid on the block," she is clear that she is experiencing and engaging in hurt and stress beyond her ability to fix. She rates this stress, however, as average rather than higher, because of how she has chosen to manage it. Her faith and reliance on God is essential toward letting go of the historical issues and trauma that she must make intentional decisions about as to not derail her focus.

Virginia F. (Group 3), former clinician and global health ambassador, indicated that the realities of the world, that were not always kind to her as a black doctor in training, were outside of her scope. There was a big transition from "Spelman College to Emory University," and she was grateful for the nurturing she had both from family, a loving partner, and through her undergraduate education to prepare her to excel and be confident toward successfully traversing professional waters. Her personal nucleus and foundation were strong, making her professional challenges easier to navigate.

Superwoman (Sojourner) Syndrome: Factors Within Her Control

Virginia F. (Group 3) indicated that, while motherhood was a choice, she is clear that "being a mom did not allow the freedom to accept all the most attractive professional opportunities" during that season in her life. She had to recognize the solid nucleus that she had through a supportive partner and family, which was more important to preserve during the brief and fleeting period of raising small children. She recognized that this was a season to be enjoyed and nurtured. She had to trust that her hard work and excellence would open other doors—and they did. She is clear that she has never had to apply for any of her dream jobs—and she has had many. She did not sacrifice the personal for the professional.

Nachae' J. (Group 1) keeps three factors in mind when rating the factors within her control in reducing the stressors of the SS and the SWS. She considers, first, whether the responsibility is related to her "calling from God." If so, it will not feel as much like work and will also sustain passion along the way. Second, she considers whether her "motivation for doing it is pure"—not primarily for her own self-promotion, but for the greater good. Third, she also feels particularly tasked when she, "from a sober perspective," feels qualified for the new responsibility. If all these things are aligned, she feels the control central to optimally managing her SS and SWS status.

Managing the Superwoman (Sojourner) Syndrome

It is important to emphasize there is more than one way to manage the SWS or the SS. Our goal is to provide suggestions for managing in a world that demands the world of AA/B women. The perspectives below were from women, at different points along the life course. They reflect introspection on themselves and not their generalization of the practices of others "like" them.

Kayla S., (Group 1), single mother and pharmacy student, stated that "she is trying to find her balance with her personal and work-related stressors." She also stated having a good support system is important when parenting and working outside of the home. Knowing she has many daily tasks, Kayla feels it is vital to schedule self-care biweekly. Securing a position as a pharmacy manager is a career goal that will allow Kayla to train and provide opportunities for other women in her field. She said this is a way she can "give back and honor those who have invested in her."

Adrienne M. (Group 2), home-care assistant, insisted that "flexibility and successful multitasking is essential for the working mother." She has implemented monthly spa days to treat herself and to manage her stress after surviving a stroke a few years ago. "Though we have routines and regularly scheduled engagements, we are not machines," Adrienne stated. We have to take care of ourselves to fulfill our life's purpose.

Beatrice J. (Group 3), retired public school teacher, heavily relies on her faith in God to cope with life's woes. She exercises and makes time for self-care activities since retiring. Her advice to women working outside the home is "select good mentors, be organized, and don't be afraid to ask for help." Overcoming the fear of asking for help can result in a freeing effect. Having to do it all and do it well becomes overwhelming. Holding others in our circle responsible for their part will allow us to focus on the tasks at hand. Strength, resilience, and survival are at the core of AA women's being. Dating back to abolitionist Sojourner Truth, AA women have taken on the role of "Superwoman" sacrificing their own needs for the betterment of others around them.

Recommendations to Live, Lead, . . . and Last

Raquel B. (Group 2) a judge and cancer-survivor, makes an effort a few times a week to exercise. She also tries to meditate and breathe. As a survivor, she recognizes that if she does not embark in these practices regularly, she could likely invite poor health and poor habits back into her life.

Martha G. (Group 3) is a retired executive who would tell her younger self to "not sweat the small stuff, continue to listen, don't take on too much and unnecessary things that are not of importance."

Nachae' J. (Group 1) strongly feels that as a millennial it is important to recognize that self-care should be a regular practice and that she must attend to the internal (physical health, emotional and spiritual health) along with the external (regular nail and hair appointments) to ensure prevention rather than treatment of burnout. Further, without getting to the root of a nearly snuffed out candle, a day of "self-care" will *not* fix the unhealthy management of the SS or SWS. She indicated the importance of "self-discipline" not just to one's field, passion, or pursuit, but to oneself.

We must be "mindful of what we are carrying" to ensure that we off-load the negative or uncontrollable and "nourish and consecrate" those gifts we carry to ensure they are best used, at the appropriate time.

The SS and SWS provide context to why AA/B women may experience certain health disparities while being in great demand, by family and their fields. Research suggests that many AA/B women inherently align with the SWS through their actions and the way they approach relationships, career, self-care, and physical and mental health. We trust that the insights detailed in this chapter, through both the literature and the voices of our sisters, serve as motivation to AA/B women to continue to accomplish their goals and as a reminder that our superpowers can move mountains when we work together and mind ourselves. Future research can consist of programs that are culturally relevant to AA/B women using the SWS framework. These programs can help AA/B women work through different coping strategies while maintaining core values.

Recommendations: Best Practices for the Sustainability of the Superwoman/Sojourner

The authors of this chapter espouse the journey toward advancing health equity through their personal and professional lives. Health equity involves the systems, settings, and context through which everyone has the opportunity to "attain his or her full health potential" and no one is "disadvantaged from achieving this potential because of social position or other socially determined circumstances" (Centers for Disease Control and Prevention, 2020). AA/B women stand in the balance—frequently described in conversations related to populations disproportionately impacted by adverse health disparities *and* a central part of the solution through their Superwoman/Sojourner identities due to their strength, resilience, and concurrent vulnerabilities. We urge all to consider the recommendations and call to action in their pursuit to live, lead, and last.

LIVE

Taking care of yourself is essential to having the physical, mental, and emotional fuel (1) to thrive in leadership and support of your family and (2) to optimally manage work- and career-related responsibilities. Self-care is broadly defined and may be a temporary or recurring "exhale" to cope with stress or reward yourself for accomplishments. Consider self-care as not a reward or response to stress but a *requirement* in order to attend to mind, body, and spirit. This "me time" can be a nap, a massage, or meditation. Make sure that whatever you choose is something *you* enjoy. Exercising is also *essential* to releasing stress, strengthening your heart and "moving" your digestive system. This, coupled with attention to a well-balanced diet, is critical to preventing the "risks for risk" for chronic diseases (i.e., diabetes and cardiovascular disease) that are among the negative consequences of the SWS/SS. Even if you are not overweight or obese, you can still be unhealthy and at risk for poorer health, so it is important to prioritize both exercise and a healthy diet, most of the time. Also central to your health is attention to your mental and behavioral health. Regular therapy, engagement with a faith- or spiritually based network and healthy social engagement are important examples of outlets and sources of fulfillment. Schedule time for these recurring activities in the same way you schedule a work meeting. They create the space to reflect, release, or have fun in order to counter the weight of the many responsibilities (whether chosen or inherited) that are required of you.

Lead

Leading is not only about your title or the power to positively influence, but the ability to govern yourself through objectively appreciating all that you do. Take the time to stay organized through writing down or electronically documenting your schedule and priorities to see all that you are responsible for daily, weekly, and monthly. Regularly assessing your "balls" in rotation or your proverbial "plate" will help you to determine whether each one is aligned with your (1) time, (2) values, and (3) gifts. Ideally, alignment with all three can help you make decisions regarding what to keep, what to delegate to another competent and responsible person, or what to bow out of. Your decision may be for the current season of your life or for good. It is also a good practice to share a general schedule with those close to you. This will provide them with some insight to your responsibilities and may inspire their support.

Recommendations and Call for Action

The AA/B Sojourner or Super women do all with good intentions, but many are gone before their time or suffer the physical, emotional, and spiritual consequences detailed in this chapter because they have not attended to self (to live) or taken the time to lead through self-awareness and the courage to (1) say no, (2) delegate, or (3) ask for help in the process. In order to last, we must also be aware of those in our circle, whether employees, family, or our social bubble who can help (and benefit from doing so). Ask for help. This may present a challenge for the Superwoman/Sojourner because she is used to carrying the weight alone or feels that she will be perceived as weak or incompetent. Nimble, discerning leaders know that soliciting help, when it can be positioned as a win-win, is often the start of a new partnership or mentoring opportunity. Each need-opportunity duo is different so should be considered through a thoughtful case-by-case approach. For the woman who may feel she has no one to call, this is just the right time for you to build up the essential village that supports and collaborates with you in ways that represent a win-win partnership for success. Take the time for this important process of building your network of support.

Resources

Being free to pursue one's dreams should be a reality that each person can experience. As we seek to empower the AA/B women and girls, we must also remember that we have allies. We are truly stronger together. The organizations described below foster an environment for strong and supported AA/B women to thrive.

Black Women's Health Imperative (BWHI). https://bwhi.org The first nonprofit organization that was created by Black women to help protect and advance the physical, mental, and spiritual health and well-being for the nation's 19.5 million African American women and girls. BWHI offers five signature programs geared toward diabetes education, advocacy and leadership, teen empowerment, HIV prevention, and reproductive health.

International Association of Women (IAW). https://iawomen.com The IAW is comprised of local chapters that are designed to connect professional women with networking opportunities, resources, and support in their careers, businesses, and work life balance. Through events hosted online and in-person, partnerships with established industry leaders, and expert content, women are equipped with the tools and connections they need to accelerate their careers and businesses.

National Association for the Advancement of Colored People (NAACP). https://naacp.org The NAACP's vison is to ensure a society in which all individuals have equal rights and there is no racial hatred or discrimination. Made up of more than two million members, the NAACP tackles issues related to race and justice, education, environment and climate justice, health and wellbeing, advocacy and litigation, Black economics, and next generation leadership.

National Coalition of 100 Black Women (NCBW). https://ncbw.org The NCBW works as change agents to influence policy that promotes gender equity in health, education, and economic empowerment. Through their initiatives, NCBW seeks to promote healthy lifestyles, eliminate disparities in education, and educate our community on financial literacy.

National Council of Negro Women (NCNW). https://ncnw.org The NCNW's mission is to lead, empower, and advocate for women of African descent, their families, and communities. NCNW promotes education with a special focus on science, technology, engineering, and math; encourages entrepreneurship, financial literacy, and economic stability; educates women about good health and HIV/AIDS; promotes civic engagement and advocates for sound public policy and social justice.

AA/B women experience the accolades and praise, but the pressures and demands of their success, coupled with the demands of cultural responsibilities as well and the newer realities of wealth can translate into poorer health, potentially challenging the degree to which they can fully experience the fruits of their personal and professional labor. We challenge them (and those who love them, collaborate with them, and champion their causes) to reconsider the innate or intentional drive to be resilient toward a higher plain. A paradigm toward bouncing forward, through understanding and awareness of how the Superwoman (Sojourner) Syndrome may show up and be reconciled in the intentional pursuit to not only live and lead, but last.

References

Adkins-Jackson, P. B., Turner-Musa, J., & Chester, C. (2019). The path to better health for Black women: Predicting self-care and exploring its mediating effects on stress and health. *Inquiry: A Journal of Medical Care Organization, Provision and Financing, 56*. https://doi.org/10.1177/0046958019870968

Allen, A. M., Wang, Y., Chae, D. H., Price, M. M., Powell, W., Steed, T. C., Rose Black, A., Dhabhar, F. S., Marquez-Magaña, L., & Woods-Giscombe, C. L. (2019). Racial discrimination, the superwoman schema, and allostatic load: exploring an integrative stress-coping model among African American women. *Annals of the New York Academy of Sciences, 1457*(1), 104–127. https://doi.org/10.1111/nyas.14188

CDC Wonder. (2020). Single-race Population Estimates, United States, 2010–2019. July 1 resident population by state, age, sex, single-race, and Hispanic origin.

Vintage 2019 estimates released by US Census Bureau on June 25, 2020. http://wonder.cdc.gov/single-race-single-year-v2019.html

Centers for Disease Control and Prevention. (2020). *Health Equity*. National Center for Chronic Disease Prevention and Health Promotion. https://www.cdc.gov/chronicdisease/healthequity/index.htm

Conway-Phillips, R., Dagadu, H., Motley, D., Shawahin, L., Janusek, L. W., Klonowski, S., & Saban, K. L. (2020). Qualitative evidence for Resilience, Stress, and Ethnicity (RiSE): A program to address race-based stress among Black women at risk for cardiovascular disease. *Complementary Therapies in Medicine, 48*, Article 102277. https://doi.org/10.1016/j.ctim.2019.102277

Dorsainvil, R. R. (2019, February 28). Black first-generation wealth builders need to put on their own financial 'oxygen masks' first. CNBC. https://www.cnbc.com/2019/02/27/the-psychology-of-first-generation-african-american-wealth-builders.html

Flynn, D. (2018, February 16). Caregiving Chronicles: African-American family caregivers face higher burdens in caring for their loved ones. Care Giving Metro West. https://www.caregivingmetrowest.org/Caregiver-Toolkit/Blog-Caregiving-Chronicles/african-american-family-caregivers-face-higher-burdens-in-caring-for-their-loved-ones#:~:text=African%2DAmerican%20caregivers%20experience%20higher,caring%20for%20their%20loved%20one

Gillett, R. (2018, August 30). 15 Important jobs women have never held. *Insider*. https://www.businessinsider.com/jobs-woman-has-never-held-2016-3

Kang, A. W., Dulin, A., Nadimpalli, S., & Risica, P. M. (2018). Stress, adherence, and blood pressure control: A baseline examination of Black women with hypertension participating in the SisterTalk II intervention. *Preventive Medicine Reports, 12*, 25–32. https://doi.org/10.1016/j.pmedr.2018.08.002

Kowitt, B., & Zillman, C. (2021, January 26). New Walgreens CEO Roz Brewer will be the only Black women chief executive in Fortune 500. *Fortune*. https://fortune.com/2021/01/26/walgreens-new-ceo-rosalind-roz-brewer-starbucks/

Lekan, D. (2009). Sojourner syndrome and health disparities in African American women. *Advances in Nursing Science, 32*(4), 307–321. https://doi.org/10.1097/ANS.0b013e3181bd994c

Martin, J., & Burns, A. (2018, May 22). Stacey Abrams wins Georgia democratic primary for governor, making history. *The New York Times*. https://www.nytimes.com/2018/05/22/us/politics/georgia-primary-abrams-results.html

Mullings, L. (2002). The Sojourner syndrome: Race, class and gender in health and illness. *Voices, 6*(1), 32–36. https://doi.org/10.1525/vo.2002.6.1.32

Mullings, L. (2005). Resistance and resilience: The Sojourner syndrome and the social context of reproduction in central Harlem. *Transforming Anthropology, 13*(2), 79–91. https://doi.org/10.1525/tran.2005.13.2.79

Sheffield-Abdullah, K. M., & Woods-Giscombe, C. L. (2021). Perceptions of superwoman schema and stress among African American women with pre-diabetes. *Archives of Psychiatric Nursing, 35*(1), 88–93. https://doi.org/10.1016/j.apnu.2020.09.011

Stanton, A. G., Jerald, M. C., Ward, L. M., & Avery, L. R. (2017). Social media contributions to strong Black woman ideal endorsement and Black women's mental health. *Psychology of Women Quarterly, 41*(4), 465–478. https://doi.org/10.1177/0361684317732330

Truth, S. (1851). Ain't I a woman. Women's Convention, Akron, OH.

Warren-Findlow, J. (2006). Weathering: Stress and heart disease in African American women living in Chicago. *Qualitative Health Research, 16*(2), 221–237. https://doi.org/10.1177/1049732305278651

Woods-Giscombe C. L. (2010). Superwoman schema: African American women's views on stress, strength, and health. *Qualitative Health Research, 20*(5), 668–683. https://doi.org/10.1177/1049732310361892

Woods-Giscombe, C., Robinson, M. N., Carthon, D., Devane-Johnson, S., & Corbie-Smith, G. (2016). Superwoman schema, stigma, spirituality, and culturally sensitive providers: Factors influencing African American women's use of mental health services. *Journal of Best Practices in Health Professions Diversity, 9*(1), 1124–1144.

Vines, A., Baird, D., McNeilly, M., Hertz-Picciotto, I., Light, K., & Stevens, J. (2006). Social correlates of the chronic stress of perceived racism among Black women. *Ethnicity and Disease, 16*(1), 101–107.

X, M. (1962, May 5). Who taught you to hate yourself? [Excerpt from a speech]. *Genius*. https://genius.com/Malcolm-x-who-taught-you-to-hate-yourself-annotated

Zaw, K., Bhattacharya, J., Price, A. Hamilton, D., & Darity, W. (2017) *Women, Race & Wealth* (Research Brief Series, vol. 1). Insight Center for Community Economic and Development. https://www.insightcced.org/wp-content/uploads/2017/01/January2017_ResearchBriefSeries_WomenRaceWealth-Volume1-Pages-1.pdf

Chapter 4

The Making of a Black American Quilt
Discussing the Threads of the Strong Black Woman Image through Family Narratives and Media Storytelling

Asha S. Winfield

She's a little piece of leather, but she's well put together.
—Donnie Elbert

Take a licking but keep on ticking.
—Mother Ozen

Black don't crack!
—Every other Black person

Phenomenal woman
—Maya Angelou

Ain't I woman?
—Sojourner Truth, maybe

> I-N-D-E-P-E-N-D-E-N-T, do you know what that mean?
>
> —Lil' Boosie

> I'm a survivor, I'm not gon give up, I'm not gon stop, I'm gon work harder.
>
> —Destiny's Child

> She's a bad mama jama.
>
> —Carl Carlton

> She's a brick house.
>
> —Rick James

> I love her cuz she got her own.
>
> —Jamie Foxx

> The most disrespected woman in America, is the Black Woman. The most unprotected person in America is the Black Woman. The most neglected person in America, is the Black Woman.
>
> —Malcolm X

Today I found myself in another departmental meeting. We gathered in an all-day event, moving in and out of Zoom sessions in attempts to prepare for another semester of unpredictable and unprecedented times. But it was our meeting with the Counseling and Psychological Services that was the most difficult for me to digest. The title of the session, "Mental health and COVID-19," positioned a middle-aged White man and young Black woman before us for a hopeful conversation. Imagine 30 graduate students who had just spent the last 11 months striving everyday to see the silver lining being told *how to be resilient* and *not take anything personal* in order to boost student morale and productivity. Though well-intended, its execution was lacking the empathy we all needed at the time. I interrupted, so politely and lovingly, *I think resilience is more nuanced for us.* For me and my other Black colleagues who had watched Black bodies be murdered in the streets, silenced in the hospitals, and forced to still show up at work—not taking something personally and bouncing back felt like a challenge we met daily, leaving us bruised for the sake of strength, for the sake of identity. *We have to be strong everyday and it's killing us*, I pleaded with our presenters. I could hear the amen corner in my direct messages telling me to *Speak on it!* But I could not hear another White man tell me to get over it and get my work done again.

    I begged them to look at resilience through an intersectional lens to capture all the ways in which Black people, and particularly Black women had been silenced again. We had watched Black women for centuries show up for every global and national movement, for every collective and individual moment styled in strength and accessorized with resilience, but what of strength and resilience to the Black woman? How do we use memory and nostalgia found in family and media stories to discuss and "empower" Black women to strive, survive, and live despite the times? What is identity to Black womanhood with/without strength after loss, and resilience after pain? And how do these responses hinder true emotionality and vulnerability? Who's telling Black women's stories? It is with those thoughts that I discuss the purpose of this essay, based on conversations birthed out of research with storytelling and identity. Adopting a Black feminist lens inside of Black feminist ethnography, I begin this discussion with my first encounters with Black women's strength.

Early Experiences with Black Feminism

Up a hill of red clay and rocks, and around another country road, I walked up the old cement steps to the porch that creaked a little to a paint-deprived wooden swing—I was at great grandmother's house, affectionately known as MaMaw. East Texas was filled with memories, history, and identity. The chains gave the swing its motion, limited but mobile, functional, and nostalgic. It was here that I would be filled with our history through narratives, centuries long in the making and pictures aged by time and weathered by storms of oppression. I had been engulfed by the stories of Black women here. From my cousins, to aunts, grandmother, and my dear mother, their stories shaped my history and my future. I aspired to be as beautiful and strong as they were, as strong as the women whose pictures decorated the walls in the small country home as reminders of our resilience throughout time.

Historical and Contemporary Storytellers

There's oral history, fables, folktales, proverbs, narrations, genealogies, songs, and more. The transmission of knowledge, history, and experience in West Africa was mainly through oral tradition and performance rather than written text (Teach Africa). From one generation to the next, oral traditions have been used to help people make sense of the world and are used to teach children and adults about their culture. Many stories told by parents and grandparents often include cultural stories. The African storyteller used more than just words—gestures, singing, facial expressions, body movements, acting, masks, costumes, riddles, myths for the event that brought families together to sit for hours. The event was a cultural transmission where the performance became about learning one's self through learning about those around you and in your community. Those traditions continued even after enslaved Africans arrived in America in 1619. With many of them not being able to read and write in the English language, the language they created was used in stories to keep them alive.

A griot or griotte (female storyteller) had an interesting task, because the stories she typically shared were at ceremonies, celebrations, and special occasions like weddings. The griotte would sing to women about their new life, their roles as women in society, and their relationships to their husbands and future families. Comparatively, the griotte reminds me of early twentieth century intellectuals who were called entertainers in the jazz, blues, literature, and gospel traditions, whose stories about Black life, in particular as a woman, were very telling. But even those songs and testimonies spoke of tragedy and the resilience to push forward.

Stories have come in many different forms: (1) church testimonies about how Black women have suffered and relied on spirituality and God in their illness (Frank, 1995); (2) life histories in beauty shops between clients and hairdressers; (3) kitchen-table talks between mothers, daughters, and granddaughters. Storying, storytelling, storymaking, and storytaking are not a new phenomenon in the research or in our communities. In fact, oral histories and storied performances have deep roots in African culture (Kouyate, 1989) and are one of the most important traditions that kept the history for many Africans and Black Americans.

According to history, the most respected person was the man or woman who held and told these stories, because they connected the past to the current and the future for the community. Stories and histories allowed for individuals to situate themselves in structures, systems, and families, through personal narratives (big or small). Black women have been storytellers or griottes of our time, telling personal narratives to reveal the Strong Black Woman in and around them; one that challenges our current ideals and stereotypes surrounding strength and vulnerability.

What Black women in my family did not share in their personal testimonies and life histories, I found in the media. Black women's biopics, for example, presented a story of history that centered Black (sometimes) women's struggles and loss as a natural part of life. These troubling elements of Black biopics gave struggle a natural place in identity. I watched *What's Love Got to Do with It, Harriet, Self-Made, Hidden Figures, Aaliyah, Whitney, CrazySexyCool, The Clark Sisters, Genius: Aretha,* and other biographical pictures and wondered why struggle and resilience along with violence and loss was so consistent thematically across these films. Alongside exceptionalism and brilliance, Black women's stories are often framed and produced in ways that alter their reality, thus impacting the Black women who are relying on the media for identity-making presentations and characterizations. Black women as an audience are the interpretive community or cultural readers who are sensitive to and protective of the stories about their population; those mediated stories will either inspire their own stories or support centuries worth of one-dimensional, stereotypical caricatures lacking the nuance to truly capture Black women's diverse identities. We *are more than our struggles, sisters.* Black women's stories are more than self-sufficient tales of survival.

The Strong Black Woman (SBW) is described as a woman of African descent in the patriarchal, sexist, and racist America, who chooses this mask "as a psychological and physical survival technique, to guard herself against all forms of additional pain and suffering by seeking love, appreciation, and respect (consciously and unconsciously) in giving of herself to the point of exhaustion and illness" (Yetunde, 2017). Unlike any other racial or ethnic group, Black women are imbued with a number of stereotypical caricatures (Bogle, 2002) like Mammy, Jezebel, Sapphire, and tragic mulatto. More recently, updated versions of these images include the hip-hop feminist, modern mammies, educated Black [queens], and Black ladies (Hill Collins, 2006). Many of these images were created to progress a narrative that made comfortable elite and racist Whites who owned Black women's bodies, raped Black women, sold their children, killed their husbands, and forced them to nurture children who would later become their master's and bosses. Yet, the SBW image is one that Black women adopted almost to ignore and avoid these travesties, to appear strong because weakness, vulnerability, and emotions were not valued. Furthermore, we still continue to see this woman referenced—she is, indeed, everywhere:

> We know that woman. She wears mighty big shoes! She's the fearless foremother. . . . She's twined throughout the branches of our family trees . . . she's your grandmother whose love seemed boundless and everlasting . . . she's that Mama men love to brag about who sacrificed all for them. . . . She's the good wife. . . . She's all around us. . . . We've named her "Strong Black Woman" . . . and [she] is here. We've been schooled by the stories about her, seen her in action, witnessed her in our sisters. (Marcia Ann Gillespie's forward, in Parks, 2010, pp. viii–ix)

It has been described as an image, stereotype, a mask, syndrome, depression, and even a burden. But what is a Strong Black Woman, and how has it affected Black women, both old and young, who have to meet/match the tacit meaning? The Strong Black Woman is a controlling image that pressures Black women to maintain a facade of strength. The image also goes by other names such as super Black woman and super-strong Black mother, but all of them are bound in the Black woman's strength and resistance to society. The image of strength prescribes an unattainable standard of invulnerability and independence that Black women are expected to uphold in their everyday lives. This representation of Black womanhood exists to maintain the Black woman's subordination, and its effects lead to stress, obesity, and depression. Black women of all ages are vulnerable to the mystification of strength. Many psychological and health studies have looked into how the image impacts individual women's interpersonal interactions and self-image.

In Jerome Bruner's (2002) *Making Stories*, he describes stories in these ways: stories are not innocent (p. 5); stories have a message (p. 5); stories help us make sense of the world (p. 7); stories helped me and others construct our realities (p. 8); and even help to shape our identities and how we describe our life to others for a number of reasons. In the same text, he uses culture as a basis of story making. Storymaking (also known as storying) is the process of structuring experiences into stories. And, much like Bruner, Banks-Wallace agrees that the process of structuring our experiences into a story is governed by culture and the rules attached to a particular culture. Storytelling is inclusive of storymaking but it establishes a common experience between teller and listener, creating a connection between them (Malong, 1994; Banks-Wallace, 2002, p.411). According to Arthur Frank, our storytelling is about relationships and meanings: "Storytelling is the recursive elaboration of the relationship between those sharing the story. Shared memories are made present, and shared futures are projected in the form of some day when stories. Stories reaffirm what people mean to each other and who they are with respect to each other" (Frank, 2000, p. 354).

Resilience in Black Women's Identity

Black women have been described through song and dance, film, theater, lyrics, and rhythm for over 100 years—all of which capture a part of their identity. Usually in narrative format with the accompaniment of music or visual, the Black woman has told her story with the key factor being her strength, or having the ability to overcome any obstacle. The Black woman's strength and resilience is significant, because the identity building process through storymaking and story sharing not only reveals self but helps to construct a similar self in others who will listen and engage. The SBW does not have to erase her own life, she is encouraged to share her testimony with others like her—which is similar to the social learning theory (Bandura, 1973) and cultural teachings that other Black women can identify with. According to Bandura's (1973) social learning theory, it involves the ability to learn by watching others engage in a behavior. As Black women share their stories, or even act out their stories, others are able to learn from them by watching the Black woman model or exhibit various behaviors, allowing the individual to pay attention to the behavior and imitate what was previously seen. "Training for the role starts at birth. Black people traditionally raise their daughters to be sensible and responsible and are often much harder on them than on their sons. . . . In American popular culture, Strong Black Women stand like friendly sentinels—reliable, warm, selfless, feisty, and funny—as saviors and fierce protectors, watching, waiting, wanting only to help" (Parks, 2010, p. 2).

In interviews with older Black women, I asked them to describe an SBW: one woman under the age of 40 stated that this image was always ready and prepared for a loss—a loss that dates back to the 17th century. During slavery, a strong Black woman was the one left to mentally, emotionally, and physically recover after losing her husband and family, and in the worst-case scenario her child. Moving forward, an SBW was described as a woman who could pick up where her husband left off, if he was ever captured, sold, lynched, or murdered. Today's SBW is met and matched by others who have lost their children and husbands to bullets—bullets by police officers and other fellow Black brothers leaving behind communities to mourn another loss. In previous studies, the SBW has never been defined as a woman who is whole, happy, or content; nor has she been described as a full person without the accompaniment or mentioning of her counterparts as representatives of her existence (her role in the family and society).

When SBW began circulating through family and friend groups, its well-intended efforts worked to silence and erase decades of pain and suffering endured at the hands of society's racist and sexist systems. What is even more interesting about Black women's storytelling traditions is how it functions as a social identity and selfhood mechanisms. When combined with images, whether stereotypical, positive, or negative, those character models shape Black women's view of heroes, villains, good stories, and strong women.

Black womanhood is strength personified. The woman is viewed as tireless, deeply caring, and seemingly invulnerable, with strength that provides a compelling story of perseverance (Beauboeuf-Lafontant, 2009, p.1). The implication of the super Black woman has affected the health practices and stories that Black women share about themselves and other Black women. A few themes are present: (1) seeing and hearing Black women and their meaningful stories is helpful in studying communication, because it impacts how scholars examine literary devices in story making; (2) investigating the intersections of race, gender, and class reveals more about how structures place Black women in society and affect identity, as well as self-perception affecting what stories are called forth as strength testimonies; (3) strength is almost always equated with struggle stories, often seen through personal and public performances where identity is supported, that is, social media, church, social organizations. Additionally, the continuation of the oral tradition of sharing life stories is continued in many ways through Black traditions in central locations: testimony services at churches; between clients and stylists in hair salons; inside the judicial system when asked to tell truthful accounts and stories to acquire freedom; and at family reunions where genealogy is reminiscent of the practices of Black ancestors.

Moving forward, it is important to examine whether *strong* is equivalent to healthy, whole, or consummated. The residue of toxic masculinity or implicit identity making has become the makeup of gender and womanhood, covering women with tasks and roles because of their identity. From infancy, Black girls have been expected to thrive without concern for details on how their successful survival came to be or even the implications of the Black woman's historical lack of care. It is apparent that the SBW identity is accomplished through her availability to men, children, and society. The interplay of Strong Black Woman and now the Black Girl Magic mystify the works of Black women and inhibit their process and healing. There is no such thing as Black girl magic; instead, survival is grounded in hard work and sacrifice, tears and discrimination—the ingredients to resilience.

Connecting Modern Day Black Women Storytellers

Today, artists like the late Aretha Franklin or today's Beyonce would be considered a national treasure. They used their bodies and creative imagination to tell themed stories through music, lyrics, instruments, video, choreography, and costume. Many of their songs birthed out of this Black feminist autoethnography of sorts centered their positions and telling their stories of love, loss, pain, and joy found in Black womanhood. Each story or song tells a deeper tale of her version of what a Strong Black Woman looks and feels like in our current times; she and other female entertainers use their platforms to continue the conversation around hip-hop feminism (Durham, 2014). Using Beyonce as one modern-day example allows scholars to explore the production of Black femininities in popular culture, as well as the production of identity through class and Black Southern respectability politics of the body through music videos as storytelling (Durham, 2012).

Conclusion: Quilted Stories of Black Women's Past

Black Women are often discussed as "objects rather than subjects," but rarely do we ever think about the objects they possessed, cared for, or curated, why they held them close, nor the stories they tell about them that recursively tell a more reflective narrative about themselves and their identity. In reflection, I think about the objects my great-grandmother possessed and shared in the private spaces of her home as a mirror to what was in her heart—the heart of a seasoned Black woman. Being a woman is like the set of quilts my great-grandmother made and passed down to us using the scraps and straps of her life—each scrap reminiscent of a lesson learned and a story told. "It's the fabric of our lives," one company would credit cotton, but, to me, it seemed that stories of trouble and triumph were the fabric of her narrative, the threads to her survival as a woman who lived during a time when the saying "the struggle is real" was an actual reflection of the era . . . real stressful, real life-threatening, real hard for those at the bottom of the American's structure, real hard for those whose labor and bodies built America (Feagin, 2016).

Black grandmothers made a quilt for everyone they loved, as if it were the lessons they learned at the sewing machine in the quiet of the day or the recipes they cooked up from whatever was left over—and yet it turned out good. It was useful. It was always themed, and I know it took a long time to "construct." Flawed but beautiful. Heavy, warm, all consuming, scented, and all mine. In this example, the quilt is a metaphor for Black women's identity—my Black Indian great-grandmother, who was born at the turn of the century, was a collection of stories whose book was never written and whose knowledge production would not have put her in the league of race women or Black public intellectuals and, yet, it is still valuable and useful to me, to scholarship.

Recommendation and Call for Action

It is encouraged that individuals, families, and communities fully embrace the lessons that elders teach in small and big ways to ultimately promote excellence.

References

Bandura, A. (1973). Aggression: A social learning analysis [review]. *Stanford Law Review, 26*(1), 239. https://doi.org/10.2307/1227918

Beauboeuf-Lafontant, T. (2009). *Behind the mask of the strong black woman: Voice and the embodiment of a costly performance.* Temple University Press.

Bogle, D. (2002). *Primetime blues: African Americans on network television.* Farrar, Straus and Giroux.

Bruner, J. S. (2002). *Making stories: Law, literature, life.* Harvard University Press.

Durham, A. (2012). "Check on It." *Feminist Media Studies, 12*(1), 35–49. https://doi.org/10.1080/14680777.2011.558346

Durham, A. S. (2014). *Home with hip hop feminism performances in communication and culture.* Peter Lang.

Feagin, J. R. (2016). *How Blacks built America: Labor, culture, freedom, and democracy.* Routledge.

Frank, A. W. (1995). *The wounded storyteller: Body, illness, and ethics.* University of Chicago Press.

Frank, A. W. (2000). The standpoint of storyteller. *Qualitative Health Research, 10*(3), 354–365. https://doi.org/10.1177/104973200129118499

Hill Collins, P. (2006). *Black sexual politics: African Americans, gender, and the new racism.* Routledge.

Kouyate, D. (1989). The role of the griot. In L. Goss & M. Barnes (Eds.), *Talk That talk: An anthology of African American storytelling* (pp. 179–181). Simon and Schuster.

Parks, S. (2010). *Fierce angels: Living with a legacy from the sacred dark feminine to the strong black woman.* One World Ballantine Books.

Yetunde, P. A. (2017). From strong Black woman to remarkably relationally resilient woman: Black Christian women and Black Buddhist lesbians in dialogue. *Buddhist-Christian Studies, 37*(1), 239–246. https://doi.org/10.1353/bcs.2017.0017

Commentary

Nothing Can Break You Unless You Give It Permission To!

Tonyka McKinney

The various forms of social stratification including, race, sexual orientation, gender, and religion have given way to my unique intersectionality as Black, lesbian, Christian woman. Raised in the deep south and as the daughter, granddaughter, and niece of pastors, there were expectations, some verbalized but most just understood. As a young girl I remember my grandmother saying, "Get in this kitchen and learn how to cook! If you don't, you'll never find a husband!" Almost as a knee jerk reaction, my subconscious screamed, "I don't want a husband ANYWAY!" However, I knew not to dare let those words escape my lips and went on to forcing myself to think and subsequently act just as I was expected to. I still remember hearing family members use derogatory terms for same-gender loving people and how frustrated my mother would get every time I gravitated to the boys clothing in the department store. My differences were evident to anyone who knew me.

By the time I was preparing to enter ninth grade, my family's patience with my "otherness" had worn thin. My mother gave me an ultimatum and stated that I was now too old to wear boy's clothes. So I proceeded to fall in line with the expectations my family had of me from that point on. As I continued through high school, college, and into my young adulthood, I was never happy. I always felt as though I was leaving part of myself out of every room I walked into and people who thought they knew me, really didn't know me at all. I experienced, what I know now, are homonegative thoughts and constant suicidal ideations. Despite those challenges, I excelled academically and professionally. As I succeeded in those other areas, I began to feel even more uncomfortable with the limitations that had been forced upon me. I'd ventured quite far away from organized religion in my early adulthood. Somehow in that departure, I found myself longing for a relationship with God, one that circumvented religion. I was fortunate to find an affirming ministry in Atlanta. This was a place where the pastor taught that the entire premise of following Christ should be based on John 3:16. God's love was created for every single "whosoever," and yes that included sexual and gender minorities. There is an immense amount of freedom that comes from having access to a place and people who love you unconditionally, just as you are. This interpretation and expression of God's love gave me the courage I needed to "come out." I shared my truth with my family of preachers and received the exact reaction I expected, rejection and denunciation. However, I continued to excel. I fell in love. I got married. No one from my family attended my ceremony. My wife and I proceeded to grow our family and, slowly but surely, most of my biological family has come around. Over those years of separation from the family I was born into, I found myself developing familial bonds with the people I'd chosen; other sexual and gender minorities became my community.

Members of the sexual and gender minority community often face challenges and barriers to accessing necessary health services, among others. As a result, they can experience poorer health outcomes. These challenges include stigma, discrimination, violence, and, in so many cases similar to mine, rejection by families and communities. Sexual and gender minorities also sometimes contend with inequality in the workplace and health insurance sectors, the provision of substandard care, and outright denial of care because of their identity. While sexual and gender minorities have many of the same health concerns as the nonminority population, they experience certain health challenges at higher rates in addition to experiencing several unique health challenges. Research suggests that some subgroups of the sexual and gender minority community are more likely to suffer from certain chronic conditions and face higher prevalence and earlier onset of disabilities compared to nonminority communities. Other major health concerns include HIV/AIDS, mental illness, substance use, and sexual and physical violence. In addition to the higher rates of illness and health challenges, some sexual and gender minority communities, specifically the trans community, are more likely to experience challenges obtaining care. Barriers include gaps in coverage for certain groups as well as cost-related hurdles and stigma, including poor treatment from health care providers. Several recent changes within the legal and policy landscape have served to increase access to care for sexual and gender minority individuals and their families. Most notably, these include the passage of the Affordable Care Act (ACA) and the Supreme Court's overturning of a major portion of the Defense of Marriage Act (DOMA) in *United States v. Windsor* and subsequent ruling in *Obergefell v. Hodges* legalizing same-sex marriage nationwide.

The adverse health outcomes experienced by sexual and gender minorities are in many cases preventable. The lack of community and acceptance have been cited in the literature to contribute to the negative mental health and common sources of HIV infection among Black gay, bisexual, and people of trans experience. Conversely, connection to affirming and accepting religious communities is cited as a protective factor against those same outcomes. Research also suggests that addressing sexual and gender minority–related stigma in the African American faith community is absolutely necessary and integral to combat the adverse health outcomes experienced by this high-risk community. As a public health scholar, this is one area I've been committed to improving through my research and evidence-based public health practice.

Even as state legislatures around the country continue to introduce anti-LGBTQIA+ bills and the deaths of our trans sisters go unsolved, we as members of sexual and gender minority communities wake up every day determined to unlearn the homonegative opinions instilled in us early on in our lives. We continue to lift our voices and fight for equity and access to so many of the public institutions we've been relegated from. This year President Biden appointed the first openly gay man, Pete Buttigieg as Secretary of Transportation and chose Rachel Levine, the first person of trans experience as his assistant US Health and Human Services Secretary. These are paramount and indications that progress is definitely being made. The work doesn't stop here.

I am determined to be the person I needed as a kid. I can only imagine that if I'd had a successful, Black, lesbian woman as a mentor, that relationship could have shown me that all was not lost. That was something I was in desperate need of while I was discovering who I was in my adolescence and may have helped me avoid many of the struggles I experienced. I'm resilient because I have to be. My life, every experience, both good and bad, can be used to lead someone else as they embark upon their journey of self-discovery. I am resilient because I have four children in my home that are learning how and how not to do life from my wife's and my example each and every day. I am resilient because this year my mother, with all her preconceived notions, attended her first family vacation with my wife, children, and myself. I am resilient because I need everyone to understand that being Black, being lesbian, and being a woman are just adjectives that society uses to check off boxes. I am not limited by these terms because they are at best insufficient to describe the totality of who I've been created to be. I am resilient because I know that nothing can ever break you unless you give it permission to.

Conversations with Thought Leaders

Beacons of Light

Annelle B. Primm, Linda Goler Blount, and Cedrice Davis

Question: What one word describes Black women to you? Why? What does that word mean to you?

SELECTED EXCERPTED RESPONSES

- Resourceful. Black women use ingenuity, creativity, and imagination at times. Whatever resources that we [Black women] have are "brought to the table" to support others.

- Fearless. We [Black women] at this moment have shown fearlessness—faced a pandemic, unstable political climate, and many oppositions to our being. Perseverance is vital to who we are. Black women have what it takes to "make it happen" and we are willing and determined to do so.

- Indomitable. We [Black women] are difficult to defeat and have withstood so much—from slavery to present day. Although we have come so far, and just elected the first Black woman VP and we have many others, for example, Oprah and Michelle Obama to look up to; the road/path was not easy.

Question: What are some of the challenges that you believe Black women must overcome in navigating through our society? How do you think we demonstrate resilience?

SELECTED EXCERPTED RESPONSES

Challenges

- The underestimation of our [Black women's] ability; negative assumptions made about our intelligence; and the misconceptions made based in part on physical attributes.
- We [Black women] consistently have to "overprove" ourselves, which unfortunately is a "bottomless pit" which may yield negative labeling, sabotage by others, and malingered/shrinking sense of self.

Resilience

- We [Black women] overcome it and demonstrate resilience through self-confidence and perseverance.
- We [Black women] establish a sense of responsibility to make changes so things don't become destructive; and we create boundaries regarding what can personally be controlled (internal locus of control) versus external locus of control.

Question: What do you believe are the most significant health concerns facing Black women and families today?

SELECTED EXCERPTED RESPONSES

- Heart disease and the (1) unrecognized risks that exist, and (2) inability to consistently engage in prevention practices that could lower risks (e.g., getting enough sleep, healthy eating, physical activity).
- Consciousness of historical underpinnings, "we know how hard [in life] it can get."

- Stress. It elevates our risk for many health problems (e.g., obesity). Stress is engendered in our daily experiences, all while we [Black women] deal with racism, sexism.

Part Two

Toward an Optimal Health Agenda: The Importance of Our Survival

Tenacity/tə'nasədē/
The quality or fact of being very determined; determination.

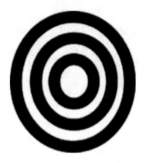

Adinkrahene
West African Adinkra Symbol for Greatness, Charisma, and Leadership

Akofena
West African Adinkra Symbol for Courage, Valor, and Heroism

86 | Part Two

Bese Saka
West African Adinkra Symbol for Power, Togetherness, and Unity

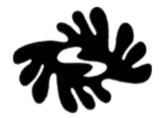

Bi Nka Bi
West African Adinkra Symbol for Peace and Harmony

Face Your Pace

ADELE BROWNE

How much time does it take to know your way,
Individualized, and subject to no one's schedule?
I never really understood why I do the things I do,
the way I've done what I am doing.
I know now, because I have had to face my pace.
Has anyone ever said to you,
You should have been . . .
You could have done, why didn't you?
I would have done it like this.
Their effort for heed did not address my need,
to know the why of my way.
I've had to face my pace.
What I do isn't fast. What I do isn't slow,
It's just that I am learning as I go.
Through valued experiences teaching me
that I can't follow.
And I needn't struggle to keep up.
You wouldn't do it this way.
I know.
I've watched you.
Seemingly targeted for success, moving about in your rhythm.
Unencumbered, undeterred, financially straight,
mentally askew?

Spiritually alive? Perhaps lacking something?
I don't know, but I understand.
I can't sing your melody,
my song is being composed now.
Each note my effort, each word by design.
Origin becomes completion in its own time.
I've finally figured it out.
It's how I must proceed.
No ease or haste.
Allowed to continue by His Grace.
Accepting full knowledge,
I have,
Faced
My Pace.

Chapter 5

The Black Women's Health Study
An Epidemiologic Snapshot of Black Women's Health

Lynn Rosenberg, Yvette C. Cozier, and Julie R. Palmer

Background

More than a quarter of a century ago, in 1993, a collaboration of breast cancer studies was established to provide a database with which to assess risk factors for that cancer (Collaborative Group on Hormonal Factors in Breast Cancer, 1996). The Collaborative Group on Hormonal Factors in Breast Cancer included 54 studies, an estimated 90% of all the world's studies, in which 53,297 women with breast cancer and 100,239 women without breast cancer were included. As large as it was, the number of Black women included in the collaboration was too small for meaningful separate analyses.

At that time, we knew, as breast cancer researchers, that US Black women were 40% more likely to die of breast cancer than White women (Miller et al., 1993). This is still the case, and the reasons have yet to be fully clarified (American Cancer Society, 2019). As cardiovascular disease researchers, we knew that cardiovascular disease also disproportionately affected Black women (Kuller, 1991). The long list of other conditions that affected Black women more than most other racial/ethnic groups included type 2 diabetes, obesity, stroke, systemic lupus erythematosus, uterine fibroids, and sarcoidosis. The list of studies of these conditions in Black women was very short. We envisioned a study focused on Black women that could informatively assess risk factors for breast cancer, all of these other conditions, and more.

Establishment of the Black Women's Health Study

In 1995, with funding from the National Cancer Institute, the largest follow-up study of Black women, the Black Women's Health Study (BWHS), was initiated. We mailed invitations to hundreds of thousands of subscribers to *Essence* magazine, which is targeted to Black women, inviting participation in a long-term study of health. The women were asked to complete and return a 14-page health questionnaire, which asked for information on demographics, reproductive history, and medical history, and included a dietary questionnaire. We also mailed to members of the Black Nurses' Association and friends and relatives of early responders. The 59,000 Black women ages 21–69 who successfully completed and returned the questionnaire comprise the cohort that has been followed for 25 years, and still counting (Rosenberg et al., 1995; Russell et al., 2001).

Information was collected at baseline in 1995 on demographic factors, height and weight, medical history, smoking and alcohol consumption, dietary intake, and many other factors. Further data have been collected every two years through mailed and online questionnaires. Importantly, information has been collected on interpersonal experiences of racism and other stressors, as well as potential coping mechanisms. Information from public sources, such as US Census data and air pollution data, has been linked to participants' addresses, making possible the study of factors such as neighborhood socioeconomic status or exposure to specific air pollutants. Validation studies have supported the usefulness of the information reported by BWHS participants (Adams-Campbell et al., 2000; Kumanyika et al., 2003; Makambi et al., 2009).

The median age of participants in 1995 was 38, making it possible to study risk factors for breast cancer among younger women who developed the disease. On the other hand, the young age of many participants also meant that it would take decades for enough cases of illnesses that affect older women, such as colorectal cancer and Alzheimer's disease, to occur.

Willingness to Participate

The Tuskegee "experiment" and other health-care abuses have resulted in suspicion among some Black Americans about participating in health studies (Byrd & Clayton, 2001). At the same time, there has been a belief among some researchers that it is difficult to obtain the participation of Black women and men in health studies, although this is not always the case (Adams-Campbell et al., 2016). Women who enrolled in the BWHS have demonstrated their eagerness to participate. Many have completed questionnaires about their health every two years, provided saliva specimens (e.g., to study the role of the oral microbiome in health), provided blood samples (e.g., to study the genetics of various diseases), allowed access to their cancer tumor samples (e.g., to study different subtypes of a particular cancer), allowed access to their mammograms (e.g., to study predictive features of the mammogram for breast cancer), and allowed access to their medical records (e.g., to learn details of the diagnoses). This willingness has made possible the collection of relevant health data every two years across the 25 years of follow-up thus far and the establishment of repositories of more than 25,000 saliva samples, 13,000 blood samples, 1,000 tumor specimens, 6,000 mammograms, and thousands of medical records. Linkage to other data, such as air pollution levels or neighborhood characteristics, has also been carried out.

Many BWHS participants have said that their willingness to participate reflects their desire to be an important part of work that will improve the health of Black women now and in future generations. To contribute to the relevance of the work, participants have their say about what should be studied through a Participant Advisory Group consisting of volunteers from the cohort, and through individual communications that they send to BWHS investigators. An External Advisory Board that includes distinguished Black women with expertise in various fields advises the BWHS investigators and has done so since the start of the study. Some of these advisors were involved in helping the investigators in the grant proposal phase. Study results are communicated to participants through twice-yearly newsletters, and a website lists publications and describes findings and relevant health news (www.bu.edu/bwhs). A series of webinars has addressed various health topics of interest to participants.

BWHS Findings

At the present time, the BWHS had contributed to more than 300 publications in medical and scientific journals. Below we give examples of the findings.

Breast cancer, the most commonly occurring cancer among American women, has been the focus of multiple studies of BWHS data alone or in collaborations. An aggressive form of breast cancer, estrogen receptor negative (ER-), which affects Black women about twice as commonly as White women and contributes to the higher breast cancer mortality in Black women, was found to differ in some risk factors from estrogen receptor positive (ER+) breast cancer. While higher parity was associated with decreased risk of ER+ breast cancer, it was associated with increased risk of ER– breast cancer, and the latter effect was counteracted by breast feeding (Palmer et al., 2011). ER– breast cancer occurred more commonly among women who lived in deprived neighborhoods, even after accounting for known risk factors (Palmer et al., 2012). This finding, seen across many countries, is as yet not fully explained. Breast cancer predisposition genes such as BRCA1, BRCA2, and PALB2 were shown to confer the same very high lifetime risk of breast cancer in Black women as had previously been shown in White women, indicating that genetic testing should be offered to Black women under the same circumstances as for White women (Palmer et al., 2020). Women who exercised regularly (Rosenberg et al., 2014) and those who ate diets high in vegetables (Boggs et al., 2010) had a lower risk of breast cancer. On the other hand, the risk was higher among BWHS participants who used menopausal hormone supplements containing both estrogen and a progestin, in agreement with randomized trial results (Rosenberg et al., 2015).

A number of factors were linked to the development of *excess weight gain and obesity*, including low levels of physical activity (Rosenberg et al., 2013) and higher intake of fast foods, fruit drinks, and soft drinks (Boggs et al., 2013). Women who lived in disadvantaged neighborhoods were at higher risk of excess weight gain and obesity even after taking into account diet and exercise, suggesting that psychosocial stressors may play a role (Coogan et al., 2010).

Type 2 diabetes, which is strongly associated with overweight and obesity, affects Black women disproportionately. In addition to obesity (Krishnan, Rosenberg, Djoussé, et al., 2007), foods with a high glycemic index (e.g., white bread) (Krishnan, Rosenberg, Singer, et al., 2007) and sugary drinks (Palmer et al., 2008) were associated with increased risk. Brisk walking was associated with a reduced risk of type 2 diabetes, whereas prolonged periods of sitting were associated with increased risk (Krishnan et al., 2009).

In 1995, when the BWHS began, many participants reported having had a *hysterectomy* (39% of women aged 45–49) (Palmer et al., 1999). Participants who lived in the South were more likely to have had a hysterectomy, as compared with participants in other regions of the US, and lower levels of education were also strongly associated with higher hysterectomy rates. At the same time, the prevalence of uterine fibroids, the primary medical indication for hysterectomy, was similar across the geographic regions. It appeared that regional differences in physician practice were behind the disproportionately high occurrence of this major surgery in the South.

Uterine fibroids are diagnosed two to three times more frequently in Black women than White women. BWHS results on menarche, parity, and lactation support the hypothesis that higher lifelong exposure to bioavailable estrogens is associated with higher risk (Wise et al., 2004), but these and other reproductive risk factors do not explain the racial difference in incidence. Higher percent African ancestry was also associated with higher risk in the BWHS, and results suggested that multiple genetic variants are involved (Wise et al., 2012).

Autoimmune diseases that affect Black women more than other population groups include sarcoidosis and systemic lupus erythematosus. In the BWHS, smoking (Cozier et al., 2019a) and several genetic variants in the MHC region (Ruiz-Narvaez et al., 2011), which is associated with several autoimmune diseases, were predictors of lupus. Obesity also appeared to play a role (Cozier et al., 2019b). Weight gain and obesity (Cozier et al., 2015) and several genetic variants (Cozier et al., 2013; Cozier et al., 2012) were associated with higher risk of sarcoidosis.

Psychosocial stressors affect Black women disproportionately. For example, Black Americans are much more likely to experience racism in their daily lives and in institutional settings (interpersonal racism) than White Americans. Evidence suggests many harmful health effects of racism. In the BWHS, frequent experiences of interpersonal racism were associated with increased weight gain and obesity (Cozier et al., 2014), asthma (Coogan et al., 2013), uterine fibroids (Wise et al., 2007), insomnia (Bethea et al., 2020), and lower rates of breastfeeding (Griswold et al., 2018). Stressors have been associated with greater cognitive decline at older ages. In line with this finding, BWHS participants who reported the highest levels of interpersonal racism also had the poorest scores on a test of memory (Coogan et al., 2020).

Black women have a shorter *life expectancy* than White women, by about 3 years (Arias & Xu, 2019). Not surprisingly, BWHS data indicate that healthy diets (Boggs et al., 2015) and exercise (Sheehy et al., 2020) lower mortality risk; even small amounts of time spent exercising appear effective. Many studies had addressed the important question of whether overweight and obesity are associated with increased mortality, but results were inconsistent. A BWHS analysis, conducted among nonsmokers so as to exclude the confounding effects of smoking, clearly demonstrated that higher weight and obesity were associated with increased risk of dying (Boggs et al., 2011).

Other research. A study of colorectal cancer, in progress, should provide informative answers to the question of whether aspirin use lowers risk. Saliva samples are being used to investigate whether the oral microbiome influences the risk of developing lung or pancreatic cancer. Genetic variants in tumor tissue are being assessed in studies of breast cancer. A study of digital mammograms in relation to breast cancer holds promise of identifying mammographic features that better predict the future occurrence of breast cancer in Black women. Likewise, a better risk prediction model for breast cancer specifically in Black women is in development A BWHS study of COVID-19 is gathering information on how this illness affects future risk of cardiovascular disease. A study of experiences of racism in relation to Alzheimer's disease is in progress. Studies of inflammatory bowel disease, kidney disease, multiple myeloma, preeclampsia, and stroke have begun. A study of methods to decrease insomnia is nearing completion.

Recommendations and Call for Action

The BWHS and other studies have reported numerous changes that would improve the health of Black women. It is not enough to convey that information to those affected, nor is it enough to make recommendations based on the findings, nor is it sufficient to present the findings in scientific articles and at scientific meetings. It takes time for new information to be absorbed by individuals and the medical/scientific community. Even then, the obstacles to change are many. Even if a suggestion, such as to substitute fruits and vegetables for meat, resonates with the recipient of the information, many individuals live in areas where healthy foods are not available or they simply cannot afford to buy these foods. The difficulty of improving diets is underscored by the difficulties that Michelle Obama's effort to improve school lunches met, with great resistance from the food industries and their supporters and lobbyists (Confessore, 2014). While suggestions to walk briskly several times a week may also resonate, women who live in areas that are unsafe, or who work two jobs, or who have pressing family responsibilities may find it difficult to find the time or place to exercise. Conveying the information to pregnant women that breastfeeding is healthy not just for the baby but also for the mother in terms of her future breast cancer risk is not enough to increase breastfeeding among Black women. Health-care providers must assist in this endeavor through information and support, and workplaces must increase that possibility for women who wish to breast feed. Even with the support of employers, it would take large changes to make this feasible. Similarly, study findings that Black women often receive less adequate care during their pregnancies than White women is not enough to change that situation—clinicians must be made aware of this reality and must be invested in improving that care (Jackson & Gracia, 2014). It is imperative that we do more to increase the diversity of the research and the health-care workforce, including doctors, nurses, and health educators.

In sum, improving health is a joint effort that involves all segments of society. It starts with obtaining knowledge about how to improve health, delivery of that information in a meaningful way to the individuals involved, the understanding and buy-in of those affected, changes from institutions and policy makers to make improvements, and the support of society at large to help the needed changes to happen. This is a difficult and long-term endeavor, well worth undertaking and fighting for with energy and dedication.

References

Adams-Campbell, L. L., Dash, C., Palmer, J. R., Wiedemeier, M. V., Russell, C. W., Rosenberg, L., & Cozier, Y. C. (2016). Predictors of biospecimen donation in the Black Women's Health Study. *Cancer Causes Control*, *27*(6), 797–803. https://doi.org/10.1007/s10552-016-0747-0

Adams-Campbell, L. L., Rosenberg, L., Washburn, R. A., Rao, R. S., Kim, K. S., & Palmer, J. (2000). Descriptive epidemiology of physical activity in African-American women. *Preventive Medicine*, *30*(1), 43–50. doi.org/10.1006/pmed.1999.0604

American Cancer Society. (2019). *Breast cancer facts and figures, 2019–2020*.

Arias, E., & Xu, J. (2019). United States Life Tables, 2017. *National Vital Statistics Reports, 68*(7).

Bethea, T. N., Zhou, E. S., Schernhammer, E. S., Castro-Webb, N., Cozier, Y. C., & Rosenberg, L. (2020). Perceived racial discrimination and risk of insomnia among middle-aged and elderly Black women. *Sleep, 43*(1). https://doi.org/10.1093/sleep/zsz208

Boggs, D. A., Ban, Y., Palmer, J. R., & Rosenberg, L. (2015). Higher diet quality is inversely associated with mortality in African-American women. *Journal of Nutrition, 145*(3), 547–554. https://doi.org/10.3945/jn.114.195735

Boggs, D. A., Palmer, J. R., Wise, L. A., Spiegelman, D., Stampfer, M. J., Adams-Campbell, L. L., & Rosenberg, L. (2010). Fruit and vegetable intake in relation to risk of breast cancer in the Black Women's Health Study. *American Journal of Epidemiology, 172*(11), 1268–1279. https://doi.org/10.1093/aje/kwq293

Boggs, D. A., Rosenberg, L., Coogan, P. F., Makambi, K. H., Adams-Campbell, L. L., & Palmer, J. R. (2013). Restaurant foods, sugar-sweetened soft drinks, and obesity risk among young African American women. *Ethnicity and Disease, 23*(4), 445–451.

Boggs, D. A., Rosenberg, L., Cozier, Y. C., Wise, L. A., Coogan, P. F., Ruiz-Narvaez, E. A., & Palmer, J. R. (2011). General and abdominal obesity and risk of death among Black women. *New England Journal of Medicine, 365*(10), 901–908. https://doi.org/10.1056/NEJMoa1104119

Byrd, W. M., & Clayton, L. A. (2001). *An American Health Dilemma: Vol. 2, Race, Medicine, and Health Care in the United States, 1900–2000* (21st ed.). Routledge.

Collaborative Group on Hormonal Factors in Breast Cancer. (1996). Breast cancer and hormonal contraceptives: Collaborative reanalysis of individual data on 53 297 women with breast cancer and 100 239 women without breast cancer from 54 epidemiological studies. *Lancet, 347*(9017), 1713–1727. https://doi.org/10.1016/s0140-6736(96)90806-5

Confessore, N. (2014, October 7). How school lunch became the latest political battleground. *The New York Times*. https://www.nytimes.com/2014/10/12/magazine/how-school-lunch-became-the-latest-political-battleground.html

Coogan, P. F., Cozier, Y. C., Krishnan, S., Wise, L. A., Adams-Campbell, L. L., Rosenberg, L., & Palmer, J. R. (2010). Neighborhood socioeconomic status in relation to 10-year weight gain in the Black Women's Health Study. *Obesity, 18*(10), 2064–2065. https://doi.org/10.1038/oby.2010.69

Coogan, P., Schon, K., Li, S., Cozier, Y., Bethea, T., & Rosenberg, L. (2020). Experiences of racism and subjective cognitive function in African American women. *Alzheimers and Dementia, 12*(1), e12067. https://doi.org/https://doi.org/10.1002/dad2.12067

Coogan, P. F., Wise, L. A., O'Connor, G. T., Brown, T. A., Palmer, J. R., & Rosenberg, L. (2013). Abuse during childhood and adolescence and risk of adult-onset asthma in African American women. *Journal of Allergy Clinical Immunology*, *131*(4), 1058–1063. https://doi.org/10.1016/j.jaci.2012.10.023

Cozier, Y. C., Barbhaiya, M., Castro-Webb, N., Conte, C., Tedeschi, S. K., Leatherwood, C., Costenbader, K. H., & Rosenberg, L. (2019a). Relationship of cigarette smoking and alcohol consumption to incidence of systemic lupus erythematosus in a prospective cohort study of Black women. *Arthritis Care and Research*, *71*(5), 671–677. https://doi.org/10.1002/acr.23703

Cozier, Y. C., Barbhaiya, M., Castro-Webb, N., Conte C., Tedeschi, S., Leatherwood, C., Costenbader, K.H., & Rosenberg, L. (2019b). A prospective study of obesity and risk of systemic lupus erythematosus (SLE) among black women. *Seminars in Arthritis and Rheumatism*, *48*(6), 1030–1034. https://doi.org/10.1016/j.semarthrit.2018.10.004

Cozier, Y. C., Coogan, P. F., Govender, P., Berman, J. S., Palmer, J. R., & Rosenberg, L. (2015). Obesity and weight gain in relation to incidence of sarcoidosis in US Black women: Data from the Black Women's Health Study. *Chest*, *147*(4), 1086–1093. https://doi.org/10.1378/chest.14-1099

Cozier, Y. C., Ruiz-Narvaez, E. A., McKinnon, C. J., Berman, J. S., Rosenberg, L., & Palmer, J. R. (2012). Fine-mapping in African-American women confirms the importance of the 10p12 locus to sarcoidosis. *Genes and Immunity*, *13*(7), 573–578. https://doi.org/10.1038/gene.2012.42

Cozier, Y., Ruiz-Narvaez, E., McKinnon, C., Berman, J., Rosenberg, L., & Palmer, J. (2013). Replication of genetic loci for sarcoidosis in US Black women: Data from the Black Women's Health Study. *Human Genetics*, *132*(7), 803–810. https://doi.org/10.1007/s00439-013-1292-5

Cozier, Y. C., Yu, J., Coogan, P. F., Bethea, T. N., Rosenberg, L., & Palmer, J. R. (2014). Racism, segregation, and risk of obesity in the Black Women's Health Study. *American Journal of Epidemiology*, *179*(7), 875–883. https://doi.org/10.1093/aje/kwu004

Griswold, M. K., Crawford, S. L., Perry, D. J., Person, S. D., Rosenberg, L., Cozier, Y. C., & Palmer, J. R. (2018). Experiences of racism and breastfeeding initiation and duration among first-time mothers of the Black Women's Health Study. *Journal of Racial and Ethnic Health Disparities*, *5*(6), 1180–1191. https://doi.org/10.1007/s40615-018-0465-2

Jackson, C. S., & Gracia, J. N. (2014). Addressing health and health-care disparities: The role of a diverse workforce and the social determinants of health. *Public Health Reports*, *129*(1, suppl. 2), 57–61. https://doi.org/10.1177/00333549141291S211

Krishnan, S., Rosenberg, L., Djoussé, L., Cupples, L. A., & Palmer, J. R. (2007). Overall and central obesity and risk of type 2 diabetes in U.S. Black women. *Obesity*, *15*(7), 1860–1866. https://doi.org/10.1038/oby.2007.220

Krishnan, S., Rosenberg, L., & Palmer, J. R. (2009). Physical activity and television watching in relation to risk of type 2 diabetes: The Black Women's Health Study. *American Journal of Epidemiology, 169*(4), 428–434. https://doi.org/10.1093/aje/kwn344

Krishnan, S., Rosenberg, L., Singer, M., Hu, F. B., Djoussé, L., Cupples, L. A., & Palmer, J. R. (2007). Glycemic index, glycemic load, and cereal fiber intake and risk of type 2 diabetes in US black women. *Archives of Internal Medicine, 167*(21), 2304–2309. https://doi.org/10.1001/archinte.167.21.2304

Kuller, L. H. (1991). Cardiovascular diseases and stroke in African-Americans and other racial minorities in the United States: A statement for health professionals. *Circulation, 83*(4), 1463–1465. https://doi.org/10.1161/01.cir.83.4.1463

Kumanyika, S. K., Mauger, D., Mitchell, D. C., Phillips, B., Smiciklas-Wright, H., & Palmer, J. R. (2003). Relative validity of food frequency questionnaire nutrient estimates in the Black Women's Health Study. *Annals of Epidemiology, 13*(2), 111–118. https://doi.org/10.1016/s1047-2797(02)00253-3

Makambi, K. H., Williams, C. D., Taylor, T. R., Rosenberg, L., & Adams-Campbell, L. L. (2009). An assessment of the CES-D scale factor structure in Black women: The Black Women's Health Study. *Psychiatry Research, 168*(2), 163–170. https://doi.org/10.1016/j.psychres.2008.04.022

Miller, B., Ries, L., Hankey, B., Kosary, C., Harras, A., Devesa, S., & Edwards, B. (1993). *SEER cancer statistics review, 1973–1990* (NIH Publication No. 93-2789). US Department of Health and Human Services.

Palmer, J. R., Boggs, D. A., Krishnan, S., Hu, F. B., Singer, M., & Rosenberg, L. (2008). Sugar-sweetened beverages and incidence of type 2 diabetes mellitus in African American women. *Archives of Internal Medicine, 168*(14), 1487–1492. https://doi.org/10.1001/archinte.168.14.1487

Palmer, J. R., Boggs, D. A., Wise, L. A., Adams-Campbell, L. L., & Rosenberg, L. (2012). Individual and neighborhood socioeconomic status in relation to breast cancer incidence in African-American women. *American Journal of Epidemiology, 176*(12), 1141–1146. https://doi.org/10.1093/aje/kws211

Palmer, J. R., Boggs, D. A., Wise, L. A., Ambrosone, C. B., Adams-Campbell, L. L., & Rosenberg, L. (2011). Parity and lactation in relation to estrogen receptor negative breast cancer in African American women. *Cancer Epidemiol, Biomarkers and Prevention, 20*(9), 1883–1891. https://doi.org/10.1158/1055-9965.EPI-11-0465

Palmer, J. R., Polley, E. C., Hu, C., John, E. M., Haiman, C., Hart, S. N., Gaudet, M., Pal, T., Anton-Culver, H., Trentham-Dietz, A., Bernstein, L., Ambrosone, C. B., Bandera, E. V., Bertrand, K. A., Bethea, T. N., Gao, C., Gnanaolivu, R. D., Huang, H., Lee, K. Y., . . . Couch, F. J. (2020). Contribution of germline predisposition gene mutations to breast cancer risk in African American women. *Journal of the National Cancer Institute, 112*(12), 1213–1221. https://doi.org/10.1093/jnci/djaa040

Palmer, J. R., Rao, R. S., Adams-Campbell, L. L., & Rosenberg, L. (1999). Correlates of hysterectomy among African-American women. *American Journal of Epidemiology, 150*(12), 1309–1315. https://doi.org/10.1093/oxfordjournals.aje.a009962

Rosenberg, L., Adams-Campbell, L., & Palmer, J. R. (1995). The Black Women's Health Study: A follow-up study for causes and preventions of illness. *Journal of the American Medical Women's Association, 50*(2), 56–58.

Rosenberg, L., Bethea, T. N., Viscidi, E., Hong, C.-C., Troester, M. A., Bandera, E. V., Haiman, C. A., Kolonel, L. N., Olshan, A. F., Ambrosone, C. B., & Palmer, J. R. (2015). Postmenopausal female hormone use and estrogen receptor-positive and -negative breast cancer in African American women. *Journal of the National Cancer Institute, 108*(4), djv361. https://doi.org/10.1093/jnci/djv361

Rosenberg, L., Kipping-Ruane, K. L., Boggs, D. A., & Palmer, J. R. (2013). Physical activity and the incidence of obesity in young African-American women. *American Journal of Preventive Medicine, 45*(3), 262–268. https://doi.org/10.1016/j.amepre.2013.04.016

Rosenberg, L., Palmer, J. R., Bethea, T. N., Ban, Y., Kipping-Ruane, K., & Adams-Campbell, L. L. (2014). A prospective study of physical activity and breast cancer incidence in African-American women. *Cancer Epdemiology, Biomarkers and Prevention, 23*(11), 2522–2531. https://doi.org/10.1158/1055-9965.EPI-14-0448

Ruiz-Narvaez, E. A., Fraser, P. A., Palmer, J. R., Cupples, L. A., Reich, D., Wang, Y. A., Rioux, J. D., & Rosenberg, L. (2011). MHC region and risk of systemic lupus erythematosus in African American women. *Human Genetics, 130*(6), 807–815. https://doi.org/10.1007/s00439-011-1045-2

Russell, C., Palmer, J. R., Adams-Campbell, L. L., & Rosenberg, L. (2001). Follow-up of a large cohort of Black women. *American Journal of Epidemiology, 154*(9), 845–853. https://doi.org/10.1093/aje/154.9.845

Sheehy, S., Palmer, J. R., & Rosenberg, L. (2020). Leisure time physical activity in relation to mortality among African American women. *American Journal of Preventive Medicine, 59*(5), 704–713. https://doi.org/10.1016/j.amepre.2020.05.013

Wise, L. A., Palmer, J. R., Cozier, Y. C., Hunt, M. O., Stewart, E. A., & Rosenberg, L. (2007). Perceived racial discrimination and risk of uterine leiomyomata. *Epidemiology, 18*(6), 747–757. https://doi.org/10.1097/EDE.0b013e3181567e92

Wise, L. A., Palmer, J. R., Harlow, B. L., Spiegelman, D., Stewart, E. A., Adams-Campbell, L. L., & Rosenberg, L. (2004). Reproductive factors, hormonal contraception, and risk of uterine leiomyomata in African-American women: A prospective study. *American Journal of Epidemiology, 159*(2), 113–123. https://doi.org/10.1093/aje/kwh016

Wise, L. A., Ruiz-Narvaez, E. A., Palmer, J. R., Cozier, Y. C., Tandon, A., Patterson, N., Radin, R. G., Rosenberg, L., & Reich, D. (2012). African ancestry and genetic risk for uterine leiomyomata. *American Journal of Epidemiology*, *176*(12), 1159–1168. https://doi.org/10.1093/aje/kws276

Chapter 6

Obesity, Heart Disease, and the Influence of Dietary Guidelines among Black Women

Jennifer Rooke

Introduction

Black women have the highest rates of obesity and heart disease in the US (Blackwell et al., 2014). While obesity is a risk factor for heart disease, there are strong independent associations between obesity, heart disease, and dietary patterns, especially meat consumption (Boutron-Ruault et al., 2017). Dietary patterns are influenced by a wide range of factors including culture, gender, age, income, social status, level of education, food policies, food industry marketing, and medical advice to patients and populations. Public health nutrition policies and health education messages are influenced by the federal *Dietary Guidelines for Americans* that have promoted consumption of "healthy lean meat, poultry and fish" for the past 40 years. United States Department of Agriculture (USDA) data indicate that Black women may be the most compliant with this advice (United States Department of Agriculture, Economic Research Service, 2012). This chapter reviews the evidence that links these foods to obesity and cardiovascular disease (CVD). Understanding these influences may be an important step toward improving the dietary guidelines and eliminating health disparities.

Dietary Guidelines for Americans

In February 1977, the first dietary guidelines—the *Dietary Goals for the United States*—were issued by the Senate Select Committee on Nutrition and Human Need. This committee had been established to address poverty and malnutrition, but after senate hearings and data collection from epidemiologists, nutritionists, and public health experts the focus shifted to nutrition, health, and obesity. Correspondence between committee members in 1976 could have been written today, one member stated: "Obesity . . . is the most serious malnutrition problem in the United States today, greatly increasing the risk of cardiovascular disease and diabetes" (Oppenheimer & Benrubi, 2014). They established six basic dietary goals: (1) Increase carbohydrate intake by increasing fruits, vegetables, and whole grains. (2) Reduce fat intake by eating less meat and increasing poultry and fish. (3) Reduce saturated fat intake and balance with polyunsaturated and monounsaturated fats. (4) Reduce cholesterol consumption by decreasing butterfat, eggs, and other high cholesterol sources, and substituting nonfat for whole milk. (5) Reduce sugar intake. (6) Reduce salt intake.

These goals were immediately opposed by the food industry, primarily meat, dairy, egg, sugar, and salt producers (Oppenheimer & Benrubi, 2014). They demanded that the guidelines be immediately withdrawn, and the senate committee disbanded. Doubt about the science supporting the guidelines was created by food industry experts and independent researchers. Health professionals also opposed the guidelines. Despite the well-documented fact that nutrition is not taught in medical schools and most physicians are ill equipped to give dietary advice (Adams et al., 2006), the American Medical Association (AMA) stated that dietary advice should be based on physician judgment and tailored to individual patients (Oppenheimer & Benrubi, 2014). Some dietitians felt professionally offended because "a Senate Committee had no business getting involved in recommendations that ought to be made by the scientific community" (Oppenheimer & Benrubi, 2014).

In December 1977, ten months after the publication of the first *Dietary Goals*, a revised version was published. The goals were essentially the same, but the wording was softened and qualified to reduce food industry opposition. Instead of advising Americans to "reduce fat intake by eating less meat," Americans were advised to "decrease consumption of animal fat, and choose meats, poultry and fish which will reduce saturated fat intake" (Senate Select Committee on Nutrition and Human

Needs, 1977). Most Americans had no idea what saturated fat was, the message was to continue to eat meat, poultry, and fish. After the revision the Senate Select Committee was disbanded and its functions were moved to a newly created Nutrition Committee in the USDA that has a dual role and conflicting interests of regulating agricultural products and promoting their sales.

The *Dietary Goals* inspired other federal agencies to publish dietary guidelines. In 1979 the Department of Health and Human Services (DHHS) produced *Healthy People: The Surgeon General's Report on Health Promotion and Disease Prevention*. In 1980 DHHS and the USDA jointly issued the first federal *Dietary Guidelines for Americans*. These guidelines are updated every five years; the most recent ninth edition was published in 2020. Updates involve review of recent nutrition research and recommendations by an expert scientific advisory panel followed by a period of oral and written public comments. Many of the panel members have ties to the food and pharmaceutical industry and potential conflicts of interest. The USDA Nutrition Committee that issues the final guidelines is heavily influenced by the food industry. Despite the passage of 43 years and strong scientific evidence about the harmful effects of meat, dairy, poultry, fish, and egg consumption, the basic 2020 *Dietary Guidelines* are essentially the same as the original *Dietary Goals*. Although these guidelines determined health policy and influenced the eating behaviors of many Americans, the most deleterious effects may have been on Black women (Sheehy et al., 2020).

Food Consumption by Gender and Ethnic Group in the US

The USDA and the DHHS collect data on food consumption patterns in the US. The Economic Research Service (ERS) and the Agricultural Research Service (ARS) in the USDA track the US food supply and collect demographic data in extensive surveys to determine consumer food preferences by age, income, region, and race/ethnicity (Sethu, 2012). The USDA and DHHS jointly administer the National Health and Nutrition Examination Survey (NHANES), an integrated program that includes both a physical examination of survey participants and a detailed interview involving a recall of everything consumed during the previous 24 hours. NHANES uses a representative sample of the US population and the data collected are widely used by scientists and medical researchers. According to USDA food consumption reports, Black people are the most compliant ethnic group with the *Dietary Guidelines* for meat consumption in the US.

In addition to advising Americans to consume animal products in the *Dietary Guidelines*, the USDA sponsors promotion programs for meat and dairy products such as the "Got Milk?" marketing campaign. Not surprisingly, in the past 40 years, overall meat consumption in the US increased (Daniel et al., 2011), mostly the recommended lean meats, poultry, and fish (figure 6.1). Since 1980 beef/red meat consumption has steadily declined (Daniel et al., 2011).

Black men and women had the highest overall meat consumption of all ethnic groups in the US (figure 6.2). Aggregated data by race and gender subgroups such as Black women were not available, but within ethnic groups food consumption patterns were the same for both genders. On average, women ate 20% less meat than men, and they were most likely to eat "healthy meats"—chicken, fish, and turkey (figure 6.2) (United States Department of Agriculture, Economic Research Service, 2012).

Evidence from recent nutrition research on obesity, chronic diseases, and dietary patterns indicates that excess meat and animal product con-

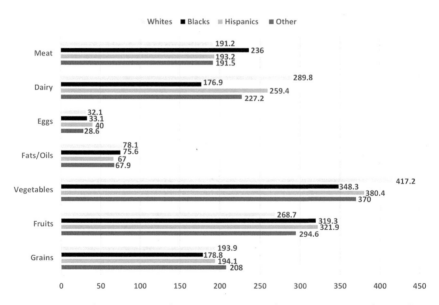

Figure 6.1. Food consumption by ethnicity. USDA, https://www.ers.usda.gov/data products/ag-and-food-statistics-charting-the-essentials/food-availability-and consumption/.

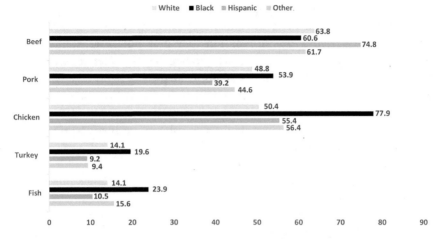

Figure 6.2. US meat consumption by ethnicity. USDA, https://www.ers.usda.gov/.

sumption are independent risk factors for both obesity and cardiovascular disease. This may be an important contributing factor to the higher rates of these and other chronic diseases among Black women.

Black Women, Obesity, and Diet

Approximately 60% of Black women in the US are considered obese (US Department of Health and Human Services, Office of Minority Health, 2017). The high rates of CVD seen among Black women is attributed to obesity, but Black men have higher rates of CVD and lower prevalence of obesity than Black women (Hales et al., 2017). Approximately 37% of Black men are obese. Excess consumption of meat and other animal products seen in USDA reports may be a common cofactor in the development of both obesity and chronic diseases such as CVD among Black women and Black men.

Obesity is defined as body mass index (BMI) of 30 kg/m^2 and above and/or waist circumference (WC) of 36 inches and above. WC is a better indicator of central obesity than BMI, which is calculated using only height and weight, but neither measurement accounts for factors such as muscle mass or total body fat distribution (Hales et al., 2017). These measurements were developed in White and European populations to accurately classify obesity-related disease risk, but they may not be as accurate for most Black women. In general, Black women have greater muscle mass and more peripheral body fat distribution in the hips and legs with less central visceral fat than White women. This decreases the risk of chronic diseases among Black women compared with White women at the same BMI (Camhi et al., 2011). Chronic disease risk among Black women may not increase until a higher BMI of 33 kg/m^2 or more and a WC of 38 inches or more (Hales et al., 2017).

Many theories have been proposed to explain the higher prevalence of obesity among Black women. Factors responsible for obesity in Black women can be grouped into social/environmental, genetic/metabolic, and behavioral/lifestyle (Agyemang & Powell-Wiley, 2013). Socially, people tend to share the eating behaviors and have similar body size and body size misperceptions as their friends and family members (Cunningham et al., 2012). Social factors such as racial discrimination, injustice, and socioeconomic inequality increase the risk of depression, which may increase the risk of obesity among Black women (Luppino et al., 2010). Black woman may self-medicate depression with high fat comfort foods instead of seeking needed mental health care. Those who want to seek mental health care may not be able to afford it or find a culturally appropriate therapist.

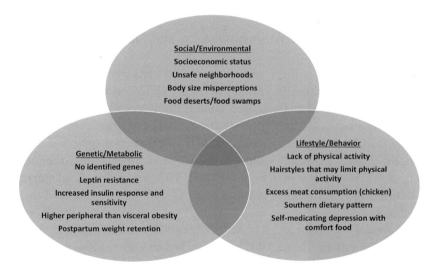

Figure 6.3. Factors underlying obesity in Black women. *Source:* Author.

Behaviorally, Black women may engage in less leisure time physical activity (Davis et al., 2015). Reasons for this may include unsafe neighborhoods (Lopez & Hynes, 2006) and concerns about maintenance of expensive hair styles (Joseph et al., 2018). Although both Black women and men tend to have jobs with higher physical demands than White women and men, the lower rates of obesity among Black men may be due to jobs with higher physical demands. Less physical activity and high consumption of meat and other animal products, fat and sugar in Southern Dietary Pattern (SDP) foods may be factors that contribute to the higher rates of obesity in Black women.

The search for obesity genes among Black women in the US has been complicated by the genetic diversity of the mixtures of races and ethnic groups that identify as Black (Agyemang & Powell-Wiley, 2013). The same problem exists with metabolism, which is genetically controlled, but there are several metabolic hypotheses. Black women may have lower resting metabolic rates and lower energy requirements than women of other ethnic groups (DeLany et al., 2014). Black women may overeat because they have fewer receptors for satiety-producing adipokines such as leptin (Khan et al., 2012). Black women may be predisposed to obesity because they produce higher levels of insulin in response to glucose and have higher levels of estrogen, which increases insulin sensitivity (Gower & Fowler, 2020). Insulin is lipogenic, so higher levels would increase fat deposition and obesity (Gower & Fowler, 2020). The researchers who proposed this theory focused on glucose/carbohydrates, forgetting that animal protein also stimulates insulin secretion (Couch et al., 2021). Animal protein may stimulate as much insulin secretion as sugar (Nuttall et al., 1984). This theory is supported by the observation that adherence to the meat-based SDP is associated with higher insulin levels and obesity while plant-based dietary patterns lower insulin levels (Gower et al., 2021) and decrease obesity. This supports a correlation between the high consumption of animal protein seen in USDA reports and the increased risk of obesity in Black women.

Conventional wisdom is that obesity is caused by eating sugar, carbohydrates, and fat, but the most obese populations around the world are those with the highest animal protein intake (Henneberg & Grantham, 2014). This may be due to the fact that carbohydrates and fat are metabolized first for energy when they are eaten with animal protein. The energy provided by animal protein may be surplus energy that is stored as fat (You & Henneberg, 2016). This is supported by the data that people and populations that eat less meat tend to be closer to ideal body weight and have lower rates of chronic diseases (You & Henneberg, 2016).

Further support comes from the European Prospective Investigation into Cancer and Nutrition-Physical Activity, Nutrition, Alcohol, Cessation of Smoking, Eating Out of Home and Obesity (EPIC-PANACEA) study, one of the largest most definitive studies on diet and obesity (Vergnaud et al., 2010). A total 373,803 participants, 103,455 men and 270,348 women aged 25–70 years old, were recruited between 1992 and 2000 in 10 European countries. Diet was assessed at baseline with the use of country-specific validated questionnaires. Weight and height were measured at baseline and self-reported annually for 5 years. Associations between the number of calories from meat per day and annual weight change in grams/year were assessed with the use of linear mixed models that controlled for age, sex, total energy intake, physical activity, dietary patterns, and other potential confounders such as initial weight, physical activity, educational level, smoking status, and total calorie intake (Vergnaud et al., 2010).

EPIC-PANACEA found that total meat consumption was positively associated with weight gain in men and women, in normal-weight and overweight subjects, and in smokers and nonsmokers (Gilsing et al., 2012). Someone eating 250 grams of meat a day (a 3.5 oz chicken breast = 100 g) will gain 422 g (0.94 pounds) a year or 2 kg (4.5 pounds) more weight after 5 years than someone eating the same number of calories but with no meat intake. This applied to red meat, poultry, and processed meat, but the strongest association was seen with chicken (Vergnaud et al., 2010). Another study found that older men and women with the highest chicken consumption, over 22 grams of chicken a day (1/4 of chicken breast) had a higher BMI (0.19–0.53 kg/m^2) than those who ate no chicken at all (Gilsing et al., 2012).

Analysis of NHANES data found a consistent positive association between meat consumption and BMI, waist circumference, obesity, and central obesity (Wang & Beydoun, 2009). Compared to the group with the lowest meat consumption, those with the highest consumption were 27% more likely to be obese and 33% more likely to have central obesity (Wang & Beydoun, 2009). Obesity and central fat distribution are associated with higher risks of chronic diseases and all-cause mortality.

Black women are often shamed for their body size and blamed for the chronic diseases that are believed to be caused by obesity. Weight loss is universally recommended by health-care professionals, but some of the recommended high protein/low carbohydrate weight loss diets may be as harmful as obesity. Adherence to any weight loss programs will usually improve glycemic control, blood pressure, and dyslipidemia, but this may not lead to the expected reduction in mortality (Køster-Rasmussen et al., 2016).

The LookAHEAD trial of a diet and exercise intervention for overweight and obese people with type 2 diabetes (T2D) was stopped early for futility after 9.6 years (Katula et al., 2017). The recommended diet was a meat-based low calorie/low fat diet that was supplemented by liquid meal replacements and weight loss medications when necessary (Katula et al., 2017). The intervention group achieved greater weight loss than the control group, but neither all-cause mortality nor cardiovascular morbidity was reduced. The Diabetes Care in General Practice study had similar findings (Køster-Rasmussen et al., 2016). In this study, successful doctor-supervised therapeutic weight loss was not associated with reduced all-cause mortality or cardiovascular morbidity/mortality after 13 years of follow-up (Køster-Rasmussen et al., 2016).

Bariatric surgery is also a challenge for Black women who have higher rates of inpatient mortality (Nguyen & Patel, 2013) and adverse events within 30 days following surgery (Stone et al., 2021). Post-surgery, Black women have less weight loss, lower comorbidity resolution, and higher all-cause mortality than other racial/ethnic groups (Hodgens & Murayama, 2019). One of the studies on the impact of bariatric surgery on Black women had an interesting finding. Black women were more likely than other ethnic groups to report better quality of life at their baseline obese weight than one year post surgery (Hodgens & Murayama, 2019).

A better understanding of the causes and consequences of obesity and the impact of weight loss programs on Black women is needed. Our society's view of obese people and the health-care profession's obsession with obesity as the cause of every chronic disease (and with weight loss in any way, at any cost) may be harmful to Black women.

Black Women, Cardiovascular Diseases, and Diet

CVDs are the most common causes of death for men and women of all races and ethnicities globally. CVDs among adults include heart attacks, stroke, hypertension, peripheral arterial disease; and deep vein thrombosis that can lead to pulmonary embolism. Eighty-five percent of CVD deaths globally are due to heart attacks and strokes (World Health Organization,

2021). The incidence of CVD among Black women in the US is not significantly different from White women, but the mortality may be 63% higher for Black women (Williams, 2009). The Centers for Disease Control and Prevention (CDC) lists deaths from heart disease and strokes separately on their leading causes of deaths list, but those conditions have the same underlying cause—atherosclerosis, commonly known as clogged arteries.

The CDC has very little about atherosclerosis on their website and the National Institutes of Health's website lists "smoking, high amounts of certain fats and cholesterol in the blood, high blood pressure, and high amounts of sugar in the blood due to insulin resistance or diabetes" as causal factors. Neither website discusses diet and atherosclerosis, which is a disservice to all Americans, but especially to Black women. The pathophysiology of atherosclerosis is well known and dietary interventions that prevent and reverse atherosclerosis are well documented (Esselstyn, 2017).

Atherosclerosis is characterized by fatty pustular abscesses in artery walls called plaques. Over time, scars form under the abscesses and artery walls harden with fibrous scar tissue. Narrowed arteries increase the pressure needed to circulate blood—this leads to hypertension. Narrowing of the arteries that supply the kidneys decreases blood flow to the kidneys, which activates the renin-angiotensin-aldosterone system (RAAS). The RAAS regulates sodium excretion and blood volume, activation of the RAAS further increases blood pressure by increasing fluid retention and vasoconstriction that further increases blood pressure (te Riet et al., 2015).

Rupture of a plaque/abscess spills pus and blood into the artery lumen. If a clot forms in an artery that supplies blood to the heart, blood flow will stop and the affected heart muscle cells will die, this is a myocardial infarct. If the area of dead heart muscle cells is large enough, the heart will not be able to beat normally, this may result in congestive heart failure or death. If the blocked vessel was supplying the brain—the affected brain cells will die resulting in an ischemic stroke. A blocked blood vessel in the brain may rupture and causing bleeding, resulting in a hemorrhagic stroke. Either way, the result may be disability or death.

Atherosclerosis is directly caused by consumption of cytotoxic cholesterol oxides, also called oxysterols, in the diet (Lizard et al., 1997; Meynier et al., 2005). *Every* animal cell contains cholesterol in the cell membrane that can become oxidized when exposed to light, heat, or processing. Oxysterols are absorbed after ingestion and may circulate freely in the blood stream or be carried by both high- and low-density lipoproteins (HDL and LDL) (Staprans et al., 2003). HDLs take them to the liver for excretion, but oxysterols oxidize LDL to become oxidized LDL (ox-LDL), a toxic substance. Oxysterols and ox-LDL have been shown to cause apoptosis or cell death when incubated with human aortic epithelial cells (Lizard et al., 1997). This triggers the inflammatory response that starts atherosclerosis in artery walls. Advice to limit saturated fat and eat "lean meats" such as chicken is counterproductive because oxysterols form in the flesh of animals, not just the fat. Avoiding cholesterol-containing foods—meat, chicken, fish, milk, cheese, butter, and eggs—prevents and reverses atherosclerosis, which prevents heart attacks and strokes.

Recommendations and Call for Action

1. The focus of health for Black women must shift away from obesity and weight loss to adopting healthy sustainable eating and lifestyle habits that build resilience and improve the overall health of Black women and their families.

2. Dietary guidelines should be evidence-based. There is an overwhelming body of strong scientific evidence that supports advice to adopt a whole-food plant-based diet for the prevention of obesity, CVD, and most chronic diseases. Given the role of the food and pharmaceutical industries in the development of the federal *Dietary Guidelines*, it is unlikely that they will ever be evidence-based or promote optimal health among Black people. Black women may have to develop their own evidence-based lifesaving dietary guidelines for their communities.

References

Adams, K. M., Lindell, K. C., Kohlmeier, M., & Zeisel, S. H. (2006). Status of nutrition education in medical schools. *American Journal of Clinical Nutrition*, 83(4), 941S–944S. https://doi.org/10.1093/ajcn/83.4.941S

Agyemang, P., & Powell-Wiley, T. M. (2013). Obesity and Black women: Special considerations related to genesis and Tterapeutic approaches. *Current Cardiovascular Risk Reports*, 7(5), 378–386. https://doi.org/10.1007/s12170-013-0328-7

Blackwell, D. L., Lucas, J. W., & Clarke, T. C. (2014). *Summary health statistics for U.S. adults: National health interview survey, 2012* (Vital and Health Statistics, series 10, no. 260). National Center for Health Statistics. https://www.cdc.gov/nchs/data/series/sr_10/sr10_260.pdf

Boutron-Ruault, M.-C., Mesrine, S., & Pierre, F. (2017). Meat Consumption and Health Outcomes. In F. Mariotti (Ed.), *Vegetarian and Plant-Based Diets in Health and Disease Prevention* (pp. 197–214). Academic Press. https://doi.org/https://doi.org/10.1016/B978-0-12-803968-7.00012-5

Camhi, S. M., Bray, G. A., Bouchard, C., Greenway, F. L., Johnson, W. D., Newton, R. L., Ravussin, E., Ryan, D. H., Smith, S. R., & Katzmarzyk, P. T. (2011). The relationship of waist circumference and BMI to visceral, subcutaneous, and total body fat: sex and race differences. *Obesity*, *19*(2), 402–408. https://doi.org/10.1038/oby.2010.248

Couch, C. A., Gray, M. S., Shikany, J. M., Howard, V. J., Howard, G., Long, D. L., McClure, L. A., Manly, J. J., Cushman, M., Zakai, N. A., Pearson, K. E., Levitan, E. B., & Judd, S. E. (2021). Correlates of a Southern diet pattern in a national cohort study of Blacks and Whites: The REasons for Geographic and Racial Differences in Stroke (REGARDS) study. *British Journal of Nutrition*, *126*(12), 1–7. https://doi.org/10.1017/S0007114521000696

Cunningham, S. A., Vaquera, E., Maturo, C. C., & Narayan, K. M. V. (2012). Is there evidence that friends influence body weight? A systematic review of empirical research. *Social Science and Medicine*, *75*(7), 1175–1183. https://doi.org/10.1016/j.socscimed.2012.05.024

Daniel, C. R., Cross, A. J., Koebnick, C., & Sinha, R. (2011). Trends in meat consumption in the USA. *Public Health Nutrition*, *14*(4), 575–583. https://doi.org/10.1017/S1368980010002077

Davis, K. K., Tate, D. F., Lang, W., Neiberg, R. H., Polzien, K., Rickman, A. D., Erickson, K., & Jakicic, J. M. (2015). Racial differences in weight loss among adults in a behavioral weight loss intervention: Role of diet and physical activity. *Journal of Physical Activity and Health*, *12*(12), 1558–1566. https://doi.org/10.1123/jpah.2014-0243

DeLany, J. P., Jakicic, J. M., Lowery, J. B., Hames, K. C., Kelley, D. E., & Goodpaster, B. H. (2014). African American women exhibit similar adherence to intervention but lose less weight due to lower energy requirements. *International Journal of Obesity*, *38*(9), 1147–1152. https://doi.org/10.1038/ijo.2013.240

Esselstyn, C. B. (2017). A plant-based diet and coronary artery disease: A mandate for effective therapy. *Journal of Geriatric Cardiology*, *14*(5), 317–320). https://doi.org/10.11909/j.issn.1671-5411.2017.05.004

Gilsing, A. M. J., Weijenberg, M. P., Hughes, L. A. E., Ambergen, T., Dagnelie, P. C., Goldbohm, R. A., van den Brandt, P. A., & Schouten, L. J. (2012). Longitudinal changes in BMI in older adults are associated with meat consumption differentially, by type of meat consumed. *Journal of Nutrition*, *142*(2), 340–349. https://doi.org/10.3945/jn.111.146258

Gower, B. A., & Fowler, L. A. (2020). Obesity in African-Americans: The role of physiology. *Journal of Internal Medicine*, *288*(3), 295–304. https://doi.org/10.1111/joim.13090

Gower, B. A., Pearson, K., Bush, N., Shikany, J. M., Howard, V. J., Cohen, C. W., Tison, S. E., Howard, G., & Judd, S. (2021). Diet pattern may affect fasting insulin in a large sample of Black and White adults. *European Journal of Clinical Nutrition*, *75*(4), 628–635. https://doi.org/10.1038/s41430-020-00762-9

Hales, C. M., Carroll, M. D., Fryar, C. D., & Ogden, C. L. (2017). Prevalence of Obesity Among Adults and Youth: United States, 2015–2016 (NCHS Data Brief, no. 288). US Centers for Disease Control and Prevention, National Center for Health Statistics.

Henneberg, M., & Grantham, J. (2014). Obesity—A natural consequence of human evolution. *Anthropological Review*, *77*(1), 1–10. https://doi.org/10.2478/anre-2014-0001

Hodgens, B., & Murayama, K. M. (2019). Not all weight loss created equal. *JAMA Surgery*, *154*(5), e190067–e190067. https://doi.org/10.1001/jamasurg.2019.0067

Joseph, R. P., Coe, K., Ainsworth, B. E., Hooker, S. P., Mathis, L., & Keller, C. (2018). Hair as a barrier to physical activity among African American women: A qualitative exploration. *Frontiers in Public Health*, *5*, Article 367. https://doi.org/10.3389/fpubh.2017.00367

Katula, J. A., Kirk, J. K., Pedley, C. F., Savoca, M. R., Effoe, V. S., Bell, R. A., & Bertoni, A. G. (2017). The Lifestyle Intervention for the Treatment of Diabetes study (LIFT Diabetes): Design and baseline characteristics for a randomized translational trial to improve control of cardiovascular disease risk factors. *Contemporary Clinical Trials*, *53*, 89–99. https://doi.org/10.1016/j.cct.2016.12.005

Khan, U. I., Wang, D., Sowers, M. R., Mancuso, P., Everson-Rose, S. A., Scherer, P. E., & Wildman, R. P. (2012). Race-ethnic differences in adipokine levels: The Study of Women's Health across the Nation (SWAN). *Metabolism*, *61*(9), 1261–1269. https://doi.org/10.1016/j.metabol.2012.02.005

Køster-Rasmussen, R., Simonsen, M. K., Siersma, V., Henriksen, J. E., Heitmann, B. L., & de Fine Olivarius, N. (2016). Intentional weight loss and longevity in overweight patients with type 2 diabetes: A population-based cohort study. In *PloS One*, *11*(1), e0146889. https://doi.org/10.1371/journal.pone.0146889

Lizard, G., Moisant, M., Cordelet, C., Monier, S., Gambert, P., & Lagrost, L. (1997). Induction of similar features of apoptosis in human and bovine vascular endothelial cells treated by 7-ketocholesterol. *Journal of Pathology*, *183*(3), 330–338. https://doi.org/https://doi.org/10.1002/(SICI)1096-9896(199711)183:3<330::AID-PATH933>3.0.CO;2-7

Lopez, R. P., & Hynes, H. P. (2006). Obesity, physical activity, and the urban environment: Public health research needs. *Environmental Health, 5*, Article 25. https://doi.org/10.1186/1476-069X-5-25

Luppino, F. S., de Wit, L. M., Bouvy, P. F., Stijnen, T., Cuijpers, P., Penninx, B. W. J. H., & Zitman, F. G. (2010). Overweight, obesity, and depression: A systematic review and meta-analysis of longitudinal studies. *Archives of General Psychiatry, 67*(3), 220–229. https://doi.org/10.1001/archgenpsychiatry.2010.2

Meynier, A., Andre, A., Lherminier, J., Grandgirard, A., & Demaison, L. (2005). Dietary oxysterols induce *in vivo* toxicity of coronary endothelial and smooth muscle cells. *European Journal of Nutrition, 44*(7), 393–405. https://doi.org/10.1007/s00394-005-0539-x

Nguyen, G. C., & Patel, A. M. (2013). Racial disparities in mortality in patients undergoing bariatric surgery in the USA. *Obesity Surgery, 23*(10), 1508–1514. https://doi.org/10.1007/s11695-013-0957-4

Nuttall, F. Q., Mooradian, A. D., Gannon, M. C., Billington, C., & Krezowski, P. (1984). Effect of protein ingestion on the glucose and insulin response to a standardized oral glucose load. *Diabetes Care, 7*(5), 465–470. https://doi.org/10.2337/diacare.7.5.465

Oppenheimer, G. M., & Benrubi, I. D. (2014). McGovern's Senate Select Committee on Nutrition and Human Needs versus the meat industry on the diet-heart question (1976–1977). *American Journal of Public Health, 104*(1), 59–69. https://doi.org/10.2105/AJPH.2013.301464

Senate Select Committee on Nutrition and Human Needs. (1977). *Dietary goals for the United States* (2nd ed). US Government Printing Office.

Sethu, H. (2012, August 23). Meat consumption patterns by race and gender. *Counting Animals: A Place for People Who Love Animals and Numbers.* https://countinganimals.com/meat-consumption-patterns-by-race-and-gender/

Sheehy, S., Palmer, J. R., & Rosenberg, L. (2020). High consumption of red meat is associated with excess mortality among African-American women. *Journal of Nutrition, 150*(12), 3249–3258. https://doi.org/10.1093/jn/nxaa282

Staprans I, Pan, X.-M., Rapp, J. H., & Feingold, K. R. (2003). Oxidized cholesterol in the diet is a source of oxidized lipoproteins in human serum. *Journal of Lipid Research, 44*(4), 705–715. https://doi.org/10.1194/jlr.M200266-JLR200

Stone, G., Samaan, J. S., & Samakar, K. (2021). Racial disparities in complications and mortality after bariatric surgery: A systematic review. *American Journal of Surgery, 223*(5), 863–878. https://doi.org/https://doi.org/10.1016/j.amjsurg.2021.07.026

te Riet, L., van Esch, J. H. M., Roks, A. J. M., van den Meiracker, A. H., & Danser, A. H. J. (2015). Hypertension. *Circulation Research, 116*(6), 960–975. https://doi.org/10.1161/CIRCRESAHA.116.303587

United States Department of Agriculture, Economic Research Service. (2012). *Commodity consumption by population characteristics.* http://www.ers.usda.gov/data-products/commodity-consumption-by-population-characteristics.aspx

US Department of Health and Human Services, Office of Minority Health. (2017). *Obesity and African Americans*. https://minorityhealth.hhs.gov/omh/browse.aspx?lvl=4&lvlid=25

Vergnaud, A.-C., Norat, T., Romaguera, D., Mouw, T., May, A. M., Travier, N., Luan, J., Wareham, N., Slimani, N., Rinaldi, S., Couto, E., Clavel-Chapelon, F., Boutron-Ruault, M.-C., Cottet, V., Palli, D., Agnoli, C., Panico, S., Tumino, R., Vineis, P., . . . Peeters, P. H. M. (2010). Meat consumption and prospective weight change in participants of the EPIC-PANACEA study. *American Journal of Clinical Nutrition*, *92*(2), 398–407. https://doi.org/10.3945/ajcn.2009.28713

Wang, Y., & Beydoun, M. A. (2009). Meat consumption is associated with obesity and central obesity among US adults. *International Journal of Obesity (2005)*, *33*(6), 621–628. https://doi.org/10.1038/ijo.2009.45

Williams, R. A. (2009). Cardiovascular disease in African American women: A health care disparities issue. *Journal of the National Medical Association*, *101*(6), 536–540. https://doi.org/https://doi.org/10.1016/S0027-9684(15)30938-X

World Health Organization. (2021). *Cardiovascular diseases (CVDs)*. https://www.who.int/news-room/fact-sheets/detail/cardiovascular-diseases-(cvds)

You, W., & Henneberg, M. (2016). Meat consumption providing a surplus energy in modern diet contributes to obesity prevalence: an ecological analysis. *BMC Nutrition*, *2*(1), Article 22. https://doi.org/10.1186/s40795-016-0063-9

Chapter 7

When Resilience Hits Its Ceiling
The Burden of the COVID-19 Pandemic

Rhonda Reid, Kristian T. Jones, Chidi Wamuo,
and Christopher Villongco

> Black women are burdened not only because they often have to take on responsibilities that are not traditionally feminine but, moreover, their assumption of these roles is sometimes interpreted within the Black community as either Black women's failure to live up to such norms or as another manifestation of racism's scourge upon the Black community.
>
> —Kimberlé Crenshaw, JD, Professor of Law, Columbia Law School

It is impossible to discuss Black women's resilience in the setting of the COVID-19 pandemic without discussing *intersectionality*, which is classically understood as the interplay between race, gender, class, and politics. When Kimberlé Crenshaw coined the term in her pivotal 1989 essay, it was a call of action for the legal community to consider societal challenges beyond the usual silos, "so that struggles are [not] characterized by singular issues." In an article published in *Stanford Law Review* two years later, Crenshaw provides three variations of intersectionality: structural, political, and representational. Structural intersectionality highlights *systems* that were created from "standards of need that are largely white and middle class." Political intersectionality asks us to interrogate whether racial or feminist *agendas and policies* are based on Black male or White female archetypes, respectively. Finally, representational intersectionality highlights the importance of examining the role of *cultural bias* in judicial decision making.

Since the term's inception, intersectionality has been applied to settings outside of the legal system, but less so within the confines of health care. After all, a body is a body. Right? Not quite. In the early 2000s, the term "social determinants of health" entered the political and clinical landscape. Like intersectionality, the social determinants of health (SDH) press us to view outcomes through a multidimensional lens. However, intersectionality can be conceptualized as *distinct-but-linked* frames of reference by which power and privilege can be afforded or withdrawn, while SDH considers the *ever-changing and cumulative* impact of biology, education, economics, and environment (among others), with the premise that health improves as positive social determinants aggregate and vice versa. Intersectionality, then, is the milieu through which the SDH exert their influences, be they positive or negative; health policy and clinical care are also subject to unjust allocation of resources, conflicting political agendas, and cultural insensitivity.

When society considers the effects of an illness, it is often reduced to its properties, intervention, or statistics, as these are measurable. These aspects of illness should not be minimized, especially when the illness is widespread, such as the COVID-19 pandemic. As of this writing, it has been found that African American patients are more likely to test positive for COVID-19, compared to White patients (Mackey et al., 2021; Magesh et al., 2021), more likely to be hospitalized due to COVID-19 infection (Muñoz-Price et al., 2020), and less likely to receive monoclonal antibodies to treat COVID-19 infection (Wiltz et al., 2022). However, it is also pertinent to examine the less tangible repercussions.

Prior to the pandemic's start, it was well established that Black women shouldered disproportionate amounts of stress/allostatic load, familial responsibility, certain medical comorbidities, and financial burden compared to their non-Hispanic White counterparts (Moore et al., 2021; Chinn et al., 2021; Simien, 2020). The COVID-19 pandemic has further illuminated these disparities. Although the effects of the COVID-19 pandemic are addressed throughout this volume, we wished to include a chapter dedicated to the pandemic's ramifications on the mental health of Black women. During our research, a few patterns emerged:

1. Most of the existing research on this topic is related to maternal health (in the peripartum period), hazards associated with frontline work, and caregiver burden. Less has been published on the educational challenges, psychological impacts, and post-COVID health concerns faced by this demographic.
2. The sample sizes in these studies were relatively small (less than 50 per study).
3. As a result of small sample sizes, the findings are not generalizable to a larger demographic, nor could the researchers explore the reasons *why* certain patterns were seen.

In this chapter, we will discuss the most studied areas of Black women's mental health in the context of the COVID-19 pandemic: maternal health, frontline work, and caregiver burden.

Maternal Health

Maternal mortality has increased in the United States, a trend not observed in other high-income countries (MacDorman et al., 2016). From 2000 to 2014, there has been a 26.6% increase in maternal mortality even after adjustments for improved data collection for maternal deaths (MacDorman et al., 2016). This concerning trend is exemplified by published data highlighting maternal death in the peripartum period being the sixth leading cause of death for women between the ages of 20 and 34 in 2014 (Heron, 2016). When examined from a racial lens, maternal mortality disproportionately impacts Black women in striking numbers, as the maternal mortality rate for Black women in 2019 was 2.5 and 3.5 times the rate for White and Hispanic women, respectively (Hoyert, 2021). The concepts of intersectionality and social determinants of health are essential themes shaping this disparity. Previous research identified implicit bias, a higher prevalence of chronic diseases, and a provision of a lower quality of care as key drivers of disparate Black maternal mortality rates (Petersen et al.,

2019). This alarming research and data point to the vulnerable position of Black maternal health even prior to the emergence of the COVID-19 pandemic in the United States. Unsurprisingly, the COVID-19 pandemic and the epidemic of Black maternal mortality have combined to create a powerful syndemic.

First coined in the 1990s and in the context of the HIV epidemic, the term *syndemic* was used to describe the larger impact of an epidemic on communities already wrestling with adverse health outcomes in other areas. For Black women, the COVID-19 pandemic caused issues that exacerbated the maternal mortality crisis. COVID-19 driven protocols that decreased prenatal physician-patient interactions and patient fear of hospital-acquired coronavirus infection were predicted to further increase Black maternal mortality rates (Minkoff, 2020). Although maternal death serves as the most lethal outcome of COVID-19 on maternal health, it is also necessary to examine COVID-19's other impacts.

It is well-known that the risk of depression and anxiety in pregnant women increases in the peripartum period, and as a result, there has been a concerted effort to increase screening for mental illness in pregnant women in psychiatric, family medicine, and obstetrics/gynecology clinics over the past few decades. The specific impact of COVID-19 on women, and specifically Black women, however, was not clear. A recent study found increased general worries from both White and Black pregnant women in the face of COVID-19; however, the specific worries differed between them (Gur et al., 2020). Black women were found to express anxiety related to financial concerns and the quality of care that would be afforded to them (Gur et al., 2020). Furthermore, self-reliance was not found to reduce the risk for depression in Black women, compared to its moderating effect in White women (Gur et al., 2020). These findings highlight the unique impact of COVID-19 on Black women. It is essential for future studies to further explore the specific factors involved with COVID-19's impact on Black maternal health, in order to devise appropriate systems-level solutions.

Frontline Workers

Being a Black woman frontline worker is a unique intersection that brings its own challenges. In general, SARS-CoV-2 prevalence of infection is higher in health-care workers (HCWs) when compared to the general population (Gómez-Ochoa et al., 2021). Regarding job classification, Black individuals are more likely to work in health-care support and personal care and services (such as psychiatric, dental, and home health aides) (HRSA, 2017). Looking at gender, women are more much more likely to be in jobs deemed essential workers such as registered nurses (9.6% men versus 90.4% women), respiratory therapists (35.4% men to 64.6% women), or medical assistants (7.8% men to 92.2% women) (HRSA, 2017). This indicates that Black women are more likely to be frontline health-care workers and thus at a higher risk of becoming infected with COVID-19.

Once infected with COVID-19, Black individuals have poorer health outcomes; a retrospective cohort study found that in a 30-day period, being Black was associated with higher mortality and higher rates of pulmonary embolisms following COVID-19 infection (Metra et al., 2021). Looking specifically at Black women, research on peripartum women and race found that Black women were at increased risk for mortality and greater length of stay when compared to their White counterparts (Tangel et al., 2019). These studies indicate that COVID-19 infections have more serious outcomes on Black women when they are infected.

Limited studies have studied the unique intersection of the COVID-19 pandemic, HCWs, and Black women specifically. Looking at minorities and Black HCWs, a study completed in the United States and the United Kingdom found Black, Asian, and minority ethnic health-care workers were at increased risk for COVID-19 infection when compared to non-Hispanic White health-care workers (Nguyen et al., 2020). However, this study did not further disaggregate to look at Black women specifically. A survey of HCWs in the UK found large concern for the lack of personal protective equipment (PPE) specifically for women, Black, Asian, and minority ethnic HCWs (Hoernke et al., 2021). Thus, even within the already at-risk group of HCWs, Black individuals are at increased risk with data suggesting limited support for minority and Black HCWs.

From a mental health standpoint, a study completed in health-care workers in China during the COVID-19 pandemic found that women, nurses, and frontline health workers experienced more severe anxiety, insomnia, and depression (Lai et al., 2020). This is combined with the fact that individuals who identify as Black or African American have a higher chance of feeling sadness, hopelessness, and worthlessness when compared to White males (CDC, 2019). From these studies, HCW Black women are at an increased risk for mental health consequences due to the COVID-19 pandemic.

Trying to contextualize the experience of Black women frontline workers, a study on Black birthworkers found that pandemic-related policies furthered racialized fear among birthworkers and their patients (Oparah et al., 2021). A qualitative study looking at Black and Latinx health care workers found that the pandemic had profound impacts not only on the job duties but also their personal lives (Rivera-Núñez et al., 2022). COVID-19 has not only a direct concern for a physical infection and mortality, but further exacerbates historical issues of racism as well as the personal lives of Black women.

Caregiver Burden

Black women successfully overcome adversity and maintain their mental health by their resilience and ability to forge social ties (Burroughs-Gardner et al., 2014). The ability to rely on family, friends, and community has been an experience that has fostered extraordinary individual and collective strengths in the Black community (Burroughs-Gardner et al., 2014). COVID-19 has disproportionately impacted the well-being of this vulnerable population (Gur et al., 2020). The ties that were vital to survival have been limited to some degree or disintegrated altogether. Many community gatherings have been canceled and church services became virtual, reducing community interaction. This change has caused even more strain on Black women, as their role in the family has to be more flexible (Burroughs-Gardner et al., 2014).

Black women have traditionally held countless roles within the family dynamic for many different reasons. One of which can be attributed to the overwhelming overrepresentation of Black men in the prison system (Burroughs-Gardner et al., 2014). A phenomenon worth highlighting is the African American Superwoman; this refers to women feeling that they must do everything for everyone (Burroughs-Gardner et al., 2014). Despite this, women have been able to balance working to financially support their family, parenting, and becoming care givers to their parents or other immediate family members. The nuclear and extended family are important in the Black community (Burroughs-Gardner et al., 2014). Traditionally, Black families are least likely to send their loved ones to assisted living or skilled nursing home facilities (Burroughs-Gardner et al., 2014). This has inevitably wedged them between taking care of those who raised them and raising their own families. The addition of the pandemic unfortunately has further exacerbated this burden. In 2020, school systems transitioned to virtual learning to decrease the chance of exposure but inevitably created a burden in some households (Oster, 2021). Not only did the children require supervision, but they also required access to tablets and computers for each child with reliable internet service.

COVID-19 has not only had a negative impact on the physical, emotional, and mental well-being of Black women, it has also created a financial burden for those caring for others (Walton et al., 2021). "As many [Black] women deal with unemployment or continue to work as 'essential workers,' the intersectionality framework sheds light on the continued legacies of racism and sexism. It asserts that targeted policy interventions are needed to mitigate the effects of COVID-19 and lessen the devastating impact(s) it has had on African American communities" (Obinna, 2021). It has been well documented that "Black Americans are more likely to move in and out of poverty due to few assets to protect them when they are unemployed" (Burroughs-Gardner et al., 2014). The COVID-19 pandemic has decimated the US economy with unemployment rates rising to 14.8% nationally in April 2020, which is the highest reported since 1948 (Patton, 2021). Historically, unemployment rates in the Black community are typically twice that of the national average (Aratani & Rushe, 2020). Sources report Black unemployment rates rising to 24% compared to 14% among White Americans (Bureau of Labor Statistics, 2021). Unemployment rates of Black women rose to 8.5% in 2020, compared to their counterparts' 5.6% (Bureau of Labor Statistics, 2021). It is important to stress that Black women are expected to be "superwomen" with significantly less finances and resources, increased familial burden, and decreased outlets to maintain their mental health.

Recommendations and Call for Action

> The precarity of Black life has been a condition of American possibility since our founding, and that equation has not changed. . . . Black people are disproportionately dying of COVID and people are okay with it.
>
> —Kimberlé Crenshaw, JD, Professor of Law, Columbia Law School

The COVID-19 pandemic is the first we have seen in a century, with consequences that are yet to be elucidated. We have covered only some of the intersecting challenges of being Black, female, and overworked in this unprecedented context. As we attempted to investigate the pandemic's impact on Black women, we were left with more questions. For instance, what are the developmental impacts on children who were born to infected mothers? How many individuals have become newly disabled due to COVID-19 infection, and will this impact their mental health? Do psychological manifestations of the pandemic differ between age groups? And can we safely assert that Black women have exhibited resilience during this pandemic? Resilience is characterized by *recovery*. Our research indicates that Black women carried an excessive load prior to COVID-19, and these responsibilities persisted during the pandemic. However, there are no indicators that a rebound is taking place. Furthermore, how do we declare recovery when the baseline is broken? Multiple factors contributed to the current state of mental health in this demographic, and it will take a multidisciplinary approach to tackle them. Solutions that consider the facets of the Black female experience—such as expansion of housing and health policies, paid sick leave, and more accessible internet service—have been suggested elsewhere (Simien, 2020). We additionally propose further studies that incorporate mixed (qualitative and quantitative) methods, larger sample sizes, greater representation of age groups, and extended follow-up intervals to address the limitations we encountered while conducting this research.

References

Aratani, L., & Rushe, D. (2020, July 1). African Americans bear the brunt of Covid-19's economic impact. *The Guardian.* https://www.theguardian.com/us-news/2020/apr/28/african-americans-unemployment-covid-19-economic-impact

Bureau of Labor Statistics. (2021). *The employment situation* (pp. 1–43). Washington, DC: US Department of Labor.

Burroughs-Gardner, T., Primm, A. B., Lawson, W. B., & Cohen, D. (2014). Issues in the assessment and treatment of African American patients. In R. F. Lim (Ed.), *Clinical Manual of Cultural Psychiatry* (2nd ed.; pp. 77–119). American Psychiatric Publishing.

Centers for Disease Control and Prevention. (2019). *Summary health statistics: National health interview survey, 2017.* Table A-7. https://www.cdc.gov/nchs/nhis/shs/tables.htm

Chinn, J. J., Martin, I. K., & Redmond, N. (2021). Health equity among Black women in the United States. *Journal of Women's Health, 30*(2), 212–219. https://doi.org/10.1089/jwh.2020.8868

Crenshaw, K. (1989). Demarginalizing the intersection of race and sex: A Black feminist critique of antidiscrimination doctrine, feminist theory and antiracist politics. *University of Chicago Legal Forum, 1989*(1), 139–167.

Crenshaw, K. (1991). Mapping the margins: Intersectionality, identity politics, and violence against women of color. *Stanford Law Review, 43*(6), 1241–1299. https://doi.org/10.2307/1229039

Gómez-Ochoa, S. A., Franco, O. H., Rojas, L. Z., Raguindin, P. F., Roa-Díaz, Z. M., Wyssmann, B. M., Guevara, S., Echeverría, L. E., Glisic, M., & Muka, T. (2021). COVID-19 in health-care workers: A living systematic review and meta-analysis of prevalence, risk factors, clinical characteristics, and outcomes. *American Journal of Epidemiology, 190*(1), 161–175. https://doi.org/10.1093/aje/kwaa191

Gur, R. E., White, L. K., Waller, R., Barzilay, R., Moore, T. M., Kornfield, S., Njoroge, W. F. M., Duncan, A. F., Chaiyachati, B. H., Parish-Morris, J., Maayan, L., Himes, M. M., Laney, N., Simonette, K., Riis, V., & Elovitz, M. A. (2020). The disproportionate burden of the COVID-19 pandemic among pregnant Black women. *Psychiatry Research, 293*, 113475. https://doi.org/10.1016/j.psychres.2020.113475

Heron, M. (2016). *Deaths: Leading causes for 2014*. National Center for Health Statistics.

Hoernke, K., Djellouli, N., Andrews, L., Lewis-Jackson, S., Manby, L., Martin, S., Vanderslott, S., & Vindrola-Padros, C. (2021). Frontline healthcare workers' experiences with personal protective equipment during the COVID-19 pandemic in the UK: A rapid qualitative appraisal. *BMJ Open, 11*(1), e046199. https://doi.org/10.1136/bmjopen-2020-046199

Hoyert, D. (2021). (rep.). *Maternal mortality rates in the United States, 2019*. National Center for Health Statistics.

HRSA. *Sex, race, and ethnic diversity of U.S. health occupations (2011–2015)*. (2017). US Department of Health and Human Services, Health Resources and Services Administration, National Center for Health Workforce Analysis.

Lai, J., Ma, S., Wang, Y., Cai, Z., Hu, J., Wei, N., Wu, J., Du, H., Chen, T., Li, R., Tan, H., Kang, L., Yao, L., Huang, M., Wang, H., Wang, G., Liu, Z., & Hu, S. (2020). Factors associated with mental health outcomes among health care workers exposed to coronavirus disease 2019. *JAMA Network Open, 3*(3), e203976. https://doi.org/10.1001/jamanetworkopen.2020.3976

MacDorman, M. F., Declercq, E., Cabral, H., & Morton, C. (2016). Recent increases in the U.S. maternal mortality rate. *Obstetrics and Gynecology, 128*(3), 447–455. https://doi.org/10.1097/aog.0000000000001556

Mackey, K., Ayers, C. K., Kondo, K. K., Saha, S., Advani, S. M., Young, S., Spencer, H., Rusek, M., Anderson, J., Veazie, S., Smith, M., & Kansagara, D. (2021). Racial and ethnic disparities in COVID-19-related infections, hospitalizations, and deaths: A systematic review. *Annals of internal medicine, 174*(3), 362–373. https://doi.org/10.7326/M20-6306

Magesh, S., John, D., Li, W. T., Li, Y., Mattingly-App, A., Jain, S., Chang, E. Y., & Ongkeko, W. M. (2021). Disparities in COVID-19 outcomes by race, ethnicity, and socioeconomic status: A systematic-review and meta-analysis. *JAMA Network Open, 4*(11), e2134147. https://doi.org/10.1001/jamanetworkopen.2021.34147

Metra, B., Summer, R., Brooks, S. E., George, G., & Sundaram, B. (2021). Racial disparities in COVID-19 associated pulmonary embolism: A multicenter cohort study. *Thrombosis Research, 205,* 84–91. https://doi.org/10.1016/j.thromres.2021.06.022

Minkoff, H. (2020). You don't have to be infected to suffer: Covid-19 and racial disparities in severe maternal morbidity and mortality. *American Journal of Perinatology, 37*(10), 1052–1054. https://doi.org/10.1055/s-0040-1713852

Moore, J. X., Bevel, M. S., Aslibekyan, S., & Akinyemiju, T. (2021). Temporal changes in allostatic load patterns by age, race/ethnicity, and gender among the US adult population; 1988–2018. *Preventive Medicine, 147,* 106483. https://doi.org/10.1016/j.ypmed.2021.106483

Muñoz-Price, L. S., Nattinger, A. B., Rivera, F., Hanson, R., Gmehlin, C. G., Perez, A., Singh, S., Buchan, B. W., Ledeboer, N. A., & Pezzin, L. E. (2020). Racial disparities in incidence and outcomes among patients with COVID-19. *JAMA Network Open, 3*(9), e2021892. https://doi.org/10.1001/jamanetworkopen.2020.21892

Nguyen, L. H., Drew, D. A., Graham, M. S., Joshi, A. D., Guo, C. G., Ma, W., Mehta, R. S., Warner, E. T., Sikavi, D. R., Lo, C. H., Kwon, S., Song, M., Mucci, L. A., Stampfer, M. J., Willett, W. C., Eliassen, A. H., Hart, J. E., Chavarro, J. E., Rich-Edwards, J. W., . . . Coronavirus Pandemic Epidemiology Consortium. (2020). Risk of COVID-19 among front-line health-care workers and the general community: A prospective cohort study. *The Lancet Public health, 5*(9), e475–e483. https://doi.org/10.1016/S2468-2667(20)30164-X

Obinna, D. N. (2021). Essential and undervalued: Health disparities of African American women in the COVID-19 era. *Ethnicity and health, 26*(1), 68–79. https://doi.org/10.1080/13557858.2020.1843604

Oparah, J. C., James, J. E., Barnett, D., Jones, L. M., Melbourne, D., Peprah, S., & Walker, J. A. (2021). Creativity, Resilience and Resistance: Black Birthworkers' Responses to the COVID-19 Pandemic. *Frontiers in Sociology, 6,* 636029. https://doi.org/10.3389/fsoc.2021.636029

Oster, E. (2021). Disparities in learning mode access among K–12 students during the COVID-19 pandemic, by race/ethnicity, geography, and grade level—United States, September 2020–April 2021. *Morbidity and Mortality Weekly Report, 70*(26), 953–958. https://www.cdc.gov/mmwr/volumes/70/wr/mm7026e2.htm

Patton, M. (2021, June 28). Pre and Post Coronavirus Unemployment Rates by State, Industry, Age Group, and Race. *Forbes*. https://www.forbes.com/sites/mikepatton/2020/06/28/pre-and-post-coronavirus-unemployment-rates-by-state-industry-age-group-and-race/?sh=6e727086555e

Petersen, E., Davis, N., Goodman, D., Cox, S., Syverson, C., Seed, K., Shapiro-Mendoza, C., Callaghan, W., & Barfield, W. (2019). Racial/ethnic disparities in pregnancy-related deaths—United States, 2007-2016. *Morbidity and Mortality Weekly Report*, 68(35), 762-765. https://doi.org/10.15585%2Fmmwr.mm6835a3

Rivera-Núñez, Z., Jimenez, M. E., Crabtree, B. F., Hill, D., Pellerano, M. B., Devance, D., Macenat, M., Lima, D., Gordon, M., Sullivan, B., Rosati, R. J., Ferrante, J. M., Barrett, E. S., Blaser, M. J., Panettieri, R. A., Jr, & Hudson, S. V. (2022). Experiences of Black and Latinx health care workers in support roles during the COVID-19 pandemic: A qualitative study. *PloS One*, 17(1), e0262606. https://doi.org/10.1371/journal.pone.0262606

Simien, E. (2020, June 9). COVID-19 and the "strong Black woman." *The Gender Policy Report* (Humphrey School of Public Affairs, University of Minnesota). https://genderpolicyreport.umn.edu/covid-19-and-the-strong-black-woman/

Tangel, V., White, R. S., Nachamie, A. S., & Pick, J. S. (2019). Racial and ethnic disparities in maternal outcomes and the disadvantage of peripartum Black women: A multistate analysis, 2007-2014. *American Journal of Perinatology*, 36(8), 835-848. https://doi.org/10.1055/s-0038-1675207

Walton, Q. L., Campbell, R. D., & Blakey, J. M. (2021). Black women and COVID-19: The need for targeted mental health research and practice. *Qualitative Social Work*, 20(1-2), 247-255. https://doi.org/10.1177/1473325020973349

Wiltz, J. L., Feehan, A. K., Molinari, N. M., Ladva, C. N., Truman, B. I., Hall, J., Block, J. P., Rasmussen, S. A., Denson, J. L., Trick, W. E., Weiner, M. G., Koumans, E., Gundlapalli, A., Carton, T. W., & Boehmer, T. K. (2022, January 21). Racial and Ethnic Disparities in Receipt of Medications for Treatment of COVID-19—United States, March 2020-August 2021. *Morbidity and Mortality Weekly Report*, 71(3), 96-102. https://doi.org/10.15585/mmwr.mm7103e1

Chapter 8

Black Women and HIV
From Surviving to Thriving

Rhonda C. Holliday, Kimberly A. Parker,
and Alyssa G. Robillard

> In the beginning, I thought it was a death sentence and now, it's like I'm starting all over. It's a new life. And I have learned to appreciate it more. I learn to love myself more.
>
> —African American woman living with HIV

Introduction

In 2009, Grammy award winning singer and actor Whitney Houston released "I Didn't Know My Own Strength," an iconic ballad chronicling the emotional journey to resiliency by overcoming darkness and despair (Warren & Foster, 2009). The chorus describes how personal strength allowed her to rebound from crashes and tumbles by proclaiming an adage familiar to Black women, she was born not to break. It is this spirit of resiliency that has been developed, fostered, reinforced, and passed down for generations among Black women. Resiliency resounds in phrases such as "what doesn't kill you will make you stronger" and "strong Black woman." Resiliency also materializes in concepts such as "Black Girl Magic." Women, especially

Black women, have commonly had to display the ability to overcome while facing adversity. A sense of resiliency may be a noble and desired outcome to adversity; subsequently, resilience is entrenched with the hardships and misfortunes commonly associated with adversity. Facing constant adversities and the fortitude to overcome these adversities, enhances the ability to bend and not break. For Black women, unfortunately, having to face increased levels of adversity is often overshadowed by limits to their ability to overcome. It is these increased levels of adversity, coupled with the persistent challenges to overcome these adversities, that place Black women at an increased risk for HIV and all too often do not center their voices in conversations about HIV prevention and care.

Black Women and the HIV Burden

In 2018, women accounted for 19% of new HIV diagnoses in the United States, with 57% of the new diagnoses being among Black women. Black women represented the fourth highest incidence of all new HIV diagnoses in 2018, surpassed only by Black, White non-Hispanic, and Hispanic/Latino men (Centers for Disease Control and Prevention, 2019a) These rates are alarming, considering Black women account for only 13% of the US population. The good news is that the rate of new HIV diagnosis among Black women decreased by 27% from 2010 to 2017. However, if we were to eliminate the disparities in incidence rates between Black women and White women, 93% of new HIV infections among Black women would not have occurred (Bradley et al., 2019). The number of Black women who are living with HIV/AIDS is also disproportionate relative to their representation in the general population. Black women living with HIV/AIDS represent well over half of all women, in the US, living with HIV/AIDS (Centers for Disease Control and Prevention, 2019a).

Despite these disparities in incidence rates for new HIV diagnosis and the prevalence rates of living with HIV/AIDS, targeted efforts to reduce the rate of new HIV infections among Black women in the United States have not always been consistently prioritized. Durvasula (2018) outlined three eras of HIV/AIDS research, early, middle, and structural. In each era, HIV/AIDS research has not adequately addressed the unique needs and concerns of women, and this is especially true for Black women. In the early era (1980s), research excluded both pregnant and nonpregnant women. During the middle era (1990s) there was inclusion of women in research, a recognition that HIV/AIDs was disproportionately affecting Black women, and acknowledgment of heterosexual contact as the primary source of new infections. The middle era saw a concerted effort to fund research focused on women. The current era is labeled as the structural era, focusing on factors that contribute to HIV in women including violence, sex trafficking, disparities in access to care and education, and poverty, to name a few.

Although there was an effort to fund HIV research focused on women during the middle era, nearly 40 years after the identification of HIV, a review of the Centers for Disease Control and Prevention (CDC) compendium for effective behavioral interventions for HIV prevention found three evidence-based interventions, meeting the current criteria for rigor, where the target population was exclusively Black adult or adolescent females. In the original compendium, which listed interventions developed between 1988 and 1996, there was an additional intervention listed, which has since been removed due to not meeting the current inclusion criteria. The lack of interventions endorsed by CDC is indicative of the lack of urgency that has been prevalent in HIV research concerning Black women in the United States. Recently, the HIV National Strategic Plan, 2021–2025, has called national attention to Black women by listing them as a priority population. Some of the key areas of focus for this plan include increased awareness and access to PrEP, and addressing stigma, discrimination, and the social and structural determinants of health. A key indicator is to increase viral suppression among Black women from 59.3% to 95% (US Department of Health and Human Services, 2021).

Black Women and Risk for HIV

Black women are at an increased risk for HIV infection for multiple reasons. Black men and women are more likely to date within their race compared to other races. Intraracial dating influences the male-female sex ratio balance for likely partners. Higher incarcerations rates for Black men inadvertently reduces the number of available partners within sexual networks. Sexual networks with higher prevalence of HIV increases the risk of transmission for Black women (Adimora & Schoenbach, 2005; Bradley et al., 2018).

The intersection of being Black and being a woman in the US amplifies these factors among Black women. Black women possess multiple identities, including race, gender, and sexual identity. Often viewed as independent correlates for health outcomes, risk for HIV infection among Black women occurs at the crossing, or intersection, of these identities (Rao et al., 2018). Intersectionality is the synergy caused by overlapping identities or personal characteristics that subsequently influence levels of privilege or oppression within society (Rao et al., 2018; Tebb et al., 2018). These multiple identities conceptualize marginalization within the unique experience of operating as a Black woman beyond the experience of isolating descriptors. Black women face a constant barrage of disadvantaged circumstances based on the intersection of multiple identities. Subsequently, resiliency is pivotal among Black women based on societal norms related to Black female bodies and hegemonic aspects of heterosexual relationships (Hill Collins, 2005). Women are often forced to operate within gender norms inequitable to those prescribed for men. This partiality leads to the hegemonic structure of heterosexual relationships; by default, men are identified as the norm and benefit from this power imbalance (Wingood et al., 2009). The manifestation of power reduces women's ability to negotiate safer sex practices and allows men to have more sexual freedom in heterosexual relationships (Frew et al., 2016; Wingood et al., 2009). The reduction of power as a societal norm, coupled with racial identity, underscores the role of intersectionality as an increased risk for HIV infection and the need for resiliency among Black women.

Historically, Black women face a greater degree of objectification compared to Black men and to women of other races and ethnicities (Hill Collins, 2005). The brutal economic practice of chattel slavery identified Black women's bodies as property to be sold, traded, and acquired as commodities for profit and capital gain. The institution of slavery produced and reinforced the hypersexed Black female moniker. Although the oversexed Black female body served a much-desired means to continue the legacy of slavery in the United States, this view of increased sexuality among Black women manifested as a characteristic commonly used to describe and stigmatize Black women (Black et al., 2015; Hill Collins, 2005). As a result, gender and race as discrete, independent identities fail to fully explain health disparities among Black women, including an increased risk for HIV infection (Bradley et al., 2018).

Black women are also likely to experience other risk dynamics for HIV infection, such as increased levels of poverty, lack of access to healthcare, victimization, and discrimination while accessing health services (McNair & Prather, 2004). Black women also must contend with racism and racist power structures that directly impact their health and well-being. Black women are often unable to access the care they need and when they are, they are often receiving care from a system that does not care about them. Racism and other structural barriers also place increased burdens on Black HIV.

Risk factors associated with HIV/AIDS carry a negative connotation that, unfortunately, is the basis for several stereotypes unfairly attributed to Black women. The labeling of Black women as hypersexual beings is often linked to unprotected sex, multiple sexual partners, and apathy toward one's own sexual health. HIV/AIDS still carries with it a sense of shame that discredits those linked to or associated with the disease. As risk factors for HIV/AIDS are ingrained in negative stereotypes used to describe Black women, the intersection of race and gender coupled with HIV-related stigma is often difficult to dispel. Distancing oneself from HIV/AIDS also places Black women at an increased risk for HIV infection and decreases engagement in care (Heller, 2015; Rao et al., 2018).

Women often face HIV-related stigma from family, friends, healthcare providers, and religious institutions (Geter et al., 2018, Fletcher et al., 2016). As a result, places where refuge may typically be sought (i.e., faith-based institutions) are not always places where support is offered (Fletcher et al., 2016). This is disconcerting, considering that faith and prayer increase resilience among Black women. When Black women have limited support, this can translate into detrimental health consequences and affect self-efficacy and self-esteem. This raises the question, How do we support and empower Black women to overcome by helping them to recognize their own strength and resilience?

Resilience

Resilience has been found to be important, particularly for Black women living with HIV (BWLH). Resilience is not always clearly defined in the literature. Resilience has been defined as one's ability to function following stressors, as multi-component, and included individual (personality characteristics), interpersonal (social support), and structural (employment, educational) level characteristics to address the reality of the breadth and number of barriers faced by people living with HIV (PLWH), particularly Black women (Dulin et al., 2018).

According to Ungar (2006), resilience is twofold: the ability to remain efficient when facing undue stress or trauma, and functioning positively following undue stress or trauma. Characterized by the capability to successfully overcome disadvantaged circumstances, resilience as a personal trait describes one's ability to overcome adversity by producing better than expected outcomes (Fletcher et al., 2020; Ungar, 2006). Resilience has been characterized as both a process and an outcome, and as a set of individual traits that serve as facilitators for the process of arriving at positive outcomes. Individuals who are resilient can achieve many positive outcomes, including behavioral, relational, physical, and psychological.

Black Women, HIV, and Resilience

The literature on Black women, HIV, and resilience has mostly focused on women who are living with HIV. Among Black women living with HIV, faith, prayer, and critical consciousness have been identified as factors that contribute to resilience (Geter et al., 2018; Kelso et al., 2014). The relationship between HIV-related stigma and depression was weaker when there were high scores on religiosity (Njie-Carr et al., 2012; Lipira et al., 2019). Resilience has been found to be related to higher self-rated successful aging, lower depressive symptoms, higher health-related quality of life, higher self-esteem, higher post-traumatic growth, lower post-traumatic cognitions, and lower trauma symptoms (Dale et al., 2015; Thurston et al., 2018; Dale et al., 2019; Rubtsova et al., 2019). As documented in qualitative interviews conducted with BWLH, resilience resources include internal strength, religion and spirituality, hopefulness about life and the future, self-awareness and self-care, social support from family and community, and health care facilities (Qiao et al., 2019; Fletcher et al., 2020). Rao et al. (2018) identified social support, self-efficacy, building trust and empowerment, spirituality, and self-esteem as resources that lead to increased resilience that helps BWLH cope with HIV related stigma.

Narratives of Resilience

To offer insight on aspects of resilience observed among Black women living with HIV in the Deep South, where the burden of HIV is higher and the context of care is complex (Centers for Disease Control and

Prevention, 2019b), the authors present findings from two independent qualitative studies. One study documented the cultural narratives of women (N = 25) over the age of 18 recruited from local HIV/AIDS service organizations using a chronological and ecological storytelling approach (Robillard, 2021). The second study collected narratives representing the lived experience of HIV positive African American women based on the discovery of one's HIV status and contrasting life experiences after diagnosis (N = 30) (Parker, 2020). In each study, participants described both emotional and HIV care-related resilience. We present findings from these two studies based on the resources for resilience described by Rao et al. (2018) earlier.

Social Support

Social support is an important aspect of well-being for women living with HIV, and it can come from varied, albeit selective, sources. Close and secure relationships are established and fortified with friends and family members who are a source of support not only emotionally, but with HIV care as well. These relationships counter stigma and provide women with validation about their experiences and create environments where emotions can be more freely expressed (Rao et al., 2018). One participant described her social support network as "small, but . . . loyal," adding: "They are very supportive. Same friends for 20 years. Nothing has changed. They motivate me, you know, they are always on top of what I know I supposed to do. Girl, you didn't take your med—you know, you got your medicine, you know, you got your prescriptions and stuff, you know, your medicine, you're good, you know, you been going to the doctor, you good everything."

This social support can also come from AIDS service organizations:

> Yes, and a lot of other things. They are more—they call you, they follow-up, you know. They have people calling you if you need anything. Meals on wheels. How you are doing. They are calling you about upcoming events. They tell you—they ask you if you need shelter, clothing, whatever you need help with. You know, they let you know. They reinforce the fact that they are there to help you where you don't feel like you are a burden to anyone.

Self-efficacy

Self-efficacy, as described by Rao et al. (2018), is the perception of having control over one's circumstances and the ability to effectively carry out actions that are in the best interest of one's own well-being. The ability to control external influences that can negatively impact emotional well-being was demonstrated by a participant who said, "If you have negativity around you and you don't want to get sicker than what you are then you need to tell whomever it might be mom, dad, uncle, and cousin, whatever. . . . I don't have time for you and your negativity I need you to move around cuz I have to stay well for me." Women living with HIV who have high self-efficacy are more likely to engage in heath-affirming activities, seek help, and practice a lifestyle that promotes/supports their HIV care (Rao et al., 2018).

Building Trust and Empowerment

A notable example of resilience is observed in the way participants in both studies described their involvement in activities designed to build trust and empowerment. These discussions highlighted ways that women created or responded to opportunities to build personal and community capacity. Support groups were described as an initial source for building trust. For many women, these groups were empowering and served as points to initiate advocacy and community engagement:

> After I came and got in support groups, and I started doing a little public speaking. . . . It was around World AIDS day. I never did any public speaking in my life. So I had these cue cards with all the stuff written down . . . 'cause I knew I was gonna be nervous. . . . And when they called me up, and when I got to the podium, when I got up and turned around to the audience, and the place was full, I thought I would die. But I was able to share my story, and after I shared that story it was like a wind blew a big block off of me.

Building trust and empowerment fosters the development and use of skills, knowledge, and resources that facilitate resilience by empowering women to face and address challenges as they arise (Rao et al., 2018).

Spirituality

Spirituality, whether formal or informal, has been found to benefit the psychological health and well-being of Black women living with HIV. For women living with HIV, this spirituality is often expressed as a source for personal meaning or purpose—a reason for living or feeling like they've been afforded a "second chance" (Rao et al., 2018). As one participant stated, "Yeah, my spirituality plays a strong key because I know God has something for me. I've been positive 25 years. . . . Spiritually I knew God had something for me when I contracted it. I know his grace was still in place for me. The grace that he had was still in place for me to be used to be—and I still believe in healing. . . ." Women described spirituality as a source of resilience, both in responding to a diagnosis of HIV and in seeking and maintaining HIV care.

Self-esteem

The overall evaluation of one's worth is another important resource to attain resilience over traumatizing experiences. "Individuals with high self-esteem may experience less stress, demonstrate adaptive coping behaviors, and seek and obtain more social support" (Rao et al., 2018). Reframing adverse narratives to benefit one's own sense of self reflects an ability to prioritize oneself as a whole person—distinct from their diagnosis; for example, "I really don't believe that [my HIV status] is something that's going to lead to death. It doesn't define me. It's just something that I happen to be diagnosed with, like when I tell people that I am diagnosed. I don't say I have HIV. I say I was diagnosed with HIV."

Conclusion

Black women living with HIV display resilience in the face of layered traumas, some of which seem nearly insurmountable. Bolstering the resources, social support, self-efficacy, building trust and empowerment, spirituality, and self-esteem, as described by Rao et al. (2018), are important if we are to have an impact on the burden of HIV among Black women. This is not only true for BWLH, but also holds for Black women at risk for HIV. This chapter presents a framework to understand resilience in BWLH and offers findings from two independent qualitative studies that speak to this framework. Concepts within this framework can be used to develop interventions that build resilience among Black women to prevent HIV and to engage in HIV care leading to viral suppression.

However, resilience alone is not enough to address this burden. While building resilience is important, it can also be viewed as having Black women do the heavy lifting once again. It is time to stop placing the burden squarely on the shoulders of Black women, asking them to bend and not break. Black Girl Magic can only take you so far. To truly tackle the burden of HIV among Black women, we must not only build, foster, and promote resilience, but we must acknowledge intersectionality and the structural inequities and systems grounded in racism that have a detrimental impact on the health of Black women. It is in this context that we offer the following recommendations to review the burden of HIV among Black women.

Recommendations and Call for Action

1. Center the voices of Black women living with HIV to better understand the mechanisms and factors that help to develop and support resilience.

2. Address the structural inequities, including poverty, education, access to healthcare, and racism that affect Black women to optimize their health and well-being.

3. Target HIV prevention, care, and treatment for Black women. The funding should be contingent on its inclusion of the voices of Black women at risk for and living with HIV and be inclusive of community based participatory research methods that engage community-based organizations.

Acknowledgments

The author received funding for this research from the Centers for Disease Control and Prevention Grant# 5 U48DP006411-01. The author(s) received no financial support from the Institute for Families in Society, University of South Carolina, for the research described in this chapter. Correspondence concerning this article should be addressed to Rhonda

Conerly Holliday, Morehouse School of Medicine, 720 Westview Dr., Atlanta, GA 30318. Email: rholliday@msm.ed.

Resources

Positive Women's Network. https://www.pwn-usa.org
SisterLove. https://www.sisterlove.org
The Well Project. https://www.thewellproject.org

References

Adimora, A. A., & Schoenbach, V. J. (2005). Social context, sexual networks, and racial disparities in rates of sexually transmitted infections. *Journal of Infectious Diseases*, *191*(suppl. 1), S115–122. https://doi.org/10.1086/425280

Black, L. L., Johnson, R., & VanHoose, L. (2015). The relationship between perceived racism/discrimination and health among Black American women: A review of the literature from 2003 to 2013. *Journal or Racial and Ethnic Health Disparities*, *2*(1), 11–20. https://doi.org/10.1007/s40615-014-0043-1

Bradley, E. L. P., Geter, A., Lima, A. C., Sutton, M. Y., & Hubbard McCree, D. (2018). Effectively addressing human immunodeficiency virus disparities affecting US Black women. *Health Equity*, *2*(1), 329–333. https://doi.org/10.1089/heq.2018.0038

Bradley, E. L., Williams, A. M, Green, S., Lima, A. C., Geter, A., Chesson, H. W., & McCree, D. H. (2019). Disparities in incidence of human immunodeficiency virus infection among Black and White women—United States, 2010–2016. *Morbidity and Mortality Weekly Report*, *68*(18), 416–418. https://doi.org/10.15585%2Fmmwr.mm6818a3

Centers for Disease Control and Prevention. (2019a). HIV Surveillance Report, 2018 (Preliminary; vol. 30). http://www.cdc.gov/hiv/library/reports/hiv-surveillance.html. Published November 2019.

Centers for Disease Control and Prevention. (2019b, September). *HIV in the Southern United States* (Issue Brief). https://www.cdc.gov/hiv/pdf/policies/cdc-hiv-in-the-south-issue-brief.pdf.

Dale, S. K., Reid, R., & Safren, S. A. (2019). Factors associated with resilience among Black women living with HIV and histories of trauma. *Journal of Health Psychology*, *26*(5), 758–766.https://doi.org/10.1177/1359105319840690

Dale, S. K., Weber, K. M., Cohen, M. H., Kelso, G. A., Cruise, R. C., & Brody, L. R. (2015). Resilience moderates the association between childhood sexual abuse and depressive symptoms among women with and at-risk for HIV. *AIDS and Behavior*, *19*(8), 1379–1387. https://doi.org/10.1007/s10461-014-0855-3

Dulin, A. J., Dale, S. K., Earnshaw, V. A., Fava, J. L., Mugavero, M. J., Napravnik, S., Hogan, J. W., Carey, M. P., & Howe, C. J. (2018). Resilience and HIV: A review of the definition and study of resilience. *AIDS Care*, *30*(suppl. 5), S6–S17. https://doi.org/10.1080/09540121.2018.1515470

Durvasula, R (2018, March). A history of HIV/AIDS in women: Shifting narrative and a structural call to arms. *Psychology and AIDS Exchange Newsletter*. https://www.apa.org/pi/aids/resources/exchange/2018/03/history-women

Fletcher, F., Ingram, L. A., Kerr, J., Buchberg, M., Bogdan-Lovis, L., & Philpott-Jones, S. (2016). "She told them, oh that bitch got AIDS": Experiences of multilevel HIV/AIDS-related stigma among African American women living with HIV/AIDS in the South. *AIDS Patient Care and STDs*, *30*(7), 349–356. https://doi.org/10.1089/apc.2016.0026

Fletcher, F. E., Sherwood, N. R., Rice, W. S., Yigit, I., Ross, S. N., Wilson, T. E., Weiser, S. D., Johnson, M. O., Kempf, M. C., Konkle-Parker, D., Wingood, G., Turan, J. M., & Turan, B. (2020). Resilience and HIV treatment outcomes among women living with HIV in the United States: A mixed-methods analysis. *AIDS Patient Care and STDs*, *34*(8), 356–366. https://doi.org/10.1089/apc.2019.0309

Frew, P. M., Parker, K., Vo, L., Haley, D., O'Leary, A., Diallo, D. D., Golin, C. E., Kuo, I., Soto-Torres, L., Wang, J., Adimora, A. A., Randall, L. A., del Rio, C., Hodder, S., & the HIV Prevention Trials Network 064 (HTPN) Study Team. (2016). Socioecological factors influencing women's HIV risk in the United States: Qualitative findings from the women's HIV SeroIncidence study (HPTN 064). *BMC Public Health*, *16*(1), Article 803. https://doi.org/10.1186/s12889-016-3364-7

Geter, A., Sutton, M. Y., & Hubbard McCree, D. (2018). Social and structural determinants of HIV treatment and care among Black women living with HIV infection: A systematic review: 2005–2016. *AIDS Care*, *30*(4), 409–416. https://doi.org/10.1080/09540121.2018.1426827

Heller, J. (2015). Rumors and realities: Making sense of HIV/AIDS conspiracy narratives and contemporary legends. American Journal of Public Health, 105(1), e43-e50. https://doi.org//10.2105/ajph.2014.302284

Hill Collins, P. (2005). *Black sexual politics: African Americans, gender, and the new racism*. Routledge.

Kelso, G. A., Cohen, M. H., Weber, K. M., Dale, S. K., Cruise, R. C., & Brody, L. R. (2014). Critical consciousness, racial and gender discrimination, and HIV disease markers in African American women with HIV. *AIDS and Behavior*, *18*(7), 1237–1246. https://doi.org/10.1007/s10461-013-0621-y

Lipira, L., Williams, E. C., Nevin, P. E., Kemp, C. G., Cohn, S. E., Turan, J. M., Simoni, J. M., Andrasik, M. P., French, A. L., Unger, J. M., Heagerty, P., & Rao, D. (2019). Religiosity, social support, and ethnic identity: Exploring "resilience resources" for African-American women experiencing HIV-related stigam. *Journal of Acquired Immune Deficiency Syndrome*, 81(2), 175–183. https://doi.org/10.1097/qai.0000000000002006

McNair, L. D., & Prather, C. M. (2004). African American women and AIDS: Factors influencing risk and reaction to HIV disease. *Journal of Black Psychology*, *30*(1), 106–123. https://doi.org/10.1177/0095798403261414

Njie-Carr, V., Sharps, P., Campbell, D., and Callwood, G. (2012). Experiences of HIV-positive African-American and African Caribbean childbearing women: A qualitative study. *Journal of the National Black Nurses Association, 23*(1), 21–28. DOI: 10.1016/j.apnu.2010.04.004

Parker, K. A. (2020) *Exploring the narratives of HIV positive African American women in the South* [Manuscript in preparation].

Qiao, S., Ingram, L., Deal, M L., Li, X., & Weissman, S. B. (2019). Resilience resources among African American women living with HIV in Southern United States. *AIDS, 33*, S35–S44. https://doi.org/10.1097/QAD.0000000000002179

Rao, D., Andrasik, M. P., and Lipira, L. (2018). HIV stigma among Black women in the United States: Intersectionality, support, resilience. *American Journal of Public Health, 108*(4), 446–448. https://doi.org/10.2105/AJPH.2018.304310

Robillard, A. (2021). *Narratives of resilience in African American women living with HIV in the South: The gendered and cultural context of motivation, management, and mastery* [Manuscript in preparation]. Institute for Families in Society, University of South Carolina.

Rubtsova, A. A., Wingood, G. M., Ofotokun, I., Gustafson, D., Vance, D. E., Sharma, A., Adimora, A. A., & Holstad, M. (2019). Prevalence and correlates of self-rated successful aging among older women living with HIV. Journal of Acquired Immune Deficiency Syndromes, *82*(2), S162–S169. https://doi.org/10.1097/QAI.0000000000002175

Tebb, K. P., Pica, G., Twietmeyer, L., Diaz, A., & Brindis, C. D. (2018). Innovative approaches to address social determinants of health among adolescents and young adults. *Health Equity, 2*(1), 321–328. https://doi.org/10.1089/heq.2018.0011

Thurston, I. B., Howell, K. H., Kamody, R. C., Maclin-Akinyemi, C., & Mandell, J. (2018). Resilience as a moderator between syndemics and depression in mothers living with HIV. *AIDS Care, 30*(10), 1257–1264. https://doi.org/10.1080/09540121.2018.1446071

Ungar, M. (2006). Resilience across cultures. *British Journal of Social Work, 38*(2), 218–235. https://doi.org/10.1093/bjsw/bcl343

US Department of Health and Human Services. (2021). HIV National Strategic Plan for the United States: A Roadmap to end the epidemic, 2021–2025. https://files.hiv.gov/s3fs-public/HIV-National-Strategic-Plan-2021-2025.pdf

Warren, D., & Foster, D. (Cowriter & Producer) (2009). I didn't know my own strength [Song]. On Whitney Houston, *I look to you*. Arista.

Wingood, G. M., Camp, C., Dunkle, K., Cooper, H., & DiClemente, R. J. (2009). The theory of gender and power: Constructs, variables, and implications for developing HIV interventions for women. In R. J. DiClemente, R. A. Crosby, & M. C. Kegler (Eds.), *Emerging theories in health promotion practice and research* (2nd ed.; pp. 393–414). Jossey-Bass.

Chapter 9

The Nexus of Chronic Stress, Autoimmune Disorders, and Black Women

Lesley Green-Rennis, Lisa Grace-Leitch, and Anika Thrower

Introduction

Autoimmune disorders are characterized as conditions in which the host's immune system mistakenly attacks itself. The overstimulated immune system attacks the very tissues, organs, and systems it is supposed to protect. The exact mechanism of autoimmune conditions is not well understood (Angum et al., 2020). One major potential contributing factor is stress. Our bodies are designed to respond to stress via a complex feedback loop involving the nervous, endocrine, and cardiovascular systems. Though intended to protect us and guarantee our survival during times of threat, the stress response can be deadly when repeatedly activated. Research has consistently documented that Black Americans are more likely to experience stressful situations and suffer the consequences of chronic exposure to stress (Williams, 2018). However, little is known about the link between stress and autoimmune disorders, and less is known about the phenomenon among Black women.

Autoimmune Disorders

Autoimmune disorders are among the least understood chronic diseases. They are often misdiagnosed, they are difficult to treat, and their unpredictable and intermittent nature make diagnosis challenging (NIH Autoimmune Diseases Coordinating Committee, 2005). Currently, there is no known cure for autoimmune disorders. The immune system is extremely complex and essential to optimal health and well-being. Like a sophisticated military force, it specializes in combat against foreign invaders. Armies of white blood cells respond to each invader with specificity. When a foreign substance invades the body, the immune system recognizes the invader's antigens and destroys them. During the process, the system memorizes the "face" of the invader. Every time it sees that face after the initial encounter, it uses the custom-made mold to recognize, capture, and destroy the invader. Breakdowns in communication and management could lead the immune system to be unnecessarily activated. In the case of autoimmune diseases, the system turns on itself. The highly effective defense system loses the ability to distinguish foreign invaders from its own rank. The result, an attack of the body's own protein structures, results in a systemic reaction that can affect one specific organ, multiple organs, or entire systems. Some describe autoimmune disorders as one disease living in different places in the body and taking on different names. It is likely that if a person has one disorder, he or she will have a second or third.

For yet to be discovered reasons, the overall incidence and prevalence of autoimmune diseases is rising, particularly in industrialized countries like the United States (Rose, 2016). Autoimmune diseases have been estimated to impact from 5% to 8% of Americans (NIH Autoimmune Diseases Coordinating Committee, 2005). According to recent National Institute of Allergies and Infectious Disease data, a quarter-million people in the US are diagnosed with one of the 80 separate autoimmune diseases each year (NIH Autoimmune Diseases Coordinating Committee, 2005; US Department of Health and Human Services, Office of Women's Health, 2021). Nine of the most common disorders account for 97% of all cases (table 9.1). Women are approximately 2.7 times more likely to be afflicted with an autoimmune disorder than men (Angum et al., 2020; US Department of Health and Human Services, Office of Women's Health, 2021).

Although the Centers for Disease Control and Prevention (CDC) (2019) has reported that for Systematic Lupus Erythematosus (SLE) minority and ethnic groups are affected more than Whites, minimal epidemiological data has been published concerning autoimmune diseases among minority populations (Roberts & Erdei, 2020). The Lupus Foundation of America (2021) states that nine out of ten adults living with lupus are minority women in their child-bearing years. Black women are three times more likely to develop lupus with 1 in every 537 having the disease (Somers et al., 2014).

Scientists have investigated the role that genetics, hormones, obesity, smoking, and low levels of vitamin D and sunlight exposure play in the development of autoimmune disorders (NIH Autoimmune Diseases Coordinating Committee, 2005). Estrogen has also been highlighted as a possible culprit. Data point to inflammation in development and progression. Recent research shows a possible relationship between autoimmune disorders and trauma or intense stress (Song et al., 2018). This is particularly relevant for Black women, who have higher stress levels than the general population (see table 9.1).

Table 9.1. Common autoimmune disorders*

Name	Percentage per population**	Name	Percentage per population
Rheumatoid arthritis	0.806%	Rheumatic fever	0.234%
Hashimoto's autoimmune thyroiditis	0.742%	Pernicious anemia/atrophic gastritis	0.141%
Celiac disease	0.703%	Alopecia areata	0.141%
Grave's disease	0.590%	Immune thrombocytopenic purpura	0.068%
Diabetes mellitus, type 1	0.450%	Multiple sclerosis	0.055%
Vitiligo	0.375%	Systematic lupus erythematosus	0.030%

*Data from the Autoimmune Registry
**Per 100,000 people
Source: Author.

Physiology of Stress

Song et al. (2018) compared more than 100,000 individuals who had stress-related disorders with 1,000,000 people without them in a population and sibling matched retrospective cohort study. Researchers found that stress was tied to a 36% greater risk of developing 41 autoimmune diseases (Song et al., 2018).

Our bodies are designed to respond to stressors through the cooperative effects of the primary stress response systems—the sympathetic nervous system (SNS) and hypothalamic-pituitary-adrenal (HPA) axis. During the stress response, also known as the "fight-or-flight" response, dozens of stress hormones flood the body in response to a real or perceived threat, preparing it to either fight back or flee. However, with exposure to chronic stress and repeated activation, the body's response becomes inefficient, resulting in an allostatic load, a biological measure of stress-mediated wear and tear on the body (McEwen & Seeman, 1999). Allostatic load may take a toll throughout the body and contribute to the development or progression of a broad range of clinical and preclinical pathological processes such as increased risks of cardiovascular, immune, and metabolic dysfunction (Khansari et al., 2009). Like the overreaction of the immune system in individuals with autoimmune disorders, the stress response system begins to destroy that which it is intended to protect.

Biological studies link psychological stress and stressful events to varying impairments of immune functioning (Glaser & Kiecolt-Glaser, 2005). Under stress, the activated autonomic nervous system might induce the dysregulation of immune function and disinhibition of inflammatory response via the inflammatory reflex (Pavlov & Tracey, 2012). Alternatively, individuals under chronic stress may be more likely to engage in behaviors such as poor sleep patterns, alcohol or substance abuse, increased smoking, and consumption of inflammatory foods, all of which have been shown to increase inflammation and may indirectly alter the risk for autoimmune diseases (Palma et al., 2006).

In this chapter, we critically examine public health data on the etiology, incidence and prevalence, symptomatology, and treatment of autoimmune disorders among Black women and what is currently known about how stress impacts such disorders. To give context and meaning to the data, a case study of a 44-year-old Black woman diagnosed with multiple autoimmune disorders is examined.

Case

Michelle, a 44-year-old Black woman currently living in North Carolina, was diagnosed with lupus and rheumatoid arthritis at the age of 32. At the time of her diagnosis, Michelle lived in New York with her husband, two teenage daughters, and two-year-old son. Michelle moved to North Carolina in search of a more sustainable and less hectic lifestyle. Michelle has struggled off and on with her weight for most of her adult life. Her medical history includes eczema since childhood and the use of the birth control Depo Provera in her early twenties. Michelle is 5 ft. 6 in. and weighs 187 lbs., with a body mass index (BMI) of 28.4.

Symptoms

Like most individuals with autoimmune disorders, Michelle initially experienced a diverse group of idiopathic symptoms. Her first clue that something might be wrong was the noticeable thinning of her eyebrows. Though tempted to attribute the spareness of hair to her heavy-handed aesthetician, she became increasingly concerned when she later realized her eyelashes were falling out as well. She also noticed but tried to rationalize her extreme exhaustion.

While some autoimmune diseases target specific organs (e.g., type 1 diabetes, Graves'), others affect the whole body. Often, the first symptoms are fatigue, muscle aches, and a low-grade fever (Angum et al., 2020; Garcia-Carretero et al., 2018). For most autoimmune diseases, these symptoms can be attributed to inflammation, the by-product of the body's immune response. When white blood cells attack foreign invaders or perceived foreign invaders, chemicals enter the blood or tissue to protect the body. This raises the blood flow to the area causing redness, swelling, heat, pain, and stiffness. Inflammation may also cause flu-like symptoms such as fever, chills, fatigue, loss of appetite, and headaches. It is normally a local and temporary event. However, disrupted innate immune regulation can result in continual pro-inflammatory cytokine activity and excessive or chronic inflammation. This state underlies the pathogenesis of a range of autoimmune disorders.

Profound and debilitating fatigue is the most common complaint reported among individuals with autoimmune disorders (Ahn & Ramsey-Goldman, 2012; Nguyen et al., 2018; American Autoimmune Related

Diseases Association, 2015). In general, fatigue is defined by debilitating periods of exhaustion that interfere with normal activities (American Autoimmune Related Diseases Association, 2015). The severity and duration of fatigue episodes vary, but as with Michelle, fatigue can cause difficulty completing the simplest of tasks and interfere with daily living. Though the multifaceted nature and broad definition of fatigue make deciphering its connection to specific autoimmune diseases difficult, studies show that fatigue can interfere with physical functioning, prevent sustained physical functioning, and worsen the condition of those with lupus and other autoimmune disorders (Sturgeon et al., 2015; Malm et al., 2017). Patients with lupus report significant disruption to their quality of life because of fatigue, including their professional relationships, self-esteem, career, ability to work, and romantic relationships (American Autoimmune Related Diseases Association, 2015). The exact mechanisms of fatigue are not well-understood. Nevertheless, physiological processes known to play a role in fatigue include oxygen/nutrient supply, metabolism, mood, motivation, and sleepiness—all of which are affected by inflammation (Morris et al., 2016). Additionally, an important contributing element to fatigue is the central nervous system—a region impacted either directly or indirectly in numerous autoimmune disorders.

Hair loss is another commonly reported autoimmune symptom. Michelle's initial symptoms, thinning and loss of eyebrow and eyelash hairs, may have been a form of alopecia areata (AA), an autoimmune disorder in which the immune system attacks the hair follicles. Alopecia can be diagnosed alone or in occurrence with other autoimmune disorders. In particular, lupus has been associated with hair loss (Parodi & Cozzani, 2014; Concha & Werth, 2018; Kridin et al., 2020). Concha & Werth (2018) found that more than half of patients experience hair loss at some point during the course of the disease. Patients have reported gradual thinning of the hair on their scalp, loss of clumps of hair, loss of eyebrows, eyelashes, beard, and body hair. Women with lupus often report weak and fragile hair along the hairline that becomes fragile and breaks off easily, leaving a ragged appearance known as frontal fibrosis alopecia (FFA), or lupus hair (Nascimento et al., 2018). FFA is also associated with loss of eyebrows and eyelashes.

Michelle also learned that a butterfly-shaped eczema patch on her chest was most likely connected to her lupus. Research (Ivert et al., 2021) has found that atopic dermatitis (a type of eczema) is significantly associated with one or more autoimmune diseases compared with controls. The association is significantly stronger in the presence of multiple autoimmune diseases versus just one. The malar rash, also known as butterfly rash, is seen in 46%–65% of lupus patients (Kumar et al., 2019) and characterized by an erythematous flat or raised rash across the bridge of the nose and cheeks, the chest, or the back. It may be transient or progress to involve other areas of the skin (Naji Rad & Vashisht, 2020). Symptoms like fatigue, hair loss, and eczema, as well as others such as joint pain and swelling, are often early signals that something has gone awry (Desai & Miteva 2021).

Diagnosis

During her initial visit to the doctor, Michelle described her symptoms and was asked about her family background. At the time, she was unaware of family members with similar symptoms. The physician ran tests, which came back positive for lupus and RA. Michelle knew little about either disease but felt devastated and overwhelmed by the diagnosis. She was certain she was dying. The doctor provided her with pamphlets and referred her to a rheumatologist. Michelle went home and searched Google for more information.

As discussed, autoimmune patients may experience a constellation of symptoms, many of which accumulate over time, occur sporadically, and can be found in patients with other chronic conditions, making diagnosis difficult (Orbai, 2021). Although laboratory tests are routinely available for the detection of some autoimmune disorders, diagnosis cannot be made from laboratory tests alone. Skilled clinicians will consider symptoms as expressed by a patient, the patient's medical and family history, and assessments (i.e., blood, urine, and biopsies) in their diagnosis (Somers et al., 2014). In the case of rheumatoid arthritis, MRI and ultrasound tests can help determine the disease's severity. A proper diagnosis of an autoimmune disease may take several months or even years to confirm. Sufferers can go for long periods free from symptoms, adding to the difficulty of making a definitive diagnosis (Somers et al., 2014). In addition, a diagnosis does not necessarily help patients understand and deal with their disease. Even after a diagnosis, autoimmune patients struggle to fully understand their disease and need ongoing support and education.

Treatment

Michelle hoped her visit with the rheumatologist would shed light on what was going on with her body. She had begun to experience more symptoms, including pain in her shoulder and hip joints, and unexplained swelling of her eyes and lips. Her rheumatologist explained that the pain was associated with inflammation and prescribed medication to help reduce it. According to Michelle, she "wasn't given much education or the type of education I needed to make decisions and take care of myself." Michelle was particularly concerned about the possible side-effects associated with long-term use of the prescribed medicine. Once again, Michelle turned to Google to gain knowledge about her disease.

Autoimmune disorders are often treated with disease-modifying antirheumatic drugs, nonsteroidal anti-inflammatory drugs (NSAIDs), corticosteroids, antimalarial drugs, and BLyS-specific inhibitors (Cleveland Clinic, 2021). Some drugs if used for long periods of time could have adverse side effects. The Mayo Clinic (2021) asserts that users may experience unwanted side effects to include high blood pressure, glaucoma, cataracts, and osteoporosis. Michelle didn't feel comfortable taking the medication and, unfortunately, she was not given the type or amount of information she needed. Not long after her visit to the rheumatologists, she stopped taking the prescribed medication and chose instead to self-medicate with the supplement black seed cumin oil. Though she experienced fewer symptoms while taking the supplement, she also discontinued its use after a few months.

STRESS

"I was under a lot of stress, a lot." Michelle recalled that during the time of her diagnosis, her life was particularly hectic. Taking care of a two-year-old and two teenagers, attending school full time, and working full time weighed heavily on Michelle. Her husband worked long hours and, though she had a support system, Michelle "didn't know exactly what I needed, so though support was there, I felt extremely overwhelmed."

Higher incidences of autoimmune diseases have been found among people previously diagnosed with stress-related disorders. Though the experience of stress is highly individual, some populations are more likely to suffer from stress-related illness. US Blacks are more likely to experience stress from a multitude of factors, including financial and material hardship, interpersonal discrimination, structural discrimination in housing and employment, and multiple caregiving roles (Geronimus et al., 2007). Geronimus et al. (2010) documented that ambient stressors in residential or work environments are further examples of stressors that can pose significant physiological challenge and to which Black Americans are disproportionately exposed, not only with greater frequency but also with greater duration and intensity than Whites. Geronimus et al. (2007) report that Blacks have higher mean allostatic load scores than Whites at all ages, and the differential in scores increases with age. Moreover, by age 30, Black women exhibit the greatest risk of having high allostatic load scores. This risk gap increases through midlife and is most severe among Black women who are poor. Burton and Whitfield (2006) found that most of the primary caregivers in their study led "highly challenging lives" and "could never get a break." Research linking stress to autoimmune disorders shows that individuals diagnosed with a stress-related disorder are more likely to be diagnosed with an autoimmune disease within one year, more likely to develop multiple autoimmune diseases, and have higher rates of autoimmune diseases at younger ages (NIH Autoimmune Diseases Coordinating Committee, 2005). Moreover, living with a chronic autoimmune disorder adds further stress to patients' lives.

Progression of Illness

Recently, Michelle was hospitalized after taking a road trip to visit her daughter and grandson. A few days after returning to North Carolina, Michelle's husband found her passed out on the bathroom floor. She was hospitalized for a week, treated with anticoagulants, and sent home to recuperate. She was also referred to a hematologist and a rheumatologist. Since then, she's returned to urgent care on a number of occasions and was most recently prescribed medication for anxiety.

Autoimmune diseases impair multiple organs and systems, typically not all at the same time. Instead, the damage is additive. As more and more symptoms occur, the dysregulation of the immune system gets more out of control. If left untreated, an autoimmune disease can result in a medical crisis, leading to organ and/or system failure or permanent damage. When patients like Michelle experience a crisis, they may become increasingly worried about their health, sometimes to the point of developing an anxiety disorder. In addition, the lack of a clear diagnosis or having multiple diagnoses may lead the patient to doubt her own experience with the disorder. As with initial symptoms, patients often make excuses for the onset of more serious symptoms and neglect seeking treatment. The inability of clinicians to fully identify and treat autoimmune disorders further adds to the patient's confusion and doubt.

Of particular concern is the link between untreated Rheumatoid Arthritis (RA) and cardiovascular disease (CVD). CVD disproportionally affects RA patients and is currently the primary cause of morbidity and mortality among RA sufferers (Urman et al., 2018). CVD accounts for nearly 40% of RA sufferers' deaths (Urman et al., 2018). Hypertension, a stress-related illness that disproportionately affects Black women, is a key factor in the development of CVD (Panoulas et al., 2007). Hypertension is a silent disease that is of particular concern for women with RA because research has shown a correlation between RA and blood clots (Kim et al., 2013). Chronic inflammation appears to be the significant underlying pathogenic factor linking RA and CVD (Urman et al., 2018).

Conclusion

Black women are at increased risk for developing autoimmune diseases, tend to develop such disorders earlier in life, experience greater disease symptoms at the time of their diagnosis, and have more severe symptoms overall than other autoimmune sufferers. Yet, they are underrepresented in clinical trials and lack representation in the medical field in general and in specialties devoted to the study of autoimmune disorders specifically. These factors, combined with the greater prevalence of stress in the lives of Black women, put them at increased risk for negative outcomes related to autoimmune disorders. The lack of culturally competent health education material specifically targeting Black women further exacerbates the problem. These issues can lead to mistrust, dissatisfaction, decreased treatment adherence, and poorer health outcomes.

Recommendations and Call for Action

Based on existing data and Michelle's case study, we recommend the following:

1. Health education material that speaks directly to the lifestyles and needs of Black women. Specifically, culturally relevant information about diagnosis, treatment, and management of autoimmune diseases, the role of stress in autoimmune disease etiology, and the importance of nutrition, diet, and self-care.

2. Training and career development opportunities for public health and medical professionals that address health disparities in autoimmune disease outcomes.

3. Initiatives that assist Black women in finding both traditional and alternative healthcare professionals who specialize in treating autoimmune diseases.

4. Increase patient and public awareness of autoimmune diseases and related available treatments.

5. Increase participation of Black women in autoimmune disorders clinical trials.

Suggested Resource

For more information about autoimmune diseases, call the Office of Women's Health Helpline at 1-800-994-9662 (TDD: 888-220-5446).

References

Ahn, G. E., & Ramsey-Goldman, R. (2012). Fatigue in systemic lupus erythematosus. *International Journal of Clinical Rheumatology, 7*(2), 217–227. https://doi.org/10.2217/IJR.12.4

Angum, F., Khan, T., Kaler, J., Siddiqui, L., & Hussain, A. (2020). The prevalence of autoimmune disorders in women: A narrative review. *Cureus, 12*(5), e8094. https://doi.org/10.7759/cureus.8094

American Autoimmune Related Diseases Association. (2015, March 23). Profound, debilitating fatigue found to be a major issue for autoimmune disease patients in new national survey. *ScienceDaily*. www.sciencedaily.com/releases/2015/03/150323105245.htm

Burton, L. M., Whitfield, K. E. (2006). Health, aging, and America's poor: Ethnographic insights on family co-morbidity and cumulative disadvantage. In J. Baars, D. Dannefer, C. Phillipson, & A. Walker (Eds.), *Aging, globalization, and inequality: The new critical gerontology* (pp. 215–230). Baywood.

Centers for Disease Control and Prevention. (2019). *Systemic lupus erythematosus (SLE)*. https://www.cdc.gov/arthritis/data_statistics/arthritis-related-stats.html

Cleveland Clinic. (2021). *Non-steroidal anti-inflammatory drugs (NSAIDs)*. https://my.clevelandclinic.org/health/drugs/11086-non-steroidal-anti-inflammatory-medicines-nsaids

Concha, J., & Werth, V. P. (2018). Alopecias in lupus erythematosus. *Lupus science and Medicine, 5*(1), e000291. https://doi.org/10.1136/lupus-2018-000291

Desai, K., & Miteva, M. (2021). Recent insight on the management of lupus erythematosus alopecia. *Clinical, Cosmetic and Investigational Dermatology, 14*, 333–347. https://doi.org/10.2147/CCID.S269288

Garcia-Carretero, R., Naranjo-Mansilla, G., Luna-Heredia, E., Arias-Baldo, P., & Beamonte-Vela, B. N. (2018). Incidental finding of a left atrial myxoma while characterising an autoimmune disease. *Journal of Critical Care Medicine, 4*(2), 64–67. https://doi.org/10.2478/jccm-2018-0009

Geronimus, A. T., Bound, J., Keene, D., & Hicken, M. (2007). Black-White differences in age trajectories of hypertension prevalence among adult women and men, 1999–2002. *Ethnicity and Disease, 17*(1), 40–48.

Geronimus, A. T., Hicken, M. T., Pearson, J. A., Seashols, S. J., Brown, K. L., & Cruz, T. D. (2010). Do US Black women experience stress-related accelerated biological aging? A novel theory and first population-based test of Black-White differences in telomere length. *Human Nature, 21*(1), 19–38. https://doi.org/10.1007/s12110-010-9078-0

Glaser, R., & Kiecolt-Glaser, J. K. (2005). Stress-induced immune dysfunction: implications for health. *Nature Reviews: Immunology, 5*(3), 243–251. https://doi.org/10.1038/nri1571

Ivert, L., Wahlgren, C.-F., Lindelöf, B., Dal, H., Bradley, M., & Johansson, E. (2021). Association between atopic dermatitis and autoimmune diseases: a population-based case-control study. British Journal of Dermatology, 185(2), 335–342. https://doi.org/10.1111/bjd.19624

Khansari, N., Shakiba, Y., & Mahmoudi, M. (2009). Chronic inflammation and oxidative stress as a major cause of age-related diseases and cancer. *Recent Patents on Inflammation and Allergy Drug Discovery, 3*(1), 73–80.

Kim, S. C., Schneeweiss, S., Liu, J., & Solomon, D. H. (2013). Risk of venous thromboembolism in patients with rheumatoid arthritis. *Arthritis Care and Research, 65*(10), 1600–1607. https://doi.org/10.1002/acr.22039

Kridin, K., Shalom, G., Comaneshter, D., & Cohen, A. D. (2020). Is there an association between alopecia areata and systemic lupus erythematosus? A population-based study. *Immunologic Research, 68*(1), 1–6. https://doi.org/10.1007/s12026-020-09115-x

Kumar, R. R., Jha, S., Dhooria, A., Dhir, V. (2019). Butterfly rash: Hallmark of lupus. *QJM: An International Journal of Medicine, 112*(11), 877. https://doi.org/10.1093/qjmed/hcz091

Lupus Foundation of America. (2021). *Lupus facts and statistics.* https://www.lupus.org/resources/lupus-facts-and-statistics

Malm, K., Bergman, S., Andersson, M. L., Bremander, A., & Larsson, I. (2017). Quality of life in patients with established rheumatoid arthritis: A phenomenographic study. *Sage Open Medicine, 5,* 2050312117713647. https://doi.org/10.1177/2050312117713647

McEwen B. S., & Seeman T. (1999). Protective and damaging effects of mediators of stress: Elaborating and testing the concepts of allostasis and allostatic load. *Annals of the New York Academy of Sciences, 896*(1), 30–47. https://doi.org/10.1111/j.1749-6632.1999.tb08103.x

Morris, G., Berk, M., Galecki, P., Walder, G., & Maes, M. (2016). The neuro-immune pathophysiology of central and peripheral fatigue in systemic immune-inflammatory and neuro-immune diseases. *Molecular Neurobioogy, 53*(2), 1195–1219. https://doi.org/10.1007/s12035-015-9090-9

Naji Rad, S., & Vashisht P. (2020). Malar Rash. In *StatPearls*. StatPearls Publishing. https://www.ncbi.nlm.nih.gov/books/NBK555981/

Nascimento, L. L., Enokihara, M. M. S. S., & Vasconcellos, M. (2018). Coexistence of chronic cutaneous lupus erythematosus and frontal fibrosing alopecia. *Anais Brasileiros de Dermatologia, 93*(2), 274–276. https://doi.org/10.1590/abd1806-4841.20186992

NIH Autoimmune Diseases Coordinating Committee. (2005, March). *Progress in autoimmune diseases research.* https://www.niaid.nih.gov/sites/default/files/adccfinal.pdf

Nguyen, M. H., Bryant, K., & O'Neill, S. G. (2018). Vitamin D in SLE: A role in pathogenesis and fatigue? A review of the literature. *Lupus, 27*(13), 2003–2011. https://doi.org/10.1177/0961203318796293

US Department of Health and Human Services, Office of Women's Health. (2021). *Autoimmune diseases.* https://www.womenshealth.gov/a-z-topics/autoimmune-diseases

Orbai, A.-M. (2021). *What are some common symptoms of Autoimmune Diseases.* Johns Hopkins Medicine. https://www.hopkinsmedicine.org/health/wellness-and-prevention/what-are-common-symptoms-of-autoimmune-disease

Palma, B. D., Gabriel, A., Jr, Colugnati, F. A. B., & Tufik, S. (2006). Effects of sleep deprivation on the development of autoimmune disease in an experimental model of systemic lupus erythematosus. *American Journal of Physiology: Regulatory, Integrative and Comparative Physiology, 291*(5), R1527–R1532. https://doi.org/10.1152/ajpregu.00186.2006

Panoulas, V. F., Douglas, K. M., Milionis, H. J., Stavropoulos-Kalinglou, A., Nightingale, P., Kita, M. D., Tselios, A. L., Metsios, G. S., Elisaf, M. S., & Kitas, G. D. (2007). Prevalence and associations of hypertension and its control in patients with rheumatoid arthritis. *Rheumatology, 46*(9), 1477–1482. https://doi.org/10.1093/rheumatology/kem169

Parodi, A., & Cozzani, E. (2014). Hair loss in autoimmune systemic diseases. *Giornale Italiano di Dermatologia e Venereologia, 149*(1), 79–81.

Pavlov, V. A., & Tracey, K. J. (2012). The vagus nerve and the inflammatory reflex—Linking immunity and metabolism. *Nature Reviews: Endocrinology*, *8*(12), 743–754. https://doi.org/10.1038/nrendo.2012.189

Roberts, M. H., & Erdei, E. (2020). Comparative United States autoimmune disease rates for 2010–2016 by sex, geographic region, and race. *Autoimmunity Reviews*, *19*(1), 102423. https://doi.org/10.1016/j.autrev.2019.102423

Rose, N. R. (2016). Prediction and prevention of autoimmune disease in the 21st century: A review and preview. *American Journal of Epidemiology*, *183*(5), 403–406. https://doi.org/10.1093/aje/kwv292

Somers, E. C., Marder, W., Cagnoli, P., Lewis, E. E., DeGuire, P., Gordon, C., Helmick, C. G., Wang, L., Wing, J. J., Dhar, J. P., Leisen, J., Shaltis, D., & McCune, W. J. (2014). Population-based incidence and prevalence of systemic lupus erythematosus: The Michigan Lupus Epidemiology and Surveillance program. *Arthritis and rheumatology*, *66*(2), 369–378. https://doi.org/10.1002/art.38238

Song, H., Fang, F., Tomasson, G., Arnberg, F. K., Mataix-Cols, D., de la Cruz, L. F., Almqvist, C., Fall, K., & Valdimarsdóttir, U. A. (2018). Association of stress-related disorders with subsequent autoimmune disease. *JAMA*, *319*(23), 2388–2400. https://doi.org/10.1001/jama.2018.7028

Sturgeon, J. A., Darnall, B. D., Kao, M. C., & Mackey, S. C. (2015). Physical and psychological correlates of fatigue and physical function: A Collaborative Health Outcomes Information Registry (CHOIR) study. *Journal of Pain*, *16*(3), 291–298.e1. https://doi.org/10.1016/j.jpain.2014.12.004

Urman, A., Taklalsingh, N., Sorrento, C., & McFarlane, I. M. (2018). Inflammation beyond the Joints: Rheumatoid Arthritis and Cardiovascular Disease. *SciFed Journal of Cardiology*, *2*(3), 1000019.

Williams, D. R. (2018). Stress and the mental health of populations of color: Advancing our understanding of race-related stressors. *Journal of Health and Social Behavior*, *59*(4), 466–485. https://doi.org/10.1177/0022146518814251

Chapter 10

Mindfulness Matters

Mental Health Risks and Protective Factors for Black Women

Kisha Braithwaite Holden, Sharon A. Rachel,
Ricardo D. LaGrange, Glenda Wrenn Gordon,
and Cynthia Major Lewis

Introduction

While several racial and ethnic minority communities suffer from disparities in prevalence of mental health disorders and access to both behavioral and physical health care (National Academies of Sciences, Engineering, and Medicine, 2017), Black women are disproportionately exposed to stressors across multiple domains that adversely affect their mental and physiological health (Holden et al., 2012). Recent estimates suggest that 60% of Black people report having a mental illness (nearly 1 in 4 report a serious mental illness) over the past year, yet the pattern of past year mental health service utilization by Black women is only 10.3%, less than half that of White women (Substance Abuse and Mental Health Services Administration, 2015). Factors including (but not limited to) racism, gender discrimination, acute life events, and socioeconomic vulnerabilities may not only be distressing for Black women, but they can lead to detrimental health outcomes. For example, research has identified strong associations between mental illness and harmful health behaviors, poor treatment adherence for comorbid chronic conditions, and lack of help-seeking and health care utilization (Sporinova et al., 2019; Lake & Turner, 2017). Other studies have identified a bidirectional relationship and increased risks that exist between selected chronic diseases like obesity, diabetes, and cardiovascular disorders and mental health problems like anxiety, depression, and post-traumatic stress disorder (PTSD) in minority populations (McGregor et al., 2020; Holden, Bradford et al., 2014).

Mental Health: A Report of the Surgeon General defined mental health as "the successful performance of mental function, resulting in productive activities, fulfilling relationships with others, and the ability to adapt to change and to successfully cope with adversity" (US Department of Health and Human Services, 1999, p. 4); conversely, it defined mental illness as "health conditions that are characterized by alterations in thinking, mood, or behavior (or some combination thereof) associated with distress and/or impaired functioning" (p. 5). A subsequent Surgeon General's report, *Mental Health: Culture, Race, and Ethnicity*, concluded that racial/ethnic minority populations, compared with the non-Hispanic White population, have less access to mental health care, are less likely to receive treatment, and, when treated, often receive poorer quality of care (US Department of Health and Human Services, 2001). Numerous psychosocial and sociocultural issues must be addressed to begin disentangling the multidimensional relationship between physical and mental health.

This chapter explores common mental health risk and protective factors among Black/African American women, complex systems in which such disorders emerge, stigma and other barriers to accessing mental health care, and strategies to help promote resiliency.

Recognizable Mental Health Concerns

Nearly one in five adults in the United States has a mental health disorder (National Institute of Mental Health [NIMH], 2021). Furthermore, data show that people suffering from mental illness experience a life expectancy that can average 25 years less than the rest of the population (Parks et al., 2006; Gilman et al., 2017). Research shows that Black women attribute causes of mental illness to personal and professional stress, trauma, substance abuse, familial influences, environmental factors, and challenges related to handling the multiple expectations and demands Black women have placed on them (Ward et al., 2013; Holden et al., 2015; Evans et al., 2017). Some of the most commonly occurring mental health disorders for Black women are anxiety, depression, and post-traumatic stress disorder (National Alliance on Mental Illness [NAMI], 2019), which we explore in further detail below.

ANXIETY

Anxiety disorders are the most common mental health conditions in the US. They are typically characterized by ongoing and disproportionate distress or nervousness in mostly benign (i.e., nonthreatening) situations. Symptoms can be both physiological (elevated heart rate, shortness of breath, gastrointestinal distress, shakiness) and emotional (feeling tense, irritable, or apprehensive). The National Institute of Mental Health reports that over 40,000,000 adults in the US have an anxiety disorder and that women are approximately 1.6 times more likely than men to suffer from this illness (NIMH, 2017). However, research has shown a much higher prevalence of anxiety among Black women; Lacey et al. (2015) estimated that over 22,000,000 (23.7%) Black women in the US have an anxiety disorder. Research into risk factors related to anxiety in Black women has shown that those who are younger, have a high school education or less, had their first child at a young age, who have experienced violence and discrimination, and who are in fair or poor health are more likely to have an anxiety disorder (Watson et al., 2012; Biaggi et al., 2016). There is a myriad of potential stressors (see table 10.1) that may occur concomitantly and increase risk for anxiety.

Table 10.1. Selected stressful anxiety-provoking issues

- Health concerns
- Individual/personal issues
- Interpersonal and intimate relationships
- Family relationships and daily demands
- Unresolved pain and trauma
- Negative life event(s)
- Confronting historical negative stereotypes and images
- Job/employment issues
- Economic and financial concerns
- Handling multiple expectations of others

Source: Author.

Depression

The World Health Organization (2020) reports that depression is a leading cause of disability and significantly affects disease burden. According to the National Institute of Mental Health (2019a), just over seven percent of US adults have had at least one depressive episode in the past year. Depression can have physical, cognitive, and emotional symptoms. People with depression may experience changes in sleep and eating patterns (i.e., sleeping or eating too much or too little), decreased energy, or physical aches and pains. They may also experience difficulties concentrating or become easily agitated. Depression is also characterized by lost interest in activities the person had previously enjoyed, feelings of guilt and hopelessness, and suicidal thoughts.

African Americans have an estimated lifetime depression prevalence rate of just over 10% and Black women experience depression at almost twice the rate of Black men (Bailey et al., 2019; Holden, McGregor et al., 2014; NIMH, 2011).

Post-traumatic Stress Disorder and Complex Trauma

Post-traumatic stress disorder (PTSD) can develop in people who have experienced shocking, scary, or dangerous events (NIMH, 2019b). While typically associated with military combat, PTSD can be caused by numerous traumatic events such as terrorism, occupational work, sexual assault, and urban trauma (Substance Abuse and Mental Health Services Administration, 2014). People with PTSD may experience chronic fear, flashbacks or nightmares about the trauma, hypervigilance or hyperarousal, or feelings of guilt or detachment (NIMH, 2019b). Some individuals may employ avoidance behaviors including avoiding thinking about the trauma or avoiding certain situations that may remind them of the trauma (NIMH, 2019b).

Black women endure the dual oppressions of racism and sexism, both of which are forms of trauma (Neal-Barnett, 2018); and a growing body of research also suggests that intergenerational trauma, or a link between genetics and PTSD, disproportionately affects Black women (Almli et al., 2013). However, PTSD does not always fully embody the symptoms that can result from the long-lasting effects of trauma stemming from slavery, racism, and discrimination, in addition to the cultural, historical, and gender-based trauma that Black women have endured. Complex trauma refers to a form of trauma that occurs repeatedly and cumulatively, usually over a period and within specific relationships and contexts, and involves a wider set of self-regulatory impairments than are exhibited by PTSD (Courtois, 2004; Ford, 2009). Relatively few researchers have focused on the relationship between Black women's experiences of complex trauma and its relationship to PTSD within specific racial, ethnic, and culturally diverse communities.

Psychosocial, Sociocultural, and Environmental Stressors

A mounting body of research indicates that perceived discrimination and oppressive systems like racism and sexism are significant contributing factors to psychological distress and a host of negative mental and physical health outcomes for Black women (Wagner et al., 2015; Belgrave & Abrams, 2016; Kershaw et al., 2016; Lewis et al., 2017). For example, Black women exposed to chronic stress related to racism may be at significantly greater risk for carotid artery blockages (Lewis et al., 2019). Additionally, Black women are uniquely vulnerable to the deleterious effects of microaggressions and covert racism because they exist within gender roles and societal norms that discourage them from critically questioning or even acknowledging the offenses. And when Black women can summon the courage necessary to confront the discrimination they face, they are told that they are too sensitive or are powerless to change things.

Mental and Behavioral Health Stigma in the Black Community

Studies over time have consistently shown that minorities stigmatize or hold negative beliefs and attitudes about mental illness and individuals who seek treatment (Silva de Crane & Spielberger, 1981; Diala et al., 2000; Eylem et al., 2020). Mental illness has been associated with shame, embarrassment, and weakness (Conner et al., 2010; Abbensetts, 2020). Ward and colleagues (Ward & Heidrich, 2009; Ward et al., 2013) found that Black women's views of mental illness included denial of a problem, perceiving mental illness as an ordinary part of life, or holding that individuals are to blame for their own mental illness because "Black people are supposed to be strong." Similarly, Waite and Killian (2008) reported that Black women believe that depression results from a "weak mind, poor health, a troubled spirit, and lack of self-love." Research has also shown a belief that mental illness can be overcome with positive thinking and prayer (Villines & Legg, 2020).

Stigma also poses a considerable barrier to African Americans accessing mental health services (US Department of Health and Human Services, 2001; Alang, 2019). As a result, mental health help-seeking uptake is low among Black women (Kalibatseva & Leong, 2014; Nelson et al., 2022). African Americans may avoid seeking help because of perceived or actual racism in mental health therapy (Villines & Legg, 2020); concerns over hospitalization, incarceration, and inappropriate medication (Bailey et al., 2011; Ward et al., 2013; Dockery et al., 2015); and the belief that, "no one outside of your family or community needs to know your business" (Watson & Hunter, 2015). Fortunately, emerging research is informing culturally competent treatment modalities and showing that stigma associated with help-seeking among Black women is beginning to abate (Ward et al., 2013; Ward and Brown, 2015; Neal-Barnett, 2018).

Promoting Resilience and Recovery

Mental health professionals may mis- or underdiagnose Black women with mental health disorders because of a dearth of culturally competent mental health assessment instruments. Moreover, "classical" symptomatology does not always apply to Black women (Holden et al., 2014; Liang et al., 2016). For example, whereas White women may report feeling worried, nervous, or afraid, or having a depressed mood or decreased energy, Black women are more likely to report feeling angry, may aggressively act out, may "keep busy" to avoid psychological distress, or may not say anything at all (Johnson, 2016; Lashley et al., 2017; Abbensetts, 2020). Mental health therapists can increase their cultural competence by familiarizing themselves with stereotypes, racism, and trauma that impact Black women's mental health, while also implementing cultural adaptations of therapeutic interventions that can enhance interventions that promote resiliency in Black women (Neal-Barnett, 2018).

Research on traumatic events suggest that trauma may shatter an individual's existing schemas, or sense of the world around them, deeply affecting their sense of purpose and meaning (Janoff-Bulman, 1992). The resultant struggle with meaninglessness can lead to neglecting existential needs, which influence how individuals cope with stress (Frankl et al., 2010). However, several potential solutions may promote resilience among Black women and mitigate the impact of psychosocial issues that increase risks for mental health disorders. Having a strong sense of mastery, self-efficacy, positive ethnic identity, and purpose in life are key psychosocial factors associated with both resilience and recovery from negative mental health events and outcomes (e.g., Harlow et al., 1986; Alim et al., 2008; Lopez et al., 2012; Zapolski et al., 2019). Research literature also supports spirituality and frequent religious service attendance as influential moderators of traumatic life events for people of color (Hickman, 2012; Staton-Tindall et al., 2013), specifically Black women (Alim et al., 2008; Drakeford, 2017). Moreover, Black women's ability to draw on key relationships with others as a resource in times of stress can facilitate resilience and has been found to buffer against the development of trauma responses (Charuvastra & Cloitre, 2008; Dale & Safren, 2018).

Black women can also employ a number of approaches to managing stress and reducing the risk for mental health problems. Self-awareness, self-care, inter- and intrapersonal restorative healing, and a redefinition of inner strength may manifest through developing a mindfulness practice for specifically targeting the contextually related factors that are thought to influence disparate outcomes for Black women (Woods-Giscombé & Black, 2010). Some personal strategies for managing stressors include developing action-oriented plans, reducing individual vulnerability and building resilience, reducing the impact of stress reactions, and utilizing strategies that support wellness goals. Learning to anticipate, recognize, and alter or remove potential stressors can prevent or mitigate risk factors for anxiety and depression.

Recently, prominent Black women figures such as world Olympic medalist Simone Biles and professional tennis player Naomi Osaka publicly demonstrated a commitment to their mental health; yet, tragically, former Miss USA Cheslie Kryst succumbed to suicide. It is important for Black women to prioritize their own needs, especially given the multiple demands placed on them by their communities. This can be accomplished by developing proactive time management and conflict resolution, communication, and assertiveness skills. Establishing attainable goals, allowing room for error, and modifying or eliminating negative self-talk and self-criticism can all help Black women cope with stress. Developing self-exploration, awareness, and renewal behaviors can help build self-confidence, and using calming and relaxation techniques such as meditation, prayer, journaling, and maintaining healthy eating, exercise, and sleeping can all help reduce stress. Even having a "me" place to go or making "me" time can ease some of the burdens that, left unchecked, can spiral into mental health disorders. Finally, leaning on social support networks, talking to trusted individuals who can offer varying perspectives, and being willing to seek professional help can all decrease feelings of stigma and isolation, and promote mental well-being.

Recommendations and Call for Action

Addressing the multi-faceted mental health needs of Black women in the United States is a complex issue that warrants attention from clinicians, researchers, scientists, public health professionals, and policy makers (Wrenn et al., 2017; Holden et al., 2019). More research is needed to develop and utilize culturally appropriate interventions that both encourage help-seeking and discourage stigma (Liang et al., 2016; Kennedy and Jenkins, 2018). Understanding the interplay between traumatic or stressful experiences and mental health disorders among Black women can help to inform methods for diagnosing and treating this population. The use of mindfulness and other mind-body practices can reduce the accumulated impact of psychological and systemic stress in vulnerable populations (Johnson et al., 2018). Researchers also argue that broader, more modern definitions of trauma and other mental health experiences are necessary to accurately reflect the experiences of diverse groups (Substance Abuse and Mental Health Services Administration, 2014; Spanierman & Poteat, 2005).

However, advancing mental health equity among Black women will necessitate a paradigm shift and take multidimensional approaches that encourage holistic wellness, proactive self-care, and reduction of stigma. Interventions within diverse communities must be culturally centered, community informed, and gender specific. Multidisciplinary professionals and community leaders can foster behavioral and mental health dialogue. Mental health care advocates can encourage receptivity among diverse communities for use of and/or adherence to psychotropic medication management as directed by their clinician. Finally, funding to improve health equity, including integrated healthcare and patient-centered medical homes, must be prioritized.

Resources

American Psychiatric Association. https://www.psychiatry.org/
American Psychological Association. https://www.apa.org/

Association of Black Psychologists. https://abpsi.site-ym.com/
Mental Health America. https://www.mhanational.org/

References

Abbensetts, R. (2020, February 1). How social anxiety can look different for Black women. *Well+Good*. https://www.wellandgood.com/social-anxiety-symptoms-black-women/

Alang, S. M. (2019). Mental health care among Blacks in America: Confronting racism and constructing solutions. *Health Services Research*, *54*(2), 346–355. https://doi.org/10.1111/1475-6773.13115

Alim, T. N., Feder, A., Graves, R. E., Wang, Y., Weaver, J., Westphal, M., Alonso, A., Aigbogun, N. U., Smith, B. W., Doucette, J. T., Mellman, T. A., Lawson, W. B., & Charney, D. S. (2008). Trauma, resilience, and recovery in a high-risk African-American population. *American Journal of Psychiatry*, *165*(12), 1566–1575. https://doi.org/10.1176/appi.ajp.2008.07121939

Almli, L. M., Mercer, K. B., Kerley, K., Feng, H., Bradley, B., Conneely, K. N., & Ressler, K. J. (2013). ADCYAP1R1 genotype associates with post-traumatic stress symptoms in highly traumatized African-American females. *American Journal of Medical Genetics Part B: Neuropsychiatric Genetics*, *162*(3), 262–272. https://doi.org/10.1002/ajmg.b.32145

Bailey, R. K., Mokonogho, J., & Kumar, A. (2019). Racial and ethnic differences in depression: Current perspectives. *Neuropsychiatric Disease and Treatment*, *15*, 603–609. https://doi.org/10.2147/NDT.S128584

Bailey, R. K., Patel, M., Barker, N. C., Ali, S., & Jabeen, S. (2011). Major depressive disorder in the African American population. *Journal of the National Medical Association*, *103*(7), 548–559. https://doi.org/10.1016/S0027-9684(15)30380-1

Belgrave, F. Z., & Abrams, J. A. (2016). Reducing disparities and achieving equity in African American women's health. *American Psychologist*, *71*(8), 723–7 33. https://doi.org/10.1037/amp0000081

Biaggi, A., Conroy, S., Pawlby, S., & Pariante, C. M. (2016). Identifying the women at risk of antenatal anxiety and depression: A systematic review. *Journal of Affective Disorders*, *191*, 62–77. https://doi.org/10.1016/j.jad.2015.11.014

Charuvastra, A., & Cloitre, M. (2008). Social bonds and posttraumatic stress disorder. *Annual Review of Psychology*, *59*(1), 301–328. https://doi.org/10.1146/annurev.psych.58.110405.085650

Conner, K. O., Copeland, V. C., Grote, N. K., Koeske, G., Rosen, D., Reynolds, C. F., & Brown, C. (2010). Mental health treatment seeking among older adults with depression: The impact of stigma and race. *American Journal of Geriatric Psychiatry*, *18*(6), 531–543. https://doi.org/10.1097/JGP.0b013e3181cc0366

Courtois, C. A. (2004). Complex trauma, complex reactions: Assessment and treatment. *Psychotherapy: Theory, Research, Practice, Training, 41*(4), 412–425. https://doi.org/10.1037/0033-3204.41.4.412

Dale, S. K., & Safren, S. A. (2018). Resilience takes a village: Black women utilize support from their community to foster resilience against multiple adversities. *AIDS Care, 30*(suppl. 5), S18–S26. https://doi.org/10.1080/09540121.2018.1503225

Diala, C., Muntaner, C., Walrath, C., Nickerson, K. J., LaVeist, T. A., & Leaf, P. J. (2000). Racial differences in attitudes toward professional mental health care and in the use of services. *American Journal of Orthopsychiatry, 70*(4), 455–464. https://doi.org/10.1037/h0087736

Dockery, L., Jeffery, D., Schauman, O., Williams, P., Farrelly, S., Bonnington, O., Gabbidon, J., Lassman, F., Szmukler, G., Thornicroft, G., & Clement, S. (2015). Stigma- and non-stigma-related treatment barriers to mental healthcare reported by service users and caregivers. *Psychiatry Research, 228*(3), 612–619. https://doi.org/10.1016/j.psychres.2015.05.044

Drakeford, N. M. (2017). *Strong Black woman: An exploration of coping, suppression, and psychological distress* [Doctoral dissertation]. University of Akron.

Evans, S., Bell, K., & Burton, N. (2017). *Black women's mental health: Balancing strength and vulnerability*. State University of New York Press.

Eylem, O., de Wit, L., van Straten, A., Steubl, L., Melissourgaki, Z., Danışman, G. T., de Vries, R., Kerkhof, A. J. F. M., Bhui, K., & Cuijpers, P. (2020). Stigma for common mental disorders in racial minorities and majorities: A systematic review and meta-analysis. *BMC Public Health, 20*(1), 879. https://doi.org/10.1186/s12889-020-08964-3

Ford, J. (2009). Neurobiological and developmental research: Clinical implications. In C. A. Courtois and J. Ford (Eds.), *Treating complex traumatic stress disorders: An evidence-based guide* (pp. 31–58). Guilford Press.

Frankl, V., Batthyany, A., & Tallon, A. (2010). *The feeling of meaninglessness: A challenge to psychotherapy and philosophy*. Marquette University Press.

Gilman, S. E., Sucha, E., Kingsbury, M., Horton, N. J., Murphy, J. M., & Colman, I. (2017). Depression and mortality in a longitudinal study: 1952–2011. *CMAJ, 189*(42), E1304–E1310. https://doi.org/10.1503/cmaj.170125

Harlow, L. L., Newcomb, M. D., & Bentler, P. M. (1986). Depression, self-derogation, substance use, and suicide ideation: Lack of purpose in life as a mediational factor. *Journal of Clinical Psychology, 42*(1), 5–21. https://doi.org/https://doi.org/10.1002/1097-4679(198601)42:1<5::AID-JCLP2270420102>3.0.CO;2-9

Hickman, E. (2012). *Religious coping, stigma, and psychological functioning among African American HIV-positive women* [Doctoral dissertation]. Catholic University of America.

Holden, K. B., Belton, A. S., & Hall, S. P. (2015). Qualitative examination of African American women's perspectives about depression. *Health, Culture and Society, 8*(1), 48–60. https://doi.org/10.5195/HCS.2015.182

Holden, K. B., Bradford, L. D., Hall, S. P., & Belton, A. S. (2014). Prevalence and correlates of depressive symptoms and resiliency among African American women in a community-based primary health care center. *Journal of Health Care for the Poor and Underserved, 24*(4 suppl.), 79–93. https://doi.org/10.1353/hpu.2014.0012

Holden, K. B., Hall, S. P., Robinson, M., Triplett, S., Babalola, D., Plummer, V., Treadwell, H., & D. Bradford, L. (2012). Psychosocial and sociocultural correlates of depressive symptoms among diverse African American women. *Journal of the National Medical Association, 104*(11–12), 493–504. https://doi.org/10.1016/S0027-9684(15)30215-7

Holden, K., McGregor, B., Thandi, P., Fresh, E., Sheats, K., Belton, A., Mattox, G., & Satcher, D. (2014). Toward culturally centered integrative care for addressing mental health disparities among ethnic minorities. *Psychological Services, 11*(4), 357–368. https://doi.org/10.1037/a0038122

Holden, K., Ofili, E., Jones, C., & Satcher, D. (2019). Transdisciplinary collaborative health policy research: Leading the creation and advancement of health equity. *Ethnicity and Disease, 29*(suppl. 2). https://www.ethndis.org/edonline/index.php/ethndis/issue/view/38

Janoff-Bulman, R. (1992). *Shattered assumptions: Towards a new psychology of trauma*. Free Press.

Johnson, C. C., Sheffield, K. M., & Brown, R. E. (2018). Mind-body therapies for African-American women at risk for cardiometabolic disease: A systematic review. *Evidence-Based Complementary and Alternative Medicine, 2018*, Article 5123217-11. https://doi.org/10.1155/2018/5123217

Johnson, J. (2016). *Dear teen self: Tips to help a teenage girl navigate through adolescence*. Jaynay Chanel Johnson.

Kalibatseva, Z., & Leong, F. T. L. (2014). A critical review of culturally sensitive treatments for depression: Recommendations for intervention and research. *Psychological Services, 11*(4), 433–450. https://doi.org/10.1037/a0036047

Kennedy, B. R., & Jenkins, C. C. (2018). African American women and depression: Promoting the need for culturally competent treatment. *BRK Global Healthcare Journal, 2*(1), 1–25. https://doi.org/10.35455/brk123456

Kershaw, K. N., Lewis, T. T., Roux, A. V. D., Jenny, N. S., Liu, K., Penedo, F. J., & Carnethon, M. R. (2016). Self-reported experiences of discrimination and inflammation among men and women: The multi-ethnic study of atherosclerosis. *Health Psychology, 35*(4), 343–350. https://doi.org/10.1037/hea0000331

Lacey, K. K., Parnell, R., Mouzon, D. M., Matusko, N., Head, D., Abelson, J. M., & Jackson, J. S. (2015). The mental health of U.S. Black women: The roles of social context and severe intimate partner violence. *BMJ Open, 5*(10), e008415. https://doi.org/10.1136/bmjopen-2015-008415

Lake, J., & Turner, M. S. (2017). Urgent need for improved mental health care and a more collaborative model of care. *Permanente Journal, 21*(4). https://doi.org/10.7812/TPP/17-024

Lashley, M., Marshall, V., & McLaurin-Jones, T. (2017). Looking through the window: Black women's perspectives on mental health and self-care. In S. Y. Evans, K. Bell, & N. K. Burton (Eds.), *Black women's mental health: Balancing strength and vulnerability*. State University of New York Press.

Lewis, J. A., Williams, M. G., Peppers, E. J., & Gadson, C. A. (2017). Applying intersectionality to explore the relations between gendered racism and health among Black women. *Journal of Counseling Psychology*, 64(5), 475–486. https://doi.org/10.1037/cou0000231

Lewis, T. T., Lampert, R., Charles, D., & Katz, S. (2019). Expectations of racism and carotid intima-media thickness in African American women. *Psychosomatic Medicine*, 81(8), 759–768. https://doi.org/10.1097/PSY.0000000000000684

Liang, J., Matheson, B. E., & Douglas, J. M. (2016). Mental health diagnostic considerations in racial/ethnic minority youth. *Journal of Child and Family Studies*, 25(6), 1926–1940. https://doi.org/10.1007/s10826-015-0351-z

Lopez, C. R., Antoni, M. H., Fekete, E. M., & Penedo, F. J. (2012). Ethnic identity and perceived stress in HIV+ minority women: The role of coping self-efficacy and social support. *International Journal of Behavioral Medicine*, 19(1), 23–28. https://doi.org/10.1007/s12529-010-9121-x

McGregor, B., Li, C., Baltrus, P., Douglas, M., Hopkins, J., Wrenn, G., Holden, K., Respress, E., & Gaglioti, A. (2020). Racial and ethnic disparities in treatment and treatment type for depression in a national sample of medicaid recipients. *Psychiatric Services*, 71(7), 663–669. https://doi.org/10.1176/appi.ps.201900407

National Academies of Sciences, Engineering, and Medicine. (2017). *Communities in Action: Pathways to Health Equity*. National Academies Press. https://doi.org/10.17226/24624

National Alliance on Mental Illness. (2019). *Mental health by the numbers*. https://www.nami.org/mhstats

National Institute of Mental Health. (2011). *Depression in women: 5 things you should know*. https://www.nimh.nih.gov/health/publications/depression-in-women/index.shtml

National Institute of Mental Health. (2017). *Any anxiety disorder*. https://www.nimh.nih.gov/health/statistics/any-anxiety-disorder.shtml

National Institute of Mental Health. (2019a). *Major depression*. https://www.nimh.nih.gov/health/statistics/major-depression.shtml

National Institute of Mental Health. (2019b). *Post-traumatic stress disorder*. https://www.nimh.nih.gov/health/topics/post-traumatic-stress-disorder-ptsd/index.shtml

National Institute of Mental Health. (2021). *Mental illness*. https://www.nimh.nih.gov/health/statistics/mental-illness.shtml

Neal-Barnett, A. (2018, April 23). To be female, anxious and Black. https://adaa.org/learn-from-us/from-the-experts/blog-posts/consumer/be-female-anxious-and-black

Nelson, T., Ernst, S. C., Tirado, C., Fisse, J. L., & Moreno, O. (2022). Psychological distress and attitudes toward seeking professional psychological services among Black women: The role of past mental health treatment. *Journal of Racial and Ethnic Health Disparities*, *9*(2), 527–537. https://doi.org/10.1007/s40615-021-00983-z

Parks, J., Svendsen, D., Singer, P., Foti, M., & Mauer, B. (2006). *Morbidity and Mortality in People with Serious Mental Illness*. National Association of State Mental Health Program Directors, Medical Directors Council.

Silva de Crane, R., & Spielberger, C. (1981). Attitudes of Hispanic, Black, and Caucasian university students toward mental illness. *Hispanic Journal of Behavioral Sciences*, *3*(3), 241–255.

Spanierman, L. B., & Poteat, V. P. (2005). Moving beyond complacency to commitment: Multicultural research in counseling psychology. *Counseling Psychologist*, *33*(4), 513–523. https://doi.org/10.1177/0011000005276469

Sporinova, B., Manns, B., Tonelli, M., Hemmelgarn, B., MacMaster, F., Mitchell, N., Au, F., Ma, Z., Weaver, R., & Quinn, A. (2019). Association of mental health disorders with health care utilization and costs among adults with chronic disease. *JAMA Network Open*, *2*(8), e199910. https://doi.org/10.1001/jamanetworkopen.2019.9910

Staton-Tindall, M., Duvall, J., Stevens-Watkins, D., & Oser, C. B. (2013). The roles of spirituality in the relationship between traumatic life events, mental health, and drug use among African American women from one Southern state. *Substance Use and Misuse*, *48*(12), 1246–1257. https://doi.org/10.3109/10826084.2013.799023

Substance Abuse and Mental Health Services Administration. (2014). *Trauma-informed care in behavioral health services*.

Substance Abuse and Mental Health Services Administration. (2015). *Racial/ethnic differences in mental health service use among adults*. https://www.samhsa.gov/data/sites/default/files/MHServicesUseAmongAdults/MHServicesUseAmongAdults.pdf

US Department of Health and Human Services. (1999). *Mental health: A report of the Surgeon General*.

US Department of Health and Human Services. (2001). *Mental health: Culture, race, and ethnicity: A supplement to mental health: A report of the Surgeon General*. http://www.ncbi.nlm.nih.gov/books/NBK44243/

Villines, C., & Legg, T. (2020, July 20). What to know about anxiety in Black communities. *Medical News Today*. https://www.medicalnewstoday.com/articles/black-anxiety

Wagner, J., Lampert, R., Tennen, H., & Feinn, R. (2015). Exposure to discrimination and heart rate variability reactivity to acute stress among women with diabetes: Racial discrimination and heart rate variability. *Stress and Health*, *31*(3), 255–262. https://doi.org/10.1002/smi.2542

Waite, R., & Killian, P. (2008). Exploring depression among a cohort of African American women. *Journal of the American Psychiatric Nurses Association*, *13*(3), 161–169. https://doi.org/10.1177/1078390307304996

Ward, E. C., & Brown, R. L. (2015). A culturally adapted depression intervention for African American adults experiencing depression: Oh Happy Day. *American Journal of Orthopsychiatry*, *85*(1), 11–22. https://doi.org/10.1037/ort0000027

Ward, E. C., & Heidrich, S. M. (2009). African American women's beliefs about mental illness, stigma, and preferred coping behaviors. *Research in Nursing and Health*, *32*(5), 480–492. https://doi.org/10.1002/nur.20344

Ward, E. C., Wiltshire, J. C., Detry, M. A., & Brown, R. L. (2013). African American men and women's attitude toward mental illness, perceptions of stigma, and preferred coping behaviors. *Nursing Research*, *62*(3), 185–194. https://doi.org/10.1097/NNR.0b013e31827bf533

Watson, K. T., Roberts, N. M., & Saunders, M. R. (2012, January 3). Factors associated with anxiety and depression among African American and White women. *International Scholarly Research Notices*, *2012*, Article 432321. https://doi.org/https://doi.org/10.5402/2012/432321

Watson, N. N., & Hunter, C. D. (2015). Anxiety and depression among African American women: The costs of strength and negative attitudes toward psychological help-seeking. *Cultural Diversity and Ethnic Minority Psychology*, *21*(4), 604–612. https://doi.org/10.1037/cdp0000015

Woods-Giscombé, C. L., & Black, A. R. (2010). Mind-body interventions to reduce risk for health disparities related to stress and strength among African American women: The potential of mindfulness-based stress reduction, loving-kindness, and the NTU therapeutic framework. *Complementary Health Practice Review*, *15*(3), 115–131. https://doi.org/10.1177/1533210110386776

World Health Organization. (2020). *Depression*. https://www.who.int/westernpacific/health-topics/depression

Wrenn, G., Muzere, J., Hall, M., Belton, A., Holden, K., Hughes-Halbert, C., Kent, M., & Bradley, B. (2017). Understanding help seeking among Black women with clinically significant posttraumatic stress symptoms. *International Journal of Psychological and Behavioral Sciences*, *11*(2), 322–326. https://doi.org/10.5281/zenodo.1339838

Zapolski, T. C. B., Beutlich, M. R., Fisher, S., & Barnes-Najor, J. (2019). Collective ethnic–racial identity and health outcomes among African American youth: Examination of promotive and protective effects. *Cultural Diversity and Ethnic Minority Psychology*, *25*(3), 388–396. https://doi.org/10.1037/cdp0000258

Chapter 11

Reckoning with Resilience
Black Breastfeeding

Kimarie Bugg, Ifeyinwa V. Asiodu, and Andrea Serano

Significance

Breastfeeding rates, measured in the categories of *initiation, exclusivity,* and *duration,* are holistic statements about many maternal and child health (MCH) outcomes. These rates are correlated with how well the prenatal providers, hospitals, and communities care for women and their babies (Walsh, 2014; Burnham et al., 2022). Considering our knowledge of the social determinants of health, and suggested by Healthy People 2030, these rates are statements concerning racism, sexism, income differences, and social and cultural norms. Lastly, for the confidence of the mother in her transition to motherhood, we in the lactation support community have long observed a mother's success in reaching her initiation and duration goals as a significant (early) accomplishment of a difficult task; consequently, this may be the first great accomplishment a woman has made, and this is especially important for the psyche of (Walsh, 2014) Black mothers and birthing people.

Seventy-five percent of Black women in the United States initiate breastfeeding (Centers for Disease Control and Prevention, 2020). While breastfeeding initiation rates among Black women have increased, the initiation and duration rates gap has changed very little in the last 30 years.

Breastfeeding women and their infants have protection from a cadre of illnesses experienced by non-breastfeeders and infants who receive no human milk. The importance of breastfeeding and its significant impact on maternal health and infant/child well-being is well documented. Yet, breastfeeding rates of duration and exclusivity for Black mothers in the United States have remained lower than for all other ethnic groups, despite the scientific evidence of its importance to the mental, physical, and emotional well-being of the woman and the developmental, nutritional, and immune protection of infants and children.

When considering all the health disparities that human milk—as the most complete "first food"—has been proven to reduce, we propose that centering first food is essential to the future health of the Black community. The act of breastfeeding reduces a woman's stress by increasing oxytocin, which is calming and stress-reducing and supports good mental health. In addition, breastfeeding strengthens the bond between mother and child. The more bonded the mother and child are, the more the child becomes a source of support for the mother (Walsh 2014).

Breastfeeding protects women against cardiac disease, hypertension, diabetes, and cancer, while some leading causes of death among Black women in the United States are (1) heart disease, 23.1%, (2) cancer, 21.8%, and (3) diabetes, 4.5% (Aune et al., 2014; Bonifacino et al., 2018). Human milk protects the infant from respiratory infections, gastrointestinal illness, asthma, sudden infant death syndrome, and childhood obesity (Bartick et al., 2017: Pérez-Escamilla, 2020)—rampant issues in Black communities. Human milk is the best preventive medicine nature provides to reduce an infant's risk of adverse health issues. Black children who experience suboptimal breastfeeding are at a greater risk for childhood disease and death than children breastfed for nine months or more (Bartick et al., 2017; Beauregard et al., 2019). We must continue to galvanize lactation support and education for communities and service providers to assure that the Black community is not marginalized but brought into the "center" by access to culturally appropriate beginning, intermediate, and expert levels of service and care (Reaching Our Sisters Everywhere [ROSE], 2019).

Historical Perspective

The history of breastfeeding in Black communities has been complicated by the history of slavery, predatory marketing of formula, and inequitable access to human milk feeding and lactation resources (Asiodu et al., 2021; Green et al., 2021). Historically, the complex relationship between Black women and breastfeeding dates to the days of slavery. During slavery, forced reproduction and wet nursing were common practices (Dunaway, 2003; Sublette & Sublette, 2015). Enslaved African women experienced a lack of reproductive autonomy as continuous breeding practices were used to increase the enslaved population and available labor workforce (Sublette & Sublette, 2015). In addition, enslaved African women were also forced to breastfeed and care for enslavers' children while their own children were left alone or tended by another lactating woman (Dunaway, 2003).

The forced reproductive labor and limited birth spacing also impacted the practice of breastfeeding (Sublette & Sublette, 2015). Thus, reproductive coercion and lactation were a few of the means by which enslaved African women's bodies were commodified during slavery, leaving a lasting negative association with breastfeeding for some Black women today. Although times have changed, this is one of many ways the historical impact of slavery has left a permanent mark on Black women and their families (Hill Collins, 2008). Black women have been dealing with a lack of resources, inequality, and poor health outcomes since the late 1600s when slavery was initiated (Dunaway, 2003). Moreover, Black women and their infants as women of color continue to experience oppression due to the historical, gender, and racial milieus in this country (Hill Collins, 2008).

As previously mentioned, Black women have exceptionally intricate relationships to infant feeding, specifically breastfeeding. Enslaved African women were sexually, reproductively, and physically exploited by enslavers (Sublette & Sublette, 2015) and, generations later, their descendants are aggressively targeted by formula companies (Green et al., 2021). These experiences may directly or indirectly impact how older generations of Black women support breastfeeding, as negative stories and experiences related to breastfeeding may have been passed down over time. Moreover, the impact of forced reproductive breeding and wet nursing remains a legacy that has limited the experiences and positive associations with breastfeeding in Black communities, potentially increasing barriers to breastfeeding. However, over the last ten years, there has been a significant shift and reclaiming of breastfeeding in Black communities.

Throughout history, breastfeeding was considered the norm, regardless of socioeconomic status, location, or education, because families depended on human milk as nutrition for their infants (Stevens et al., 2009). This dependence on breastfeeding changed in the early 1900s with the advent of medical and pharmaceutical advances. Sensing a shift in public perception, formula companies capitalized on these advances and began to market artificial infant formula as a superior method of feeding newborns. Consequently, infant formula was seen as a high commodity and a status symbol for wealthy families or those with discretionary incomes (Stevens et al., 2009). Families with moderate to low incomes, notably families of color, were left to purchase evaporated milk-based products or breastfeed, thereby further perpetuating the negative stigma of breastfeeding developed during slavery (Barness, 1987).

In the 1950's there was an increased push from the makers of infant formula to market their products as similar to if not better than breastfeeding and evaporated milk products (Stevens et al., 2009). After successfully capturing upper- to middle-class mothers, infant formula companies quickly turned their attention to moderate- to low-income women (Stevens et al., 2009; Barness, 1987). Formula companies began giving free samples of their products to hospitals (to distribute to new mothers upon discharge) and partnered with the Special Supplemental Nutrition Program for Women, Infants, and Children (WIC), a government nutrition program, primarily used by low-income women and families of color. Decades ago, women had very few choices or limited resources for infant feeding methods; their options included breastfeeding, evaporated milk products, or organic means (Stevens et al., 2009). Now there are several different brands and consistencies to choose from, and if they qualify, women can receive free infant formula vouchers from the WIC program. With the increased accessibility of infant formula, lack of breastfeeding normalization, and limited lactation resources and equitable access to lactation support persons, many mothers have forgone exclusive breastfeeding for supplementation with formula.

It is important to note that presently Black women and families are still burdened with the highest breastfeeding inequities and disparities in the United States.[1] Racism, bias, lack of equitable access and resources, and exposure to systemic and structural barriers have been driving these inequities and disparities for decades (Asiodu et al., 2021). These challenges are not only relegated to breastfeeding when compared to other populations; we see similar if not worse inequities and disparities related to maternal mortality and morbidity, preterm birth, access to respectful maternity care practices, reproductive health services such as contraception and abortion care, and preventative services such as pap smears and mammograms

(Julian et al., 2020). These issues are all connected, and highlight the importance and need to contextualize health disparities data through the lens of those affected and impacted by Black women who want to breastfeed. As described later in this chapter, community-led efforts have led to great strides related to breastfeeding in Black communities. These endeavors have led to significant increases in breastfeeding initiation, duration, and exclusivity (Centers for Disease Control and Prevention, 2020, 2010, 2017). In the last 10 years, the number of Black infants receiving human milk has grown, as has the opportunity for Black women to experience the short-term and long-term benefits of breastfeeding.

As we look to the future, we cannot forget our past. We have endured the inhuman treatment of enslaved Africans, oppressive and anti-Black racism associated with Jim Crow laws, redlining, civil rights movement, war on drugs, mass incarceration, gentrification, and yet we still rise (Dunaway, 2003; Sublette & Sublette, 2015; Wildeman & Wang, 2017; Smith et al., 2020). More and more Black women are standing up to say we deserve maternity care practices that support breastfeeding in our communities. We need to see lactation support providers that look like us and have similar lived experiences. We want to see community-engaged research and diverse research teams. We demand a health-care workforce that understands the impact of social and structural determinants of health on our abilities to breastfeed and be healthy. To achieve breastfeeding equity in this country, we must continue building off of the momentum of the past decade and speak truth to power. It is time that we truly invest in our communities. It is time that we trust and listen to Black women. It is time that we dismantle the systems of inequities that perpetuate existing breastfeeding disparities. The time is now.

African American Breastfeeding Blueprint

Reaching Our Sisters Everywhere (ROSE) was cofounded in July 2011 by a women's health nurse practitioner, a pediatric nurse, and an expert community partner. The vision for ROSE began at a spaghetti dinner at the home of a founder, an opportunity that was held to build a local network focused on addressing breastfeeding disparities for Black families. The cofounders mentored many young women and provided them with breastfeeding support. Other advocates at the dinner shared similar experiences of feeling siloed and challenged by the systemic inequities in health care and social support systems that impact Black women and their ability to meet their breastfeeding goals.

ROSE was created to address both the systemic inequities that prevented the diversification of lactation support providers and the problems that contributed to the lack of quality, accessible, and culturally centered lactation care. ROSE's inaugural 2012 Breastfeeding Summit: Reclaiming an African American Tradition, held at Morehouse School of Medicine, launched their work in both areas. The event featured a keynote presentation by the 16th surgeon general of the United States and former director of the Satcher Health Leadership Institute, Dr. David Satcher. Presentations centered on the 2011 Surgeon General's Call to Action to Support Breastfeeding, which highlighted mothers and their families, communities, health care, employment, research and surveillance, and public health infrastructure (Centers for Disease Control and Prevention, 2011). In addition, attendees learned about exemplary breastfeeding projects, fatherhood initiatives, the Baby-Friendly Hospital Initiative, anthropological perspectives on Black breastfeeding, the continuum of care from hospital to neighborhood, and reducing disparities. An invitation-only second-day catered to deeper conversations on action planning and discipline-specific topics were covered.

The action agenda developed from ROSE's first summit created the framework for how the organization would move forward and structure its mission. The cornerstone of ROSE's organizational strategy consisted of community-centered needs assessments and programs informed by the communities most impacted by systemic racism in maternal and infant health care. This perspective is clear in ROSE's initial mission "to enhance the overall mental and physical health of African American women, babies, and their families by working collaboratively to encourage, promote, support, and protect breastfeeding throughout the United States by training health-care providers on culturally sensitive techniques."

ROSE has now held ten national Breastfeeding and Equity Summits and several regional forums with participants including parents, community health workers, medical providers, researchers, and government staff. Presenters and participants have shared valuable perspectives and contributed to improving health inequities.

ROSE expanded its staff in 2013 after being awarded a W. K. Kellogg Foundation grant to support the creation of ROSE Community Transformers, a program designed to increase access to evidence-based breastfeeding resources within communities. This program centers the lived experience of women and their breastfeeding journey while equipping them with the tools for supporting other women to meet their breastfeeding goals. The program was modeled from the Women, Infant, and Children (WIC) Breastfeeding Peer Counselor model. ROSE felt it essential to create a program that expanded across socioeconomic statuses, as data related to breastfeeding rates demonstrated racial inequities even among women with high socioeconomic status. ROSE offered its first Community Transformer Training in December of 2013, training 13 Black women in Georgia. Through collaborative relationships, such as partnerships with Boston Medical Center's Communities and Hospitals Advancing Maternal Practices (CHAMPS), state breastfeeding coalitions, county health departments, and community-based organizations, ROSE has gone on to conduct Community Transformer Training in nine states plus virtual sessions during the pandemic, training 563 women as community-based breastfeeding peer counselors.

In 2014, significant discussions were had on the lack of diversity among certified lactation support providers. These complex but necessary discussions were had in spaces like United States Breastfeeding Committee annual conferences, ROSE Breastfeeding and Equity Summits, and similar spaces where members of the field would gather. A part of this discussion centered on how the formal field of lactation was created and where fissures of inequities grew within this work. In response, ROSE collaborated with Bright Future Lactation Resource Centre to host a Master Train the Trainer Initiative. This initiative aimed to train International Board-Certified Lactation Consultants (IBCLCs) of color to facilitate lactation management training for those seeking lactation-specific education credits. ROSE engaged 14 IBCLCs of color that identified as Black, Indigenous, and Latinx from around the country. Several of the master trainers, including ROSE staff, have focused their training on women from historically marginalized communities, including one training by the DC Breastfeeding Coalition conducted in American Sign Language. The number of individuals that have benefited from these master trainers has far surpassed the initial goal of 150.

> In 2018 Reaching Our Sisters Everywhere, Incorporated (ROSE) expanded its mission to include building equity in maternal and child health through culturally competent training, education, advocacy, and support. ROSE is committed to working in 5 areas, including: empowering a growing cadre of advocacy-oriented "Community Transformers"; pursuing and maintaining a seat at the table of leaders who are developing policies for health care

services that support breastfeeding activities through private and public health sectors; providing education and training for agencies to enhance Steps 3 and 10 of the Baby-Friendly Hospital Initiative; establishing and implementing national and regional initiatives that will enhance and strengthen family and community breastfeeding programs; and training health care providers to manage lactation. ROSE also builds mutually beneficial relationships with national policy-making organizations.

Reaching Our Brothers Everywhere (ROBE) became one of ROSE's first expanded programs, centering efforts to educate, equip, and empower men to reduce infant mortality by increasing knowledge on safe sleep practices and supporting breastfeeding. ROBE recognizes that fathers, grandfathers, brothers, sons, cousins, and uncles all contribute to the cause of protecting breastfeeding. ROBE began with town halls and engaging with men directly to learn of their experiences in the upbringing of children. Much of those candid conversations lent themselves to the development of ROBE toolkits and initiatives such as Hoop Therapy.

In 2018, ROSE set out to create the African American Breastfeeding Blueprint, a national report addressing African American breastfeeding determinants and an action plan to achieve health equity. One of the most jarring statistics that came from the Pregnancy Risk Assessment Monitoring System (PRAMS) data review was that breastfeeding rates amongst African American/Black women decreased by 21% each week after birth for the first 4 weeks (ROSE, 2019). In addition, there was a significant difference in the degree of breastfeeding inequity by geography, with the Southern States region having the most significant disparity gap between African American/Black women and all women in terms of breastfeeding initiation rates. The importance of representation of providers is a vital element that contributes to respectful care. This blueprint has guided us to continued growth through building significant partnerships with agencies, organizations, and individuals.

From Representation to Power

To create a culture of sustainability, strong partnerships must be developed and nurtured. We must gleefully curate and mentor up-and-coming lactation support providers at every level and work diligently to motivate allies to aid us in dismantling racism, decolonizing research, and disseminating best practices and policy impacts based on findings from deep community engagement and leadership (filtered through the rigidity of research-based academic requirements).

When ROSE began in 2011, the lactation support field was pregnant with possibility, expectancy, and need for a national networking presence in the Black community. The conception of the ROSE partnership came from the San Diego lactation program. In 1989, a ROSE cofounder was part of a team chosen as one of the 10 teams picked from each public health region to be funded and trained in San Diego by the leading national experts on lactation management. Each team consisted of a pediatric physician, an obstetrician, a nurse, and a dietician. The team had to be associated with an academic center and hospital. Our team consisted of two Black physicians, one from Morehouse School of Medicine, the other from Emory School of Medicine, a Black nurse from Grady Memorial Hospital, and a White dietician. We were the *only* team with Black participants. We were asked to participate and assemble and send a second team.

To address the persistent disparity in breastfeeding rates, an integrative approach (considering social, behavioral, and psychological factors) is needed to address cultural breastfeeding barriers identified by formative research. We have worked with a three-pronged method that includes (1) a grassroots community-based approach to share and disseminate information and resources; (2) Baby-Friendly Hospital Initiative (BFUSA) to impact policy of birthing centers and to train health care professionals; and (3) impacting the skills, knowledge, and attitudes of public health providers, academia, and leadership through interdisciplinary professional education (IPE) (CHAMPS) (Burnham et al., 2022; Gambari et al., 2022).

Partnerships

We have had working relationships with the National Medical Association, American Academy of Pediatrics, Satcher Community Health Leadership Institute, Academy of Breastfeeding Medicine, United States Breastfeeding Committee, Concerned Black Clergy (CBC), Office on Women's Health (OWH), Centers for Disease Control and Prevention (Division of Nutrition, Physical Activity, and Obesity), Baby-Friendly USA, National Institute for Children's Health Quality (NICHQ), Communities and Hospitals Advancing Maternal Practices (CHAMPS), and others. In addition, we have worked in partnership with numerous cultural coalitions and long-standing community-based organizations, Black Greek organizations, Black barbershops, fatherhood organizations, federal, state, and local MCH government agencies, and the Black faith community to disseminate education and information on lactation management.

Mentorship

Mentoring and training is the only way to promote and protect sustainability. We have mentored ROSE Community Transformers, peer counselors, community health workers, public health practitioners, allied health-care providers, dieticians, nurses, physicians, students, and *everybody else* to sustain momentum and increase breastfeeding duration and exclusivity. Our ROSE board of directors led us in developing a breastfeeding medicine rotation for residents, which we intend to expand. We mentored several pediatric residents to attain the International Board-Certified Lactation Consultant (IBCLC) designation. We are in the process of setting up a community lactation certificate program with a local historically Black college and university (HBCU). This must be done with a willing spirit and the mentality that we, as mentors, will also learn valuable lessons from our mentees.

Allies

From our inception, we have stated that we desire that *all* babies receive human milk. We do not apologize for our focus on Black families. We have had allies from every ethnicity alongside us every step of the way. The fantastic Dr. Audrey Naylor, the founder of WellStart, the San Diego lactation program, was a key advisor and component of the beginning and shaping of ROSE. Allies call out racism, help us show up to spaces we did not know existed, learn from us about their microaggressions and actively work to change them, help us find funds and fund projects and programs, make room at tables that have traditionally not embraced Black women and our families, and so much more. We recognize allies several times a year, especially at our annual summit with a William Lloyd Garrison Ally Award.

Decolonizing Breastfeeding

Decolonization calls for the decentering of colonial ideologies and Western or European ways of being that are incorporated into all aspects of life, as these thoughts and practices are rooted in White supremacy and racism (Asiodu et al., 2021). The current health-care workforce does not represent the communities most impacted by health inequities and disparities (Hardeman & Kozhimannil, 2016). Unfortunately, this is by design. Historically, Black communities were excluded from attending White institutions of higher education or engaging in the professionalization of health-care providers (e.g., physicians, nurses, midwives, International Board Certified Lactation Consultants) (Gasman et al., 2017; Miles & Drew, 2020). The lack of diversification of the health-care workforce perpetuates harm, bias, and disparate care (Greenwood et al., 2020). Historically Black colleges and universities and apprentice training methods have provided the greatest opportunities to diversify the health-care workforce (Gasman et al., 2017). Utilizing a decolonizing framework calls for more significant investment in HBCUs and community-led efforts to diversify the health-care workforce, specifically, lactation support providers.

Currently, the majority of both lactation support providers holding the International Board-Certified Lactation Consultant designation and of lactation researchers self-identify as White. Representation matters. Decolonizing the current lactation workforce will help efforts to normalize breastfeeding in Black communities and increase breastfeeding initiation, duration, and exclusivity rates. In addition, decolonizing breastfeeding demands that we reimagine the current ways in which research is conducted. More Black, Indigenous, and people of color (BIPOC) led research teams are needed. Black women need greater access to lactation support providers and maternity care practices supporting breastfeeding. The Black Mamas Matter Alliance, Center for Social Inclusion, Reaching Our Sisters Everywhere, and others have called for new approaches and innovative practices to providing perinatal care and reproductive health-care services (ROSE, 2019; Black Mamas Matter Alliance Research Working Group, 2020; Center for Social Inclusion, 2015). It is time to take heed and listen.

Recommendations and Call for Action

The elements of the African American Breastfeeding Blueprint have significantly impacted ROSE's work in how the organization designs and improves programming. We believe in community leadership and not just community engagement. There is not enough culturally appropriate lactation support and information available in the Black community. Pregnant and parenting Black women need access to evidence-based, culturally relevant, and convenient breastfeeding information, education, and support. This information needs to be available at a convenient facility in the neighborhood, in the woman's home, by face time or internet connection, or by telephone or text. Their support people, partners, grandparents, and friends also need accurate, culturally appropriate breastfeeding information to help protect their decision and encourage them to extend breastfeeding.

References

Asiodu, I. V., Bugg, K., & Palmquist, A. E. L. (2021). Achieving breastfeeding equity and justice in Black communities: Past, present, and future. *Breastfeeding Medicine*, *16*(6), 447–451. https://doi.org/10.1089/bfm.2020.0314

Aune, D., Norat, T., Romundstad, P., & Vatten, L. J. (2014). Breastfeeding and the maternal risk of type 2 diabetes: A systematic review and dose-response meta-analysis of cohort studies. *Nutrition, Metabolism and Cardiovascular Diseases*, *24*(2), 107–115. https://doi.org/10.1016/j.numecd.2013.10.028

Barness, L. A. History of infant feeding practices. *American Journal of Clinical Nutrition*, *46*(1), 168–170. https://doi.org/10.1093/ajcn/46.1.168

Bartick, M. C., Jegier, B. J., Green, B. D., Schwarz, E. B., Reinhold, A. G., & Stuebe, A. M. (2017). Disparities in breastfeeding: Impact on maternal and child health outcomes and costs. *Journal of Pediatrics*, *181*, 49–55. https://doi.org/10.1016/j.jpeds.2016.10.028

Bartick, M. C., Schwarz, E. B., Green, B. D., Jegier, B. J., Reinhold, A. G., Colaizy, T. T., Bogen, D. L., Schaefer, A. J., & Stuebe, A. M. (2017). Suboptimal breastfeeding in the United States: Maternal and pediatric health outcomes and costs. *Maternal and Child Ntrition*, *13*(1), Article e12366. https://doi.org/10.1111/mcn.12366

Beauregard, J. L., Hamner, H. C., Chen, J., Avila-Rodriguez, W., Elam-Evans, L. D., & Perrine, C. G. (2019). Racial disparities in breastfeeding initiation and duration among US infants born in 2015. *Morbidity and Mortality Weekly Report*, *68*(34), 745–748. https://doi.org/10.15585%2Fmmwr.mm6834a3

Black Mamas Matter Alliance Research Working Group. (2020). Black maternal health research re-envisioned: Best practices for the conduct of research with, for, and by Black Mamas. *Harvard Law and Policy Review*, *14*, 393–415.

Bonifacino, E., Schwartz, E. B., Jun, H., Wessel, C. B., & Corbelli, J. A. (2018). Effect of lactation on maternal hypertension: A systematic review. *Breastfeeding Medicine*, *13*(9), 578–588. https://doi.org/10.1089/bfm.2018.0108

Burnham, L., Knapp, R., Bugg, K., Nickel, N., Beliveau, P., Feldman-Winter, L., & Merewood, A. (2022). Mississippi CHAMPS: Decreasing Racial Inequities in Breastfeeding. *Pediatrics, 149*(2), Article e2020030502. https://doi.org/10.1542/peds.2020-030502

Center for Social Inclusion. (2015). Removing Barriers to Breastfeeding: A Structural Race Analysis of First Food. https://www.raceforward.org/system/files/pdf/reports/2015/CSI-Removing-Barriers-to-Breastfeeding-REPORT.pdf

Centers for Disease Control and Prevention. (2010). *Breastfeeding report card—United States, 2010.* https://www.cdc.gov/breastfeeding/pdf/breastfeedingreportcard2010.pdf

Centers for Disease Control and Prevention. (2011). *The Surgeon General's call to action to support breastfeeding.* https://www.cdc.gov/breastfeeding/resources/calltoaction.htm

Centers for Disease Control and Prevention. *Breastfeeding among U.S. children born 2010-2017, CDC National Immunization Survey.* https://www.cdc.gov/breastfeeding/data/nis_data/results.html

Centers for Disease Control and Prevention. (2020). *Breastfeeding report card United States, 2020.* https://www.cdc.gov/breastfeeding/pdf/2020-Breastfeeding-Report-Card-H.pdf

Dunaway, W. A. (2003). *The African-American family in slavery and emancipation.* Cambridge University Press.

Gambari, A., Burnham, L., Berger, J., Annapragada, B., Bugg, K., Serano, A., & Merewood, A. (2022). A qualitative assessment of mothers' perspectives on hospital and community breastfeeding support in Mississippi. *Journal of Neonatal Nursing.* Advance online publication. https://doi.org/10.1016/j.jnn.2022.02.004

Gasman, M., Smith, T., Ye, C., & Nguyen, T. H. (2017). HBCUs and the Production of Doctors. *AIMS Public Health, 4*(6), 579–589.

Green, V. L., Killings, N. L., Clare, C. A. (2021). The historical, psychosocial, and cultural context of breastfeeding in the African American community. *Breastfeeding Medicine, 16*(2), 116–120. https://doi.org/10.1089/bfm.2020.0316

Greenwood, B. N., Hardeman, R. R., Huang, L, & Sojourner, A. Physician-patient racial concordance and disparities in birthing mortality for newborns. *Proceedings of the National Academy of Sciences, 117*(35), 21194–21200. https://doi.org/10.1073/pnas.1913405117

Hardeman, R. R., & Kozhimannil, K. B. (2016). Motivations for entering the doula profession: perspectives from women of color. *Journal of Midwifery and Women's Health, 61*(6), 773–780.

Healthy People 2030. US Department of Health and Human Services. Office of Disease Prevention and Health Promotion. https://health.gov/healthypeople/search?query=breastfeeding

Hill Collins, P. (2008). *Black feminist thought: Knowledge, consciousness, and the politics of empowerment.* Routledge.

Julian, Z., Robles, D., Whetstone, S., Perritt, J. B., Jackson, A. V., Hardeman, R. R., Scott, K. A. (2020). Community-informed models of perinatal and reproductive health services provision: A justice-centered paradigm toward equity among Black birthing communities. *Seminars in Perinatology, 44*(5), Article 151267. https://doi.org/10.1016/j.semperi.2020.151267

Miles, P. N., & Drew, M. (2020, October 22). Constructing the modern American midwife: White supremacy and White feminism collide. *Nursing Clio.* https://nursingclio.org/2020/10/22/constructing-the-modern-american-midwife-white-supremacy-and-white-feminism-collide/

Pérez-Escamilla, R. (2020). Breastfeeding in the 21st century: How we can make it work. *Social Science and Medicine, 244*, Article 112331. https://doi.org/10.1016/j.socscimed.2019.05.036

Reaching Our Sisters Everywhere. (2019). *Saving tomorrow today: An African American breastfeeding blueprint.* www.breastfeedingrose.org/aablueprint/

Smith, G. S., Breakstone, H., Dean, L. T., Thorpe, R. J., Jr. (2020). Impacts of gentrification on health in the US: A systematic review of the literature. *Journal of Urban Health, 97*(6), 845–856. https://doi.org/10.1007/s11524-020-00448-4

Stevens, E. E., Patrick, T. E., & Pickler, R. (2009). A history of infant feeding. Journal of Perinatal Education, *18*(2), 32–39.

Sublette, N., & Sublette, C. (2015). The American Slave Coast: A history of the slave-breeding industry. Chicago Review Press.

Walsh, E. (2014, July 29). The collective impact approach to breastfeeding support. *Breastfeeding Medicine.* https://doi.org/10.1089/bfm.2014.0091

Wildeman, C., & Wang, E. A. (2017). Mass incarceration, public health, and widening inequality in the USA. Lancet, *389*(10077), 1464–1474. https://doi.org/10.1016/S0140-6736(17)30259-3

Chapter 12

The Color Line of Infertility

Reproductive Disparities in Black Women

Yoann Sophie Antoine, Blessing Chidiuto Lawrence, Shubhecchha Dhaurali, Beverly Udegbe, Lauren Cohen, Paige E. Feyock, Mildred Watson-Baylor, and Ndidiamaka Amutah-Onukaga

Selected theoretical frameworks of intersectionality state that there are multiple axes of power and social divisions that appear to be mutually exclusive but are deeply interconnected with one another (Bowleg, 2012). For example, class, gender, and race are three critical axes of social division, but they are not the only ones. Nationality, sexuality, age, ability, and citizenship are perhaps even more salient axes of power in a given situation. This chapter utilizes intersectionality to analyze the experiences of Black women navigating infertility. These interlocking forms of domination all have critical implications on health and wellness outcomes (Caldwell, 2017). While several White women during the women's rights movement and Black men during the civil rights movement may have experienced gender and racial inequality as separate issues, Patricia Hill Collins, a leading intersectionality and critical social theory scholar, refuses to place one struggle over the other (Harnois, 2010). Hill Collins asserts that the "lived conditions" of Black women generate an intersectional understanding of oppression (Harnois, 2010).

It is evident that systemic racism continues to persist in American society, and it has adverse health consequences for those who experience it. In fact, microaggressions have been broken down into three forms of behavior: microassault, or explicit discrimination meant to hurt the victim; microinsult, or insensitive communication; and microinvalidation, or unconscious exclusionary practices that overlook an individual's feelings (Bleich, 2015; Miller & Peck, 2019). In a recent study, over 50% of Black Americans reported experiencing microaggressions and discrimination (Bleich et al., 2019). Moreover, Black Americans who have chronic stress stemming from institutional and interpersonal racial discrimination are at a higher risk for mortality, hypertension, anxiety, depression, and diet-related diseases (Bleich et al., 2019; Ibrahim & Zore, 2020). Discrimination in healthcare led to worse prenatal outcomes for Black women compared with White women (Slaughter-Acey et al., 2019).

Black women have experienced discrimination and racism in the form of reproductive health disparities and medical mistreatment for centuries (Prather et al., 2018). The only "health care" that enslaved women received between 1619 and 1865 was experimentation without anesthesia. From Jim Crow through the civil rights era, medical students performed unnecessary hysterectomies on Black women for practice (Prather et al., 2018). Many forms of birth control were first tested in Black communities, and the high levels of hormones increased risk of hypertension and stroke (Prather et al., 2018; Feagin & Bennefield, 2014). Such examples demonstrate that Black women are treated merely as bodies to be used in the hopes of advancing medicine without careful thought to how they are adversely impacted. Another related and well-known example of mistreatment involves Henrietta Lacks, an African American woman who unknowingly donated cells that were used in medical research that yielded remarkable and groundbreaking findings.

Unfair treatment of Blacks in healthcare may be due, in part, to lack of representation. In 2018, only 5% of physicians in the country were Black, while 75% were White (Ibrahim & Zore, 2020; Feagan & Benenfield, 2014). Therefore, provider-patient relationships may often be at risk for being racialized; and additionally, many Black Americans likely receive health information from White doctors (Feagin & Bennefield, 2014). Patients of color are less likely than their White counterparts to receive quality care and communication from their medical providers (Miller & Peck, 2019). An implicit association test revealed that 70% of physicians unconsciously preferred Whites to Blacks. White doctors and nurses believed that Black patients did not experience racism in medicine, instead blaming the patients for being passive, not following medical advice, or having less intelligence than White patients. On the other hand, Black physicians are more likely to perceive race as important in medical treatment (Feagin & Bennefield, 2014). Black women still bear the brunt of the gross injustices, inequities, and biases of the American healthcare system.

Socioeconomic status (SES) is a major determinant of health outcomes (Phelan & Link, 2015). Respondents to the University of Michigan Health and Retirement Survey who self-reported excellent health had 2.5 times as much household income and 5 times as much household wealth as respondents with poor health (Smith, 1998). Recent data on median household income indicates that Black individuals earn 59 cents for every dollar earned by White individuals (Williams et al., 2019). While it is clear that race and SES are interrelated, it is important to note that race is still a key factor in health outcomes that should be acknowledged. Since the civil rights movement, Black individuals have experienced a significant amount of socioeconomic mobility, although an increase in wealth does not necessarily ameliorate racial disparities in health care (Hill, 2016). Given the intersection of disadvantaged and privileged statuses, wealthy Black individuals still suffer from the consequences of a racialized social system (Lewis & Van Dyke, 2018).

The Strong, Fertile Black Woman

Though slavery ended in 1865, institutionalized racism continues to contribute to the marginalization of Black women. Racism is a core determinant of health inequities among people of color and its effects are specifically seen among Black women, who disproportionately experience higher rates of maternal mortality, infant mortality, sexually transmitted infections, and HIV (Prather et al., 2018). Common and well-rooted practices of sexual violence, medical exploitation, and health-care marginalization reinforced the intergenerational transmission of adverse sexual and reproductive health outcomes among Black women (Prather et al., 2018). The literature shows that stereotypes toward Black women are in part due to their intersecting race and gender identities that disproportionately contribute to high rates of adverse sexual and reproductive health outcomes in the United States (Rosenthal & Lobel, 2016). Compared to their White counterparts, Black women are stereotyped as stronger and more domineering, which is consistent with the Sapphire archetype where they are portrayed as "Angry Black Women" (Rosenthal & Lobel, 2016). Black women are also stereotyped as individuals who are poor and uneducated, and who purposefully have children to take advantage of the public welfare system (Windsor et al., 2011). Such stereotypes are consistent with the Welfare Queen archetype based on racist assumptions that Black women are lazy and are constantly taking advantage of the welfare system (Windsor et al., 2011). The Superwoman notion bolsters Black women's efforts to transform the stereotypes attributed to them by highlighting their resilient nature despite oppression and adversity (Woods-Giscombé, 2010). For Black women, the Superwoman notion is a method of survival as they are repeatedly faced with limited health-care resources, systemic racism, and gender-based discrimination.

Racial and ethnic minorities are more likely to experience infertility in the United States, though there is limited research on these populations (Ceballo et al., 2015). Stereotypes such as the motherhood mandate, which suggests that all women should be mothers, and the Black fertility mandate, which assumes that all Black women are fertile, have prompted Black women dealing with infertility to be silent about the issue and eventually isolate themselves from family and friends (Ceballo et al., 2015). As some celebrities such as former First Lady Michelle Obama and Chrissy Teigen have been transparent about their infertility experiences, Black women's struggle with infertility is gradually coming to light. Nonetheless, due to limited research and resources available, the average Black woman's infertility woes and experiences with infertility treatments are different from that of celebrities (Ceballo et al., 2015). In addition, Black women are faced with physicians' assumptions about their inability to pay for services or support a child (Ceballo et al., 2015). Even so, Black women have substantially proven to be resilient in spite of repeated adversities. However, the stereotypes and discrimination toward Black women must be addressed, as they are not only wrong and harmful, but they also hinder Black women's access to equitable sexual and reproductive care.

Infertility Does Not Discriminate

Infertility, the inability to conceive within one year of unprotected sex, impacts 80 million individuals of reproductive age worldwide (Luke, 2017). Infertility remains a public health issue in the United States, as 12% of reproductive women, regardless of marital status, experience infertility (Wiltshire et al., 2019). Despite the classification of infertility as a disease stemming from the reproductive system, less than 50% of infertile women receive medical services for this illness (Chin et al., 2015; Greil et al., 2016). Infertility can be classified as either primary infertility, referring to women who have never been pregnant, or secondary infertility, the inability to conceive even after conceiving one or more children (Greil et al., 2016). Causes of infertility range from a number of comorbidities to gynecological risk factors, mainly uterine fibroids and polycystic ovarian syndrome, resulting in additional physiological and psychological impacts (Wellons et al., 2008). Despite the numerous symptoms and factors that contribute to infertility, there are successful treatment options that range from medical procedures like assisted reproductive technologies to counseling and education. Infertility exists as a medicalized phenomenon where access to treatment is at the core of understanding the illness.

Assisted reproductive technologies (ART) provide infertile women alternative options to biologically conceive; the most effective and commonly used ART is in vitro fertilization (IVF) (Resilient Sisterhood Project, n.d.). However, not all technologies assist equitably. Black women who use ART have lower live-birth rates and higher rates of spontaneous abortion, and are underrepresented in ART utilization (Seifer et al., 2008). The process of IVF is emotionally and physically draining as well as costly and complex. Disparities in coverage, education, and income contribute to racial and ethnic risk factors in IVF failure (Humphries et al., 2016). In fact, those most successful with IVF are White, highly educated women with middle to high income. Indeed, systemic racism, not race itself, drives disparities in health outcomes. IVF implantation and clinical pregnancy rates for Black women are about three times lower than for White women. Black women often require more aggressive ovarian stimulation, present a longer period of infertility, have higher tubal disease incidence, higher BMI, and have 2.6-fold decreased odds of becoming pregnant than White women (Wiltshire et al., 2019; Humphries et al., 2016; Seifer et al., 2008).

Uterine fibroids disproportionately contribute to infertility issues among Black women. Fibroids are benign tumors found in the lining of the uterus in 70%–80% of American women (Noel et al., 2019). Approximately 2%–10% of all infertility cases are due to uterine fibroids being the primary reason for reproductive complications (Dillard, 2016; Laughlin-Tommaso et al., 2016). Over the years, uterine fibroid growth has declined in White women, while it presents an increasing burden of disease for Black women. Black women develop fibroids earlier, have larger and often multiple fibroids, and suffer more severe symptoms (Noel et al., 2019; Dillard, 2016). Little has been done to understand the vast disparity of fibroid incidence in Black women, especially considering Black women only comprise 15% of women in fibroid-specific studies (Laughlin-Tommaso et al., 2016).

Polycystic ovarian syndrome (PCOS) disrupts ovulation, causing a number of consequences for hormonal and metabolic systems due to the abnormal number of cysts and sacs that form in the ovaries. Due to disruptions in the menstrual cycle and resulting reproductive health problems, PCOS is the leading cause of infertility in women and there is no current cure (Ogunbiyi, 2019). PCOS affects all races and ethnicities of women, but Black women shoulder the burden of this disease. Black women with PCOS have increased rates of hirsutism (higher testosterone produced in females causing rapid hair growth), risk of cardiovascular disease and metabolic syndromes, and higher infertility (Black Women's Health Imperative, 2017). Early intervention strategies and advocacy of ART therapies are critical for PCOS high-risk populations experiencing infertility.

The use of ART has risen in the past two decades; examining its shortcomings and working to make this technology more equitable is crucial for the future of reproductive health (Luke, 2017). Certain organizations, many championed by women with similar experiences, work to make fertility accessible and affordable for Black and Brown women; these organizations, by providing emotional, mental, and community support, promote resiliency for Black and Brown women.

ART is riddled with highs and lows for the women struggling to conceive, which can take a physiological and psychological toll. This becomes even more apparent when discussing Black women's challenges conceiving, given that Black women undergoing IVF tend to have lower success rates than White women (McQueen et al., 2015). Therefore, it is imperative to understand that resiliency may play a major role in how Black women living with infertility and mental health challenges experience the reproductive health-care system. These varied encounters may lead to mental health concerns that may arise due to engagement in treatment, physical demands, lack of resources, and inadequate support. Closer attention needs to be paid to the psychological stress endured by Black women undergoing IVF and infertility issues. Although the IVF success rate is low, some Black women continue to seek treatment, which speaks to the importance of resiliency factors. The willingness to forge

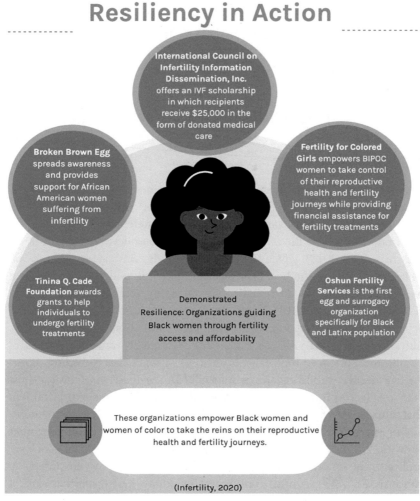

Figure 12.1. Resiliency in action.

ahead after a failed IVF cycle or eventually deciding to make a difficult choice regarding a change to their reproductive story showcases women's strengths (Jaffe & Diamond, 2010).

Reproductive specialists and therapists should avoid minimizing Black women's experiences, as they may feel a sense of inadequacy. Normalizing Black women's experiences may decrease the sense of isolation and shame (Ceballo et al., 2015). Other relevant salient factors include sense of self, and positive social and familial support when working with Black infertility clients (Ceballo et al., 2015). Drawing from infertility stress and coping theory, it is essential to recognize that infertility can be both uncontrollable and controllable (Stanton, 1991). This approach could help Black women with infertility issues foster effective coping skills and garner support.

Yes, Black Women Are Resilient. Now What?

Need for Research

A quick search of notable medical search engines reveals the persistent scarcity of research on infertility among Black women. Moreover, researchers have often neglected to examine demographic differences across infertility experiences as well as Black women's knowledge on infertility (Riegle, 2015; Wiltshire et al., 2019). Given the existence of a discriminatory pathway via which race impacts the health of Black people, it is evident that there is a need for additional studies on Black women's experiences with infertility (Lewis & Van Dyke, 2018). These studies need to take on a multifactorial approach in examining and addressing Black women's struggles with infertility. As Black women are at a higher risk for sexually transmitted diseases and have experienced high rates of medical misdiagnosis regarding reproductive health, studies regarding infertility in the Black community must take such factors into account (Prather et al., 2018). Likewise, it is imminent that future research acknowledges how the intersection of multiple identities at the micro level predisposes Black women to adverse health outcomes (Bowleg, 2012). It is essential that mental health professionals take a closer look into the emotional distress endured by Black women with infertility concerns. So, while we must continue to highlight where disparities exist, it is equally important that interventions seek to address the underlying causes of these disparities. Owing to the limited information on Black women's infertility treatment, future research on Black infertility and resilience from a strengths-based approach is warranted.

Understanding Cultural Factors: Why Representation Matters

While we have called for increased research on Black women's experiences with infertility and expansion of coverage for fertility care, these efforts will be moot if attempts are not made to understand the historical and cultural factors that influence Black people's relationship with public health systems. Even in states with comprehensive insurance plans that cover infertility services, the individuals who access infertility services the most are highly educated and wealthy White women, revealing the presence of additional factors contributing to high rates of infertility among Black women (Missmer et al., 2011). Equal access to state-mandated coverage for IVF does not equate to equal use of this service by Black and non-Black women, further depicting the need for a greater evaluation of how cultural and social cues affect this condition (Missmer et al., 2011). Rather than striving for equal access to infertility treatments and assistance, there needs to be a shift to an emphasis on equity. The social stigma surrounding infertility in the Black community needs to be addressed, as that looming stigma serves as a barrier toward Black women receiving the same equitable access as White women to proper and early diagnosis.

As a byproduct of the motherhood mandate, Black women are less likely to confide in friends and family about infertility issues, thus cutting off an avenue of support and creating a particularly distressing experience for Black women (Riegle, 2015). In dismantling the Black fertility mandate, there should be resounding conversations on infertility and its effects. To that end, efforts to overturn media practices that make some hypervisible and others invisible need to be initiated (Jones, 2020). Social depictions of infertility should be reflective of all women. Furthermore, there should be more informal pathways to receiving education and referrals for clinical assistance (Missmer et al., 2011). The lack of diversity in medicine and science continues to aggravate the Black community's distrust of healthcare providers. Increased representation of Black Americans as physicians and leaders in science and medicine would circumvent the discomfort that Black Americans feel regarding confiding in a medical professional. This translates to increased funding of pipeline programs that encourage Black children to pursue related careers as well as lowering the financial burden of obtaining this education. Considering the benefits of physician-patient racial and gender concordance, these long-term strategies can improve the face of Black women's experiences with reproductive health services (Wiltshire et al., 2018).

Conclusion

Facing the effects of systemic racism and sexism, Black women have displayed resilience while navigating these systems of oppression. Understanding the experiences of Black women requires a multidimensional approach and it is pertinent that we understand the layered existence of Black women through employing an intersectional framework. Further research, stronger policies, and cultural competency training for health-care professionals are necessary to properly address the scarcity of resources available to them to alleviate such burdens. Black women have no other choice but to be resilient, as the system was never structured to care for them. We must eliminate cultural biases and stereotypes, strengthen representation in medicine, and use a holistic approach to dismantle a system that has proven to be detrimental in improving the health of Black women.

Recommendations and Call for Action

The US experience with HIV/AIDS prevention reveals that the historical practice of shaping health policy from the perspective of the White middle class does not amount to improved health outcomes for minority groups (Bowleg, 2012). Therefore, to eliminate disparities in health outcomes, efforts should be made to design policies from the viewpoint of historically oppressed populations. This calls for an in-depth examination of the policies that perpetuate the mutually reinforcing dimensions of social deprivation, economic disadvantage, and democratic disqualification of Black communities (Razza, 2018). To effectively structure policies from the perspective of Black women and repair the harm done to Black communities, stakeholders and grassroots organizations must be involved in the design and implementation of policies.

Accordingly, we need to teach Black history—beyond slavery—and augment curricula at all levels of education to demonstrate the resilience of Black people despite structures in place to limit their progress. This would inform people's ability to name racism, overcome the shortcomings of implicit bias training, and help mitigate racism denial (Green & Hagiwara, 2020; Jones, 2020). Several studies have documented the role that racism and bias in health-care delivery plays in limiting the health of minorities, so it is high time that experts investigate innovative ways to hold providers accountable (Ibrahim & Zore, 2020; Lewis & Van Dyke, 2018). To narrow the gap in access to fertility care, steps should be taken to augment collaboration initiatives with pharmaceutical and insurance companies. Lobbying of state officials needs to be enhanced as we advocate for insurance coverage of assisted reproductive technologies and provision of therapies to historically underserved populations (Ibrahim & Zore, 2020).

Selected Resources

Mildred Watson-Baylor, PsyD, LPC
Ferris Healthcare Group
Website: www.ferrishealthcaregroup.com
P: 770.203.0842
Maternal Outcomes for Translational Health Equity Research (MOTHER) Lab
Website: motherlab.org
Email: info@motherlab.org

References

Black Women's Health Imperative. (2017, August 1). What is PCOS? Understanding polycystic ovary syndrome. https://bwhi.org/2017/08/01/pcos-understanding-polycystic-ovary-syndrome/

Bleich, M. R. (2015). Microaggression and its Relevance in health care. *Journal of Continuing Education in Nursing*, 46(11), 487–488. https://doi.org/10.3928/00220124-20151020-13

Bleich, S. N., Findling, M. G., Casey, L. S., Blendon, R. J., Benson, J. M., & Steelfisher, G. K. (2019). Discrimination in the United States: Experiences of black Americans. *Health Services Research*, 54(suppl. 2), 1399–1408. https://doi.org/10.1111/1475-6773.13220

Caldwell, K. L. (2017). Black women's health activism and the development of intersectional health policy. In *Health Equity in Brazil: Intersections of Gender, Race, and Policy* (pp. 44–64). University of Illinois Press.

Ceballo, R., Graham, E. T., & Hart, J. (2015). Silent and infertile: An intersectional analysis of the experiences of socioeconomically diverse African American women with infertility. *Psychology of Women Quarterly*, 39(4), 497–511. https://doi.org/10.1177/0361684315581169

Chin, H. B., Howards, P. P., Kramer, M. R., Mertens, A. C., & Spencer, J. B. (2015). Racial disparities in seeking care for help getting pregnant. *Paediatric and Perinatal Epidemiology*, 29(5), 416–425. https://doi.org/10.1111/ppe.12210

Dillard, S. (2016). Abnormally normal uteri: Exploring the meaning of fibroid tumors among African American women in the United States. *Women's Reproductive Health*, 3(2), 117–134. https://doi.org/10.1080/23293691.2016.1196087

Feagin, J., & Bennefield, Z. (2014). Systemic racism and U.S. health care. *Social Science and Medicine, 103*, 7–14. https://doi.org/10.1016/j.socscimed.2013.09.006

Green, T. L, & Hagiwara, N. (2020, August 28). The problem with implicit bias training. *Scientific American.* https://www.scientificamerican.com/article/the-problem-with-implicit-bias-training/

Greil, A. L., McQuillan, J., & Sanchez, D. (2016). Does fertility-specific distress vary by race/ethnicity among a probability sample of women in the United States? *Journal of Health Psychology, 21*(2), 183–192. https://doi.org/10.1177/1359105314524970

Harnois, C. (2010). Race, gender, and the Black women's standpoint. *Sociological Forum, 25*(1), 68–85. https://doi.org/10.1111/j.1573-7861.2009.01157.x

Hill, S. A. (2016). Race, racism, and health outcomes. In Inequality and African-American health: How racial disparities create sickness (pp. 15–28). Bristol University Press.

Humphries, L. A., Chang, O., Humm, K., Sakkas, D., & Hacker, M. R. (2016). Influence of race and ethnicity on in vitro fertilization outcomes: Systematic review. *American Journal of Obstetrics and Gynecology, 214*(2), 212.e1–212.e17. https://doi.org/10.1016/j.ajog.2015.09.002

Ibrahim, Y., & Zore, T. (2020). The pervasive issue of racism and its impact on infertility patients: What can we do as reproductive endocrinologists? *Journal of Assisted Reproduction and Genetics, 37*, 1563–1565. https://doi.org/10.1007/s10815-020-01863-x

Jaffe, J., & Diamond, M. O. (2010). *Reproductive trauma: Psychotherapy with infertility and pregnancy loss clients.* American Psychological Association.

Jones, C. P. (2020, August 25). Seeing the water: Seven values targets for anti-racism action. Center for Primary Care, Harvard Medical School. https://info.primarycare.hms.harvard.edu/review/seven-values-targets-anti-racism-action

Laughlin-Tommaso, S. K., Jacoby, V. L., & Myers, E. R. (2016). Disparities in fibroid incidence, prognosis, and management. *Obstetrics and Gynecology Clinics, 44*(1), 81–94. https://doi.org/10.1016/j.ogc.2016.11.007

Lewis, T. T., & Van Dyke, M. E. (2018). Discrimination and the health of African Americans: The potential importance of intersectionalities. *Current Directions in Psychological Science, 27*(3), 176–182. https://doi.org/10.1177/0963721418770442

Luke, B. (2017). Pregnancy and birth outcomes in couples with infertility with and without assisted reproductive technology: With an emphasis on US population-based studies. *American Journal of Obstetrics and Gynecology, 217*(3), 270–281. https://doi.org/10.1016/j.ajog.2017.03.012

McQueen, D. B., Feinberg, E. C., Lee, S. M., Schufreider, A., & Uhler, M. (2015). Racial disparities in in vitro fertilization (IVF). *Fertility and Sterility, 104*(2), 398–402. https://doi.org/10.1016/j.fertnstert.2014.07.938

Miller, L. R., & Peck, B. M. (2019). A prospective examination of racial microaggressions in the medical encounter. *Journal of Racial and Ethnic Health Disparities, 7*, 519–527. https://doi.org/10.1007/s40615-019-00680-y

Missmer, S. A., Seifer, D. B., & Jain, T. (2011). Cultural factors contributing to health care disparities among patients with infertility in Midwestern United States. *Fertility and Sterility*, 95(6), 1943–1949. https://doi.org/10.1016/j.fertnstert.2011.02.039

Noel, N. L., Gadson, A. K., & Hendessi, P. (2019). Uterine fibroids, race, ethnicity, and cardiovascular outcomes. *Current Cardiovascular Risk Reports*, 13(9), 1–7. https://doi.org/10.1007/s12170-019-0622-0

Ogunbiyi, O. (2019, June 27). PCOS: Black women are being let down by the NHS. *Stylist*. https://www.stylist.co.uk/life/pcos-polycystic-ovary-syndrome-symptoms-treatment-black-women-misdiagnosed-nhs/275704

Phelan, J. C., & Link, B. G. (2015). Is racism a fundamental cause of inequalities in health? *Annual Review of Sociology*, 41(1), 311–330. https://doi.org/10.1146/annurev-soc-073014-112305

Prather, C., Fuller, T. R., Jeffries, W. L., IV, Marshall, K. J., Howell, A. V., Belyue-Umole, A., & King, W. (2018). Racism, African American women, and their sexual and reproductive health: A review of historical and contemporary evidence and implications for health equity. *Health Equity*, 2(1), 249–259. https://doi.org/10.1089/heq.2017.0045

Razza, C. M. (2018). *Social exclusion: The decisions and dynamics that drive racism*. Demos. https://www.demos.org/research/social-exclusion-decisions-and-dynamics-drive-racism

Resilient Sisterhood Project. (n.d.). *Black women and infertility*. https://rsphealth.org/infertility/

Riegle, A. L. (2015). *Economic and racial differences in women's infertility experiences* [Doctoral dissertation, Iowa State University]. ProQuest Dissertations Publishing.

Rosenthal, L., & Lobel, M. (2016). Stereotypes of Black American women related to sexuality and motherhood. *Psychology of Women Quarterly*, 40(3), 414–427. https://doi.org/10.1177/0361684315627459

Seifer, D. B., Frazier, L. M., & Grainger, D. A. (2008). Disparity in assisted reproductive technologies outcomes in black women compared with white women. *Fertility and Sterility*, 90(5), 1701–1710. https://doi.org/10.1016/j.fertnstert.2007.08.024

Slaughter-Acey, J. C., Sneed, D., Parker, L., Keith, V. M., Lee, N. L., & Misra, D. P. (2019). Skin tone matters: Racial microaggressions and delayed prenatal care. *American Journal of Preventive Medicine*, 57(3), 321–329. https://doi.org/10.1016/j.amepre.2019.04.014

Smith, J. P. (1998). Socioeconomic status and health. *American Economic Review*, 88(2), 192–196. http://www.jstor.org/stable/116917

Stanton, A. L. (1991). Cognitive appraisals, coping processes, and adjustment to infertility. In A. L. Stanton & C. Dunkel-Schetter (Eds.), *Infertility: Perspectives from stress and coping research* (pp. 87–108). Plenum Press.

Wellons, M. F., Lewis, C. E., Schwartz, S. M., Gunderson, E. P., Schreiner, P. J., Sternfeld, B., Richman, J., Sites, C. K., & Siscovick, D. S. (2008). Racial differences in self-reported infertility and risk factors for infertility in a cohort of Black and White women: The CARDIA Women's Study. *Fertility and Sterility*, *90*(5), 1640–1648. https://doi.org/10.1016/j.fertnstert.2007.09.056

Williams, D., Priest, N., & Anderson, N. (2019). Understanding associations between race, socioeconomic status, and health: Patterns and prospects. In J. Oberlander, M. Buchbinder, L. Churchill, S. Estroff, N. King, B. Saunders, R. P. Strauss, & R. L. Walker (Eds.), *The Social Medicine Reader* (3rd ed., Vol. 2, pp. 258–267). Duke University Press.

Wiltshire, J., Allison, J. J., Brown, R., & Elder, K. (2018). African American women perceptions of physician trustworthiness: A factorial survey analysis of physician race, gender and age. *AIMS Public Health*, *5*(2), 122–134. https://doi.org/10.3934%2Fpublichealth.2018.2.122

Wiltshire, A., Brayboy, L.M, Phillips, K., Matthews, R., Yan, F., & McCarthy-Keith, D. (2019). Infertility knowledge and treatment beliefs among African American women in an urban community. *Contraception and Reproductive Medicine*, *4*(1), Article 16. https://doi.org/10.1186/s40834-019-0097-x

Windsor, L. C., Dunlap, E., & Golub, A. (2011). Challenging controlling images, oppression, poverty and other structural constraints: Survival strategies among African American women in distressed households. *Journal of African American Studies*, *15*(3), 290–306. https://doi.org/10.1007/s12111-010-9151-0

Woods-Giscombé, C. L. (2010). Superwoman schema: African American women's views on stress, strength, and health. *Qualitative Health Research*, *20*(5), 668–683. https://doi.org/10.1177/1049732310361892

Commentary

Abortion Is a Reproductive Justice Issue for Black Families and Communities

JOIA CREAR-PERRY, NIA MITCHELL, DONNA L. BRAZILE, AND RACHEL VILLANUEVA

Black Mamas Matter Alliance * Black Women's Health Imperative * In Our Own Voice: National Black Women's Reproductive Justice Agenda * National Birth Equity Collaborative * SisterSong Women of Color Reproductive Justice Collective

There have always been those who have stood in the way of our exercising our rights, who tried to restrict our choices. There probably always will be. But we who have been oppressed should not be swayed in our opposition to tyranny, of any kind, especially attempts to take away our reproductive freedom. You may believe abortion is wrong. We respect your belief and we will do all in our power to protect that choice for you. You may decide that abortion is not an option you would choose. Reproductive freedom guarantees your right not to. All that we ask is that no one deny another human being the right to make her own choice. That no one condemn her to exercise her choices in ways that endanger her health, her life.

—*We Remember: African American Women for Reproductive Freedom*

> We are engaged in every aspect of the decision-making process about this struggle against eugenics and for human rights, providing a context for our abortion decisions by telling our stories and validating the trust of our communities. We always resist. Our opponents would do well to never forget that. Trust Black Women.
>
> —Loretta Ross, *Radical Reproductive Justice: Foundation, Theory, Practice, Critique* (Ross et al., 2017)

Over 30 years ago, 16 Black women courageously led a movement for reproductive freedom with the release and distribution of the seminal brochure *We Remember: African American Women for Reproductive Freedom* in 1989. In response to the US Supreme Court decision to uphold Missouri's restrictions to abortion in the *Webster v. Reproductive Health Services* case, the brochure was a reminder that when abortions are made illegal or restricted, Black women disproportionately suffer life-threatening complications and even death. Furthermore, it placed Black women's struggle for reproductive freedom in historical context—our struggle against intersecting oppressions during enslavement, Jim Crow, and the War on Drugs—and defined what reproductive freedom meant to Black women.

We reflect on their legacy in this moment when the US Supreme Court ruled on another case, *Dobbs v. Jackson Women's Health Organization*, seeking to restrict abortion in Mississippi and overturn *Roe v. Wade* during the COVID-19 pandemic, an ongoing maternal health crisis, and sanctioned actions that disproportionately take the lives of Black people. Transnationally, cases such as this impact funding and policies toward abortion in other countries. While many countries are moving toward the liberalization of abortion laws, the US is moving in the opposite direction, toward restriction. The purpose of this call to action is (1) to situate the current struggle for abortion rights within our broader struggle for reproductive justice, (2) to uplift the leadership and activism of Black reproductive justice organizations working to safeguard affordable and accessible abortions, and (3) to provide actions the White House can take that will contribute to Black people, families, and communities' sexual and reproductive health and well-being, which includes but is not limited to abortion. Several national organizations have supported efforts to strategically uplift the need for reproductive justice to be prioritized in the U.S.

Coined by US Black women in 1994, reproductive justice, or the human right to maintain personal bodily autonomy, have children, not have children, and parent the children we have in safe and sustainable communities, is rooted in our experiences with and resistance to reproductive oppression. We have experienced forced pregnancy and childbearing, involuntary sterilization, restrictions to abortion and contraception, and policies and environments that endanger and take away our children. Reproductive justice captures the complexities of our lives as well as our activism. As a framework and a movement, it centers communities disproportionately impacted by reproductive oppression as well as uplifts our leadership and organizations. It is intersectional and it works to shift power (e.g., structures, policies, institutions).

Equitable access to safe and legal abortion is a reproductive justice issue. All people regardless of their backgrounds and circumstances have the right to decide when and how they want to have a child, and we trust their ability to make the best decisions for themselves and their families. Although the US Supreme Court legalized abortion in 1973 when it overturned Texas's attempt to criminalize abortion, it upheld the Hyde Amendment in 1980, preventing low-income individuals from using Medicaid to pay for abortions. *Harris v. McRae* is one of many Supreme Court decisions that have eroded *Roe v. Wade* and compromised the reproductive freedom of groups and communities that have been and continue to be marginalized (e.g., Black and Brown people, immigrants, LGBTQIA+ people, people with disabilities, young people). As a result, these groups and communities are susceptible to higher rates of unsafe abortions that may result in life-threatening complications and even death. Furthermore, US domestic policies impact access to abortion in other countries. For example, the so-called Global Gag Rule, which was expanded under the Trump administration, prohibited any form of US assistance to nongovernmental organizations providing or advocating for abortions in other countries where there is already limited or no access to contraception and abortion, as well as high rates of unintended pregnancy and unsafe abortions.

Uplifting the Activism and Leadership of the Black Reproductive Movement

Despite these challenges and restrictions to safe and legal abortion, Black reproductive justice organizations have resisted attempts to control the reproductive decision-making of communities and limit their access to health care. This was true when 12 Black women formed Women of African Descent for Reproductive Justice in 1993 as a response to President Bill Clinton's Health Security Act, which would have neglected the health-care needs of low-income individuals. It was also true in 2010 when anti-abortion billboards were placed in our communities declaring Black children an endangered species in hopes of garnering support for anti-abortion legislation rooted in racism and sexism. Under the leadership of Loretta Ross and then of Monica Simpson, SisterSong Women of Color Reproductive Justice Collective led a national coalition of Black reproductive justice organizations demanding our communities to "Trust Black Women," and defeated local and state legislation (Ross et al., 2017). Similar efforts led by other Black reproductive justice activists and organizations have been conducted throughout the US in response to similar campaigns, while In Our Own Voice: National Black Women's Reproductive Justice Agenda works with its state partners to focus its efforts to change policies at the regional and national levels. For Black reproductive justice organizations, our priority is making sure our families are safe and have the resources and decision-making power to do what is best for them.

Recommendations and Call for Action

Although our communities and organizations will continue to fight for, serve, hold, and uplift our families and communities during this difficult time, increased funding and changes in legislation are essential to ensure all people continue to have not only access to safe and legal abortion but everything required for their sexual and reproductive health and well-being. As a result, we recommend the following:

1. increased funding and support to Black reproductive justice organizations working to ensure equitable access to safe and legal abortion, health care, and other needed services in our communities,

2. the establishment of a White House Office of Sexual and Reproductive Health and Well-Being that can push forward a federal strategy for promoting equitable sexual and reproductive health and well-being through a human rights, gender, and racial equity lens, and

3. the incorporation of reproductive justice values into foreign policy, which includes ratifying human rights treaties that protect sexual and reproductive health and rights (e.g., the Convention on the Elimination of All Forms of Discrimination against Women).

Black reproductive justice organizations are on the front line, advocating for and supporting our families and communities. Many of them are underfunded and lack the infrastructure needed to adequately respond to the challenges our communities navigate daily. Specialized funding to these organizations is necessary to ensure that they can continue to do the work. Moreover, the establishment of a White House Office of Sexual and Reproductive Health and Well-Being is imperative. The office would work in tandem with these organizations to realize holistic sexual and reproductive health services and social support policies, regulations, and funding streams. It would also work to remedy those policies, regulations, and funding streams that are currently siloed, disjointed, and ill-suited for ensuring that federal agencies, states, and health-care systems address systemic racism. The office will provide a permanent infrastructure to (1) develop a federal strategy for promoting equitable sexual and reproductive health and well-being through a human rights, gender, and racial equity lens, and (2) better coordinate the actions of the many departments and agencies whose actions in both domestic and foreign policy contexts impact sexual and reproductive health and well-being of people in the US and around the world, including the Departments of Defense, Education, Health and Human Services, Homeland Security, Labor, Housing and Urban Development, Treasury, and Veterans Affairs, and the Office of Personnel Management. Lastly, the US must ratify human rights treaties that protect sexual and reproductive health and rights. The US's continued restriction to abortion access and erosion of abortion rights violates many of these treaties and compromises the health and well-being of many of its people.

In the midst of a global pandemic and with maternal mortality rates at the highest they have been in decades, we cannot possibly afford to turn back the clock or reverse policies that protect the reproductive freedoms of every individual. As we approach the 50th anniversary of *Roe v. Wade*, we ask our allies in government to lead from the front. We ask them to see that it is imperative that we stand firmly in our convictions, hold the line, and refuse to back down from the fight—especially given its inevitable impact on our community specifically. We, the signers of this document, stand firmly on the shoulders of the warriors who came before us and declare that the next generation of women and pregnant people will be spared the indignity of having others legislate away their bodily autonomy. Our legacy will be one of liberation, enlightenment, and empowerment and we will *not* relent until that also includes the irrevocable right to have or not have an abortion.

References

Ahmed, Z. (2020). The unprecedented expansion of the global gag rule: trampling rights, health and free speech. *Guttmacher Policy Rev, 23*, 13–18.

Amnesty International. (2005, August 25). *A fact sheet on CEDAW: Treaty for the rights of women.* https://www.amnestyusa.org/files/pdfs/cedaw_fact_sheet.pdf

Center for Reproductive Rights. (2010, September 13). *Whose choice? How the Hyde Amendment harms poor women.* https://www.reproductiverights.org/sites/crr.civicactions.net/files/documents/Hyde_Report_FINAL_nospreads.pdf

Center for Reproductive Rights. (2021, July 22). *Mississippi abortion ban case before the U.S. Supreme Court poses a direct challenge to Roe v. Wade.* https://reproductiverights.org/case-scotus-mississippi-abortion-ban-roe-wade-challenge/

Center for Reproductive Rights. (2007, July 1). *Roe v. Wade—Then and now.* https://reproductiverights.org/roe-v-wade-then-and-now/

Howell, M. (2019, November 14). *Written statement of Marcela Howell: Examining state efforts to undermine access to reproductive health care.* In Our Own Voices: National Black Women's Reproductive Justice Agenda. http://blackrj.org/wp-content/uploads/2019/11/IOOV-Examining-State-Efforts-to-Undermine-Access-to-Reproductive-Health-Care.pdf

Kortsmit, K., Jatlaoui, T. C., Mandel, M. G., Reeves, J. A., Oduyebo, T., Petersen, E., & Whiteman, M. K. (2020). Abortion surveillance—United States, 2018. *Morbidity and mortality weekly report, 69*(7), 1–29. https://doi.org/10.15585/mmwr.ss6907a1

National Birth Equity Collaborative. (2021, March 8). *Office of Sexual Reproductive Health and Well-Being Sign On Letter.* https://birthequity.org/wp-content/uploads/2021/09/OSRHW-Sign-on-Letter-3.8.21-1.pdf

Rhodes A. M. (1989). Webster versus Reproductive Health Services. *MCN: The American Journal of Maternal Child Nursing, 14*(6), 423.

Ross, L., Derkas, E., Peoples, W., Roberts, L., & Bridgewater, P. (Eds.). (2017). *Radical reproductive justice: Foundation, theory, practice, critique.* Feminist Press at CUNY.

United Nations, Office of the High Commissioner for Human Rights. 2020. *Abortion.* https://www.ohchr.org/Documents/Issues/Women/WRGS/SexualHealth/INFO_Abortion_WEB.pdf

You know your body best
If you experience something that seems unusual or is worrying you, don't ignore it.

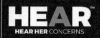

Learn about urgent warning signs and how to talk to your healthcare provider.

During Pregnancy
If you are pregnant, it's important to pay attention to your body and talk to your healthcare provider about anything that doesn't feel right. If you experience any of the urgent maternal warning signs, get medical care immediately.

After Pregnancy
While your new baby needs a lot of attention and care, it's important to remain aware of your own body and take care of yourself, too. It's normal to feel tired and have some pain, particularly in the first few weeks after having a baby, but there are some symptoms that could be signs of more serious problems.

Tips:
- Bring this conversation starter and any additional questions you want to ask to your provider.
- Be sure to tell them that you are pregnant or have been pregnant within a year.
- Tell the doctor or nurse what medication you are currently taking or have recently taken.
- Take notes and ask more questions about anything you didn't understand.

Learn more about CDC's Hear Her Campaign at www.cdc.gov/HearHer

---- Tear this panel off and use this guide to help you start the conversation: ----

Urgent Maternal Warning Signs
If you experience any of these warning signs, get medical care immediately.

- Severe headache that won't go away or gets worse over time
- Dizziness or fainting
- Thoughts about harming yourself or your baby
- Changes in your vision
- Fever of 100.4° F or higher
- Extreme swelling of your hands or face
- Trouble breathing
- Chest pain or fast-beating heart
- Severe nausea and throwing up (not like morning sickness)
- Severe belly pain that doesn't go away
- Baby's movement stopping or slowing down during pregnancy
- Vaginal bleeding or fluid leaking during pregnancy
- Heavy vaginal bleeding or leaking fluid that smells bad after pregnancy
- Swelling, redness or pain of your leg
- Overwhelming tiredness

This list is not meant to cover every symptom you might have. If you feel like something just isn't right, talk to your healthcare provider

Use This Guide to Help Start the Conversation:
- Thank you for seeing me.
  I am/was recently pregnant. The date of my last period/delivery was _____ and I'm having serious concerns about my health that I'd like to talk to you about.

- I have been having _____ (symptoms) that feel like _____ (describe in detail) and have been lasting _____ (number of hours/days)

- I know my body and this doesn't feel normal.

Sample questions to ask:
- What could these symptoms mean?
- Is there a test I can have to rule out a serious problem?
- At what point should I consider going to the emergency room or calling 911?

Notes:

Learn more about CDC's Hear Her Campaign at www.cdc.gov/HearHer

Figure C.1. Maternal health fact sheet. Hear Her Campaign, Centers for Disease Control and Prevention, https://www.cdc.gov/hearher/index.html. Public domain.

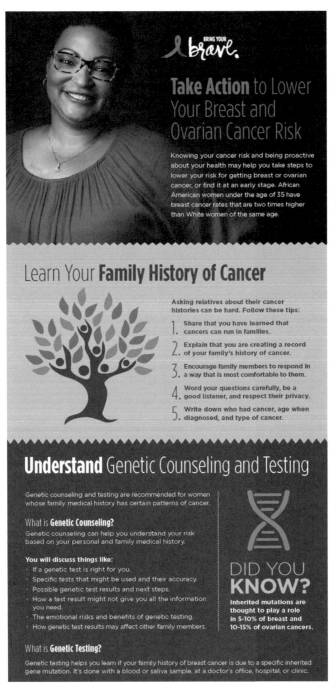

Figure C.2a. Cancer fact sheet. Bring Your Brave Campaign, Centers for Disease Control and Prevention, https://www.cdc.gov/cancer/breast/young_women/bringyourbrave/index.htm. Public domain.

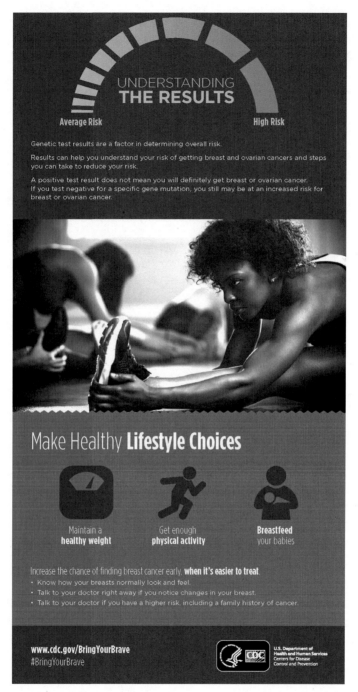

Figure C.2b. Cancer fact sheet. Bring Your Brave Campaign, Centers for Disease Control and Prevention, https://www.cdc.gov/cancer/breast/young_women/bringyourbrave/index.htm. Public domain.

Conversations with Thought Leaders

Beacons of Light

HENRIE M. TREADWELL, HELENE D. GAYLE, AND GAIL E. WYATT

Question: What one word describes Black women to you? Why? What does that word mean to you?

SELECTED EXCERPTED RESPONSES

- Vigilant. I think we are always having to survey the scene, survey the environment. Whether it's for us, our family, or for our community benefit, so we are always out there sensing what it is that's going on and responding to it. Vigilant to me says it's more than just looking. It means you're looking with insight.

- Resilient. I think that Black women have weathered a lot of storms. We often have a lot thrown at us. But I think despite it all we rally and rise to the occasion. Resilience, because no matter what happens we understand that in many ways we are the strength, the pillar, and the backbone for our families and our communities, so we get back up and keep going. If it's our families, if it's our profession, whatever it is, we've got to continue along our path and seek our purpose, whatever that may be.

- Flexible. We hold our own in terms of what we bring to relationships, what we bring to society, and what we bring to children. What we bring to ourselves is where I think we need to work.

Question: How do you feel about Black women's position or status in today's society?

SELECTED EXCERPTED RESPONSES

- I believe Black women have started and energized many of the social movements. Nevertheless, the work that we do and stimulate sometimes gets hijacked by others. Black women need to figure out how to put the work more firmly in their hands and within their power.

- Black mothers really cannot step away from their role. Even if you look at the construct of the Black family today, so often it is the woman who is in the position of trying to move things along not for any other reason other than the way the society has treated the African American male in so many ways.

- The most obvious and recent examples are our elections; and the power of one woman who did not get the governor's seat but then created a movement that helped to elect our current president, vice president, and two senators who shifted what could have been the balance of the senate. That was a very clear example of resilience. She could have licked her wounds and gone home, but she believed she could have an even bigger purpose, and that was much greater than any one office she could have gotten herself. That's a current example of this notion of resilience mixed with purpose and intentionality.

- It is well documented that African descended women are at the bottom of any ranking when it comes to beauty, desirability, and when it comes to sexuality we're at the top. This is all borne out of stereotypes. It's not certainly not borne out of any data, our bodies don't do anything different. It's just that people think they own our bodies.

Question: What do you believe are the most significant health concerns facing Black women and families today?

SELECTED EXCEPTED RESPONSES

- Both mental and physical health. We are totally uneducated, uninformed, and exploited; you name it, large corporations, music, it's just everywhere, and it has not changed.

- I put stress way at the top of my list and then that can be related to hypertension, diabetes, preterm labor, obesity. But also I'd have to include in there infectious diseases, because we are not protected in so many ways from those things that come to us.

- COVID-19 is impacting our communities more and Black women are at the forefront of caregiving.

Part Three

Journey to Wellness and Community Healing

Fortitude/fôrdə͵t(y)o͞od/
Strength of mind that enables a person to face adversity with courage

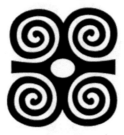

Dwennimmen
West African Adinkra Symbol of Humility together with Strength

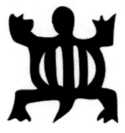

Denkyem
West African Adinkra Symbol of Adaptability

214 | Part Three

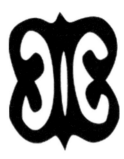

Hye Won Hye
West African Adinkra Symbol for Endurance

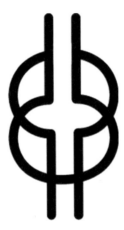

Nyansapo
West African Adinkra Symbol for Wisdom, Ingenuity, and Patience

Corona Reflections

Threading the Needle All the Way Through

Tamia A. McEwen

Something old, Something new
Something broken, Something borrowed
Something repaired something blue
I often wonder just what to do
With all of these discarded pieces that may just need some glue.
Or perhaps they need a match like my favorite pair of socks
That once were two but now the other I haven't got.
Or my favorite earrings with all of the Adinkra symbols
I wore them boldly and proud.
Until I looked and was only wearing one,
The other could not be found.
I was overcome with grief. I mean I looked everywhere
Only to see it months later ground up in pieces underneath my driver's chair.
The iPad I adored, after 4 years fell on its face. Crack!
I lost my creative luster for a moment.
It took almost two years to get it back.
On the issues of things broken, things borrowed, repaired or blue
Of the things that are old and of those that are new.
New and shiny is fresh, feels so good on our skin.
But new only last for a moment, until the wears of life set in.
Borrowed has a certain flavor, special sentiments sometimes.

But borrowed things go back to the owner
bringing joy—but it's theirs, not mine.
Old things carry wisdom and stories of all that they've endured.
And still show their regal value,
existing longer than some thought they should.
Blue sometimes represents sadness, but I equate blue to the sea.
Carrying the emotions of life that are sure to come to you and me.
That leaves us with the last quality, that was not originally there
And that is of those things that are in need of or have been repaired.
Every broken bone is not useless, every cracked pot is not done.
Every shattered mirror is not bad luck nor is every lost victory a bad run.
The blessing of being broken is the awareness it can bring.
Awareness that life is sometimes simply filled with a multitude of things.
Things that come and things that go.
Things that we create and things we do not own.
In our times of uncertainty, we can remember this one truth:
Sometimes the difference between lost and won is
simply threading the needle all the way through.

Chapter 13

On the Frontlines

Stressors of Black Women Caring for Children of Incarcerated Parents

SHENIQUE THOMAS-DAVIS, VIVIAN C. SMITH, AND BAHIYYAH M. MUHAMMAD

The intersecting oppression Black women confront daily is structurally rooted in the fabric of our hegemonic, racist, patriarchal society. The social, economic, gendered, and political injustices facing Black women are part of a longstanding legacy embedded in customs and cultural norms that have historically stratified Black women to the lowest tier of institutional power and citizenship. Yet, Black women are relied on as the "backbone of our democracy" and expected to hold and sustain the frontline (Harris, 2020). Despite the consistent instrumental contributions and unrelenting devotion of Black women as caregivers of families, communities, and this nation, the stories and lived experiences validating their mere existence often are left untold, unacknowledged, and repudiated. Black women are bequeathed to navigate untenable social positions.

"Black women—feel responsible for the world" (Scott, 1991, p. 8). A fundamental lesson and skill that many Black women receive is to tend to the world first and themselves last—habits of surviving (Scott, 1991). "Surviving" surfaces in varied forms, including but not limited to denial, detachment, ceaseless accommodations for others, ardent religiosity/

spirituality, extreme self-reliance, and regulation. Scott's (1991) research finds that Black women teach these habits of surviving to each other, often without verbal descriptions, but through demonstrations of lived experiences. Habits are adaptive movements likened to that of "dance steps," "that we practice and perfect through continual use" (p. 7). These routinized responses affirm that Black women are apt to exercise control in chaos. Ultimately, the habits become intergenerational coping strategies, deeply rooted in culture and tradition. Considering that families act as agents of socialization and serve as symbolic resources through which norms and relationships develop and thrive, these habits transmit across generations. In the face of obstacles, the custom of the "dance" demarcates the lines between livelihood and annihilation. Life is a series of rehearsals where Black women learn to perfect their performance in survival mode.

Coping mechanisms, habits, and dance steps masked as resilience have sustained Black women amid adversity. Resiliency as a process is the ability to adapt, cope, and manage when encountering adverse events such as trauma, tragedy, threats, or significant sources of stress (American Psychological Association, 2012; Ungar et al., 2013). This qualitative work advances scholarship on the disruptive impact of familial incarceration on Black women by delineating strategies employed to anticipate, react to, and cope with cumulative stress.

Under Siege: Black Communities and Incarceration

In his seminal work, epidemiologist Ernest Drucker (2011) deemed mass incarceration a public health threat, invoking the term "plague of prisons." Mass incarceration is part of a racialized experiment and deeply immersed in the lives of Black Americans (Clear & Frost, 2014). Set in motion under the Nixon administration, punitive policies inundated with racist tactics targeted communities as pathogens and Black people as contaminants and carriers of criminality. To be explicit, Drucker (2011) calls this outbreak a chronic contagious condition with potentially long-term effects. This process has undoubtedly ravaged neighborhoods and families with profound implications for the livelihood, individual trajectories, and routine activities of Black people (Burt et al., 2012; Muhammad, 2019). Recently, the lack of urgency to respond to the widespread incidence of the COVID-19 virus in carceral facilities made the intention of the human experiment increasingly clear. These actions have been purposive in their selection of targets and persistent in their dehumanization and second-class citizenship designation of marginalized groups (Alexander, 2010; Wilkerson, 2020).

An estimated 1,400,000 persons were incarcerated in state and federal prisons at year-end 2019 (Carson, 2020). Black men were six times more likely to be incarcerated than their White and Hispanic counterparts and Black women were imprisoned at a rate of 1.7 times that of White women (Sentencing Project, 2013, 2020). People under correctional supervision are embedded in larger intricate family systems. We must consider those left behind.

Parental incarceration, estimated to affect approximately 3,000,000 minor children, forces parents to rely on others to render childcare (Western & Pettit, 2010). Usually, grandparents, extended kin, or other legal guardians assume caregiving responsibilities. Forty-two percent of mothers in state prisons identified the child(ren)'s grandmother(s) as the current sole caregiver and 37% listed the child(ren)'s other parent(s) (Glaze & Maruschak, 2008). In stark contrast, 88.4% of fathers in state prison reported the child(ren)'s mother(s) as the current caregiver and 12% relied on grandmother caregivers. Unfortunately, these data are not systematically collected to enumerate impact. Taking into account incarceration trends and Black families' traditional prioritization of extended family and kinship care, Black women tend to acquire these additional parental roles/responsibilities (Luckey, 1996).

Interaction with the carceral state radiates out to create "multilayered burdens for adult female family members of the incarcerated" (Arditti et al., 2020, p. 102). Research on connectedness to imprisoned individuals finds that Black women disproportionately experience incarceration of an acquaintance, family member, neighbor, or trusted person compared to Black men and White women and men; pointedly, 50% have at least one imprisoned family member (Lee et al., 2015). This oversaturation in Black women's networks may result in multidimensional "spillover effects" that perpetuate further collective harm in the form of decreased social capital, economic distress, and other physical or psychological consequences (Lee & Wildeman, 2011; Patterson et al., 2020; Schnittker et al., 2015). Parental incarceration has serious implications for children, in the form of enduring trauma and of psychological, emotional, developmental, and behavioral challenges (Kjellstrand et al., 2018; Murray et al., 2012; Turney, 2018; Wakefield & Wildeman, 2014). Children face stigmatization, and their teachers have lower expectations of competency, skills, and educational attainment (Dallaire et al., 2010).

Spillover effects permanently percolate in the lives of Black women required to perform what Gurusami (2019) defines as "motherwork"—the ways and process that "mothers on the margins support their families under carceral infrastructures" (p. 132)—or what Collins (1994) termed "othermothers," women who share the mothering of the community. Incarceration criminalizes family networks, contaminates relationships, and creates undue compounding stress. Scant research addresses the link between incarceration and health outcomes (Drucker, 2011; Kjellstrand et al., 2018; Lee et al., 2015, 2014; Schnittker et al., 2015). In this chapter we center Black women who care for children left behind as they encounter significant, persisting life changes, increasing ambiguity, and burgeoning obligations. Our analysis, framed by stress adaptation and resilience literature, seeks to explore the stress-resilience paradox.

Methods

Through a qualitative methodological approach, the study works to contextualize the lived experiences of Black women navigating carceral crisis. Drawn from in-depth interviews of caregivers in a larger ethnographic study on children of persons incarcerated (Muhammad, 2011), the current sample includes twelve Black women caregivers, recruited from community organizations providing mentoring services for children in their care. Interviews prompted participants to reflect on life, relationship, and caregiving changes and challenges, and necessary adjustments.

Caregivers, ranging in age from 30 to 61 years ($M = 41.2$) included mothers (7), grandmothers (3), an aunt, and a sister; 33 children were under their care. On average, women solely supported three children (range 1–8 children), ages 6 months to 20 years old. Fifty-five percent of the caregivers were unemployed and 75% indicated severely restricted incomes. Six incarcerated parents permanently lost custodial rights and two households had foster care involvement.

Analysis sought to "uncover and explicate" the ways in which participants understood, experienced, and negotiated their lives as caregivers connected to the carceral state (Van Maanen, 1979, p. 540). Narratives presented an opportunity to process and validate the authentic accounts of Black women navigating racism, sexism, and classism, magnified by familial imprisonment. Further, these stories are "both social products and socially productive," meaning, they can be culturally transformative and inform systemic change (Wilkins, 2012, p. 175). Data revealed a litany of integrative themes anchored in survival, despair, burdened, physical distress, taxed, grief, social isolation, embattled, sacrifice, turmoil, disappointment, adjustment/coping, faith, and resilience. The variation suggests that caregivers contend with an overwhelming myriad of stressors.

Findings

Narrative analysis indicated that being thrust into the role of sole caregiver negatively affected participants' well-being. Nevertheless, caregivers emphasized their continued will, commitment to their family, trust/faith in divinity, and hope for better days. Despite their circumstances, participants refused to abandon their care-work obligations. Collectively, caregivers expressed improved life opportunities for children in their care as fuel for their persistence, perseverance, and faith; yet, it was evident that caregivers often took minimal regard for their own physical and psychological well-being in order to maintain stability with the familial unit. Within this analytic scheme, we explore the emergent themes of surrender, strain, and resilient faith: surrender, the act of halting current and future lives to provide care for the child(ren); strain, expressed as feeling taxed and overwhelmed with increased labor and responsibilities; and resilient faith, the process of growth/adaptation due to compounding stressors and adversity through fervent reliance on religiosity.

Surrender

> I'm living life on life's terms right now. That's all I can do. I've been trying to show my kids that I'm not a weak person and things happen in life and you just have to deal with it. . . . I'm mentally drained right now and—but I'm a survivor so I always bounce back from anything, actually.
>
> —Sharon, 36

> At the end of the day, I have to suck up my feeling and deal with the hand I was dealt. What else can I do?
>
> —Jada, 30

Caregivers unconsciously operate in survival-resilience mode even when experiencing feelings of drain and longing to escape. By living in a constant survival state and facing the world as a "warrior," caregivers did not foresee alternative options. Scott (1991) elaborates: "In this mode, we can never let down our guard (even to ourselves). In the warrior mode, many Back women's individual and group responsibilities are distorted, personal and political boundaries are blurred, and personal and community priorities are unbalanced. . . . In this way, the warrior mode is an additional obstacle—along with all the 'isms' that black women have to overcome" (p. 8).

Participants, compelled into "crisis mother work," abruptly relinquished their plans in order to fulfill familial duties (Gurusami, 2019). Strategies used to confront and adapt to crises are said to be influenced by family background variables and are positioned to establish the family's future defining characteristics (Helms & Demo, 2005; Karney & Bradbury, 1995).

Caregivers' identities have been defined by their responses to constantly evolving, complicated obligations. Here, Jada, a 30-year-old mother described her constant wrestle: "I felt like running at one point. But I needed a couple of days to gather my thoughts together and I knew that running away would not solve anything. If I ran away, the children would have no one. . . . It took a lot of patience. . . . I had to put my wants and needs on the backburner. . . . Their issues are more important than mine."

Jada embraced a period of internal reflection, grappled with thoughts of fleeing, and gradually processed this significant life change—performing as sole caretaker. In doing so, Jada acknowledged the dilemma, cultivated a response, and, in that pivot, worked to increase her resilience muscle.

Caregivers surrendered and abandoned their dreams, hopes, goals, wants, and needs, reminisced of past lives, and reckoned with how the criminal legal system's imposition on their family altered their outlook and trajectory. In a sense, caregivers grieved their future lives. Sunny, a 61-year-old grandmother, expressed, "It's not an easy task to be a grandmother with kids as young as they are, because there's a lot of things they want to do that I don't feel like doing. . . . Because sometimes I feel like getting up and running somewhere and not coming back. But you know what? These kids is here and I don't want nothing to happen to them." Caregivers loved the children and preferred kinship care rather than foster care exposure/state placement; however, they discussed feelings of regret, guilt, and emotional withdrawal. Fifty-six-year-old Jill raised three sets of grandchildren. She explained, "I had the first set of grandchildren in

1993, and I had them until 2002, and then I got another set. . . . At one time, I had all nine of them." Jill further conveyed,

> I have to do everything. I had to make all changes in my life to watch my grandson. I don't have a chance to live. I have been working all my life. I am so tired of working, but I cannot quit because this is the only income that I have. I can't be tired. I have to keep working even though I am tired. I can't just get up and go. I have to make arrangements. I have to find a babysitter. I don't have the money to get a babysitter, and nobody wants to babysit. I used to work dayshift, now I have to work nightshift. . . . I am hanging in there with all this. If I don't do it, nobody will.

In between the brief periods of (non–)care work, Jill enjoyed her autonomy—dating and entertaining friends. She anticipated devoting time to her dream and goal of writing; instead, her son's recent incarceration necessitated modifications to her lifestyle. Without a doubt, the women adore the children in their care, but the responsibility culminates in diminished social capital and reduces their quality of life.

Strain

Our analysis revealed that connection to an incarcerated parent and care work elicited increased feelings of worry, anger, anxiety, and stress. Participants reported severe financial hardship, resource deprivation, child behavioral challenges, and difficulty managing childcare. Caregivers relied on limited income, with more than half on public assistance, impeding the ability to afford basic needs like rent. Households were transient, as families moved on average four times per year due to eviction, resulting in increased levels of strain. Despite barely providing for themselves and children, caregivers also extended their crowded homes to others.

Though money seemed to be a problem, caregivers accepted parents' collect calls and frequently added funds to commissary accounts. Limited income created tenuous situations as arguments ensued when the children were denied material requests. Caregivers revealed being burdened as the sole caretakers and unsure of how to best fill the void. Tasha, a 43-year-old mother, speaks to the role duality and says, "I am the mommy and daddy now. . . . Being a woman daddy is a lot of heartache and pain."

Ruby, a 57-year-old grandmother further describes the struggles with negotiating multiple and conflicting positions. "I have never been able to just be the grandmother. I have been the mother, the father, and the grandmother. . . . It is a lot on one person to be three people." Difficult to pinpoint and name, caregivers emphasized various health-related outcomes. On average, each caregiver managed three health-related-issues. Presenting problems included hypertension, diabetes, and mood/anxiety disorders. More serious diseases included cancer, heart disease, seizures, and sleeping conditions.

Many of the developmental, socio-emotional, and physical conditions of the children predate caregivers. Specifically, grandmothers underscored the multiple layers they contend with daily—limited resources and network, controlling messaging about parental absence, shame/stigma, post-traumatic stress reactions, and management of their own and the child's health. As one grandmother observed, "Jason takes medication for ADD, and has been diagnosed as having emotional problems; Ronny has deep depression, he does not sleep at night; Franky has ADD; and Kenya has her own stuff."

Table 13.1. Reported health outcomes/conditions

Caregiver	Asthma Anxiety disorders Cancer Diabetes Digestive conditions Heart disease High blood pressure High cholesterol Sleep apnea
Child	Attention-deficit hyperactivity disorder Anxiety Disruptive mood dysregulation disorder Enuresis Fetal alcohol/Neonatal abstinence syndrome Substance abuse Mental health comorbidity Physical disability

Source: Author.

Tasha offered the following when describing the exhausting task of supporting herself and children: "I'm hurting right now because I am not used to doing things on my own.... He misses his father, so it takes a toll on me.... He tells me that every second he get a chance." Likewise, informing the children about parents' whereabouts proved to be a point of internal contention. Ruby remembered, "It was hard for me to tell my grandson where his dad was. He [dad] would be with them all the time, so I knew it would be hard on them.... I told him right away..."

Tasha adds, "I didn't want to tell the kids about their dad. I didn't want to listen to myself say it out loud. I waited a while before I told them. I didn't know how. I didn't know where to start. I felt like the bad one, because I was the one delivering the news. I cried a lot over it. I prayed over it. I was so unhappy, bitter, and stressed that I started having nightmares about it. I had to just tell them." These predicaments culminate in the form of impractical demands and accommodations, disruption of parent-child bonds, management of child welfare, scarce financial and material resources, diminished human capital, and emotional labor. Parental imprisonment has significant punitive consequences, extending beyond the prison walls, that undermine familial relationships and create complicated conditions that force Black women into precarious mother work (Gurusami, 2019). It is crucial to consider the disparate, critical impact of the intersection of gender-racialized marginalization coupled with systems of carcerality as these structures reinforce the overreliance on, yet undervalued instrumental labor of, Black women.

Resilient Faith

Incarceration is a toxin for those left behind. The carceral crisis, coupled with caregiving duties, leads to emotional and physical labor, exhaustion, and distress. Caregivers were wary of sharing their tribulations with others for fear of scrutinization, distrust, and lack of empathy. Consequently, they drew on and prioritized their relationship with God through incessant prayer and meditation. The majority of caregivers explicitly indicated their dependence on, connection with, and confidence in God. The following excerpts illustrate their reliance: "God is who I call on, who I talk to when things are going wrong, and things are always going wrong. God is my best friend. My only friend" (Sunny). "I am great when it comes to my spiritual health. That is the only part of my life that has not been destroyed or broken. It seems to have gotten stronger through all this. Thank the Lord. Praise the Lord" (Jada).

Aligned with resilience concepts, caregivers maintained a positive outlook reinforced by their spiritual connection and capacity to identify supportive networks. As evident from the study recruitment strategy, caregivers exercised agency by enrolling children in mentoring programming to strengthen positive socialization while simultaneously taking advantage of a short reprieve from care work.

Black women have grown accustomed to unduly accepting challenges and making sacrifices for the greater good and family legacy (Giddings, 1984). While contemplating their expanded caregiving responsibilities, participants engaged in patterns of productive processing, careful to not ruminate on negative thoughts or become engulfed in pessimism. Instead, these caregivers, without clear viable alternative options, kept "dancing" and performing as taught—the habits of surviving. The collective sentiment of the caregivers was articulated by one grandmother: "God makes a way." Spiritual faith provides continued strength and resilience but the ingrained, learned habits sustains them.

Conclusion

The emergence of and exposure to the carceral state cuts deeper for and has had far-reaching collateral consequences for Black families (Coates, 2015). The additional layer of disproportionate incarceration rates exacerbates existing challenges within these vulnerable communities and has intergenerational social and health implications. Dialogues on carceral impacts rarely address the plight of women left to perform as sole caregivers—mothers, grandmothers, aunts, sisters, and other extended kin. Grandmothers described the experience of starting over as a new parent, at the age of 60. They vehemently expressed grieving their past and future lives. In spite of being relegated these arduous tasks with few instrumental assets, participants were compelled to enact parental duties given their profound commitment to preserve their families and communities.

Black women are well acquainted with struggle. Resilience has long been part of the Black experience, as it remains necessary to navigate racism, sexism, and classism. In this study, emergent themes included surrender, strain, and resilient faith. The process of surrendering led the caregivers to succumb to their current life predicament triggered by familial carceral bondage. Surrendering produced additional strains, manifesting as financial, emotional, social, and physical troubles. The implementation of the habits alongside unrelenting faith contributed to participants' invulnerable resilience. This union of habits and resilient faith did not mute the spillover effects of familial incarceration; however, they worked to mediate the impact. Research linking incarceration and health disparities merits further consideration. Historically, Black families have been known to gain their strength from the family matriarch. The self-sacrificing labor of Black women caregivers to children of persons incarcerated should be acknowledged and their selfless contributions championed and heralded.

Recommendations and Call for Action

Based on our findings, we recommend that public health professionals, clinicians, and policymakers:

1. Advocate for structural changes to disrupt and dismantle systems that perpetuate racism.
2. Become educated on, adopt, and implement an anti-racist, culturally responsive, trauma-informed culture of care.
3. Collaborate and coordinate with systems that families tend to navigate, such as public schools, social services, child welfare, and others to facilitate interventions.
4. Require systematic tracking of familial incarceration trends to better inform policies and service delivery.
5. Encourage cross-disciplinary collaboration between researchers and practitioners in social and health sciences. Ground research to center and amplify counternarratives.
6. Provide supportive spaces, such as group therapy (in venues like beauty salons) for families to share experiences, as they can be catalysts for micro/macro-level changes.
7. Implement in-home, family-based, and child-centered interventions for those connected to an incarcerated member.

Resources

For more information about families affected by incarceration, visit these resources:

Child Welfare Information Gateway. https://www.childwelfare.gov/topics/supporting/support-services/incarceration/
National Resource Center on Children and Families of the Incarcerated. https://nrccfi.camden.rutgers.edu/resources/directory/

References

Alexander, M. (2010). *The new Jim Crow: Mass incarceration in the age of colorblindness*. New Press.
American Psychological Association. (2012). *Building your resilience*. https://www.apa.org/topics/resilience/building-your-resilience
Arditti, J. A, Christian, J. C., & Thomas, S. S. (2020). Mass incarceration and Black families. In A. G. James (Ed.), *Black families: A systems approach*. Cognella Academic.
Burt, C. H., Simons, R. L., & Gibbons, F. X. (2012). Racial discrimination, ethnic-racial socialization, and crime: A micro-sociological model of risk and resilience. *American Sociological Review, 77*(4), 648–677. https://doi.org/10.1177/0003122412448648
Carson, E. A. (2020, October). *Prisoners in 2019* (Bureau of Justice Statistics Bulletin). Department of Justice, Office of Justice Programs.
Clear, T. R., & Frost, N. A. (2014). *The punishment imperative: The rise and failure of mass incarceration in America*. New York University Press.
Coates, T.-N. (2015, October 15). The black family in the age of mass incarceration. *The Atlantic*. https://www.theatlantic.com/magazine/archive/2015/10/the-black-family-in-the-age-of-mass-incarceration/403246/
Dallaire, D. H., Ciccone, A., & Wilson, L. C. (2010). Teachers' experiences with and expectations of children with incarcerated parents. *Journal of Applied Developmental Psychology, 31*(4), 281–290. https://doi.org/10.1016/j.appdev.2010.04.001
Drucker, E. (2011). *A plague of prisons: The epidemiology of mass incarceration in America*. New Press.
Giddings, P. (1984). *When and where I enter: The impact of Black women on race and sex in America*. Morrow.
Glaze, L. E., & Maruschak, L. M. (2008). *Parents in prison and their minor children* (Bureau of Justice Statistics Special Report). Department of Justice, Office of Justice Programs.

Gurusami, S. (2019). Motherwork under the state: The maternal labor of formerly incarcerated Black women. *Social Problems, 66*(1), 128–143. https://doi.org/10.1093/socpro/spx045

Harris, K. (2020, November). Vice-presidential acceptance speech. MSNBC.

Helms, H. M., & Demo, D.H. (2005). Everyday hassles and family stress. In P. C. McKenry and S. J. Price, *Families and change: Coping with stressful events and transitions* (3rd ed., pp. 375–378). Sage.

Karney, B. R., & Bradbury, T. N. (1995). The longitudinal course of marital quality and stability: A review of theory, method, and research. *Psychological Bulletin, 118*(1), 3–34. https://doi.org/10.1037/0033-2909.118.1.3

Kjellstrand, J. M., Reinke, W. M., & Eddy, J. M. (2018). Children of incarcerated parents: Development of externalizing behaviors across adolescence. *Children and Youth Services Review, 94*, 628–635. https://doi.org/10.1016/j.childyouth.2018.09.003

Lee, H., McCormick, T. H., Hicken, M. T., & Wildeman, C. (2015) Racial inequalities in connectedness to imprisoned individuals in the United States. *DuBois Review, 12*(2), 1–14. https://doi.org/10.1017/S1742058X15000065

Lee, H., & Wildeman, C. (2011). Things fall apart: Health consequences of mass imprisonment for African American women. *Review of Black Political Economy, 40*(1), 39–52. https://doi.org/10.1007/s12114-011-9112-4

Lee, H., Wildeman, C., Wang, E. A., Matusko, N., & Jackson, J. S. (2014). A heavy burden: The cardiovascular health consequences of having a family member incarcerated. *American Journal of Public Health, 104*(3), 421–427. https://doi.org/10.2105/AJPH.2013.301504

Luckey, I. (1996). African American elders: The support network of generational kin. *Families in Society, 75*(20), 82–89. https://doi.org/10.1177/104438949407500203

Muhammad, B. (2011). *Exploring the silence among children of Prisoners: A descriptive study* (Doctoral dissertation, Rutgers University Graduate School–Newark).

Muhammad, K. G. (2019). *The condemnation of Blackness: Race, crime, and the making of modern urban America* (with new preface). Harvard University Press.

Murray, J., Farrington, D. P., & Sekol, I. (2012). Children's antisocial behavior, mental health, drug use, and educational performance after parental incarceration: A systematic review and meta-analysis. *Psychological Bulletin, 138*(2), 175–210. https://doi.org/10.1037/a0026407

Patterson, E. J., Talbert, R. D., & Brown, T. N. (2020). Familial incarceration, social role combinations, and mental health among African American women. *Journal of Marriage and Family, 83*(1), 86–101. https://doi.org/10.1111/jomf.12699

Schnittker, J., Uggen, C., Shannon, S. K., & McElrath, S. M. (2015). The institutional effects of incarceration: Spillovers from criminal justice to health care. *Milbank Quarterly, 93*(3), 516–560. https://doi.org/10.1111/1468-0009.12136

Scott, K. Y. (1991). *The habit of surviving: Black women's strategies for life.* Rutgers University Press.

The Sentencing Project. (2013). *Report of the Sentencing Project to the United Nations Human Rights Committee: Regarding racial disparities in the United States criminal justice system.* https://www.sentencingproject.org/publications/shadow-report-to-the-united-nations-human-rights-committee-regarding-racial-disparities-in-the-united-states-criminal-justice-system/

The Sentencing Project. (2020). *Fact sheet: Incarcerated women and girls.* https://www.sentencingproject.org/publications/incarcerated-women-and-girls/

Turney, K. (2018). Adverse childhood experiences among children of incarcerated parents. *Children and Youth Services Review, 89,* 218–225. https://doi.org/10.1016/j.childyouth.2018.04.033

Ungar, M., Ghazinour, M., & Richter, J. (2013). Annual research review: What is resilience within the social ecology of human development? *Journal of Child Psychology and Psychiatry, 54*(4), 348–366. https://doi.org/10.1111/jcpp.12025

Van Maanen, J. (1979). The fact of fiction in organisational ethnography. *Administrative Science Quarterly, 24*(4), 539–549.

Wakefield, S., & Wildeman, C. (2014). *Children of the prison boom: Mass incarceration and the future of American inequality.* Oxford University Press.

Western, B., & Pettit, B. (2010). Incarceration and social inequality. *Daedalus, 139*(3), 8–19. https://doi.org/10.1162/DAED_a_00019

Wilkerson, I. (2020). *Caste: The origins of our discontents.* Random House.

Wilkins, A. C. (2012). Becoming Black women: Intimate stories and intersection identities. *Social Psychology Quarterly, 75*(2), 173–196. https://doi.org/10.1177/0190272512440106

Chapter 14

Resilience, Recovery, and Resistance
Black Women Overcoming Intersectional Complex Trauma

BRENDA INGRAM AND AMORIE ROBINSON

> You may shoot me with your words, you may cut me with your eyes, you may kill me with your hatefulness, but still, like air, I'll rise.
>
> —Maya Angelou, "Still I Rise" (1978, p. 197)

Black women have a long history of being resilient and surviving in the face of adversity and trauma. However, this process can take its toll on their well-being due to the overwhelming nature of enduring traumatic experiences. Black women live at the intersection of sexism and racism, which leaves them at risk for trauma. Their multiple sociocultural identities—for example, LGBTQ+,[1] socioeconomic status, immigration status, physical abilities, and age—intersect with their gender and racial identities (Crenshaw, 1994), increasing their risk of trauma responses (Sue, 2006). These multiple factors combine to create a type of complex trauma that will be referred to as *intersectional complex trauma* in this chapter. Such trauma contributes to significant health and social disparities for Black women, impacting their overall well-being (Comas-Diaz et al., 2019). To reduce these concerns, Black women need to build resilience, support networks, recovery skills, and resistance to trauma and oppression. Mental health providers working with Black women should emphasize their strengths such as self-efficacy and perseverance, to amplify their resilience and develop social activism that increases overall well-being. This chapter will discuss intersectional complex trauma and describe strategies that mental health providers can utilize to mitigate traumatic impacts at the micro and macro levels.

Improving the overall well-being of Black women means more than just the absence of mental and physical health illnesses. It includes emotional, physical, social, workplace, and societal well-being (Davis, 2019). The Full Frame Initiative, a national organization that focuses on equity and social justice approaches to achieve well-being, characterizes it as social connectedness, safety, stability, mastery, and meaningful access to resources (Full Frame Initiative, 2020). To achieve well-being, individuals must:

- have quality social relationships that nurture individuals and communities;
- be free from harm and feel safe in neighborhoods, homes, and institutions;
- have stability and predictability in all aspects of living;
- have mastery over ones' life which includes self-efficacy and empowerment to make decisions; and
- have access to the relevant resources that address basic living needs, such as food, healthcare, and shelter.

These domains of human life are interrelated and require a holistic and systemic approach to achieving well-being. One cannot "fix" one area without addressing the impact on another area. For example, a poor Black woman with children who is living with an abusive partner cannot be "pushed" to leave that relationship and home, unless the lack of affordable nondiscriminatory housing is addressed, or else that Black family faces the trauma of homelessness.

Given that Black women's well-being is rooted in sociocultural interconnectedness based on intersecting identities, it is important to explore the theory of intersectionality originally coined by Kimberlé Crenshaw in 1989 and further discussed in the essay, "Mapping the Margins" (1994): "The experiences of women of color are frequently the product of intersecting patterns of racism and sexism . . . the interests and experiences of women of color are frequently marginalized within both . . . and . . . the intersection of racism and sexism factors into Black women's lives in ways that cannot be captured wholly by looking at the woman's race or gender dimensions of those experiences separately." These processes of intersectionality and marginalization further include identities across attractional orientation and gender identity. The health concerns of Black women and girls who are lesbian-identified are even more overlooked or marginalized (Stansbury et al., 2010;), especially those lesbians who are "masculine-identified" (Robinson, 2010; Moore, 2011). Most Black women, including poor Black women, Black cisgender lesbians[2], and Black transgender women, are at high risk for developing complex traumatic responses due to intersections of racism, sexism, gendered racism, classism, heterosexism, homophobia, and transphobia within the context of systemic powerlessness and oppression (Bowleg et al., 2003; Grant et al., 2011; Greene, 1996; Lewis et al., 2013).

Risk factors affecting the well-being of Black women starts in childhood. Due to their gender, girls are rendered an oppressed and subordinate identity because they exist within a patriarchal system in which men dominate women, and what is considered as masculine is valued over what is considered feminine (De La Rue & Ortega, 2019). For example, girls born and raised in highly sexist states carry those beliefs throughout their lives regardless of where they live or their educational attainments in adulthood, and these beliefs interfere with their economic aspirations (Charles et al., 2018). This includes girls who are lesbian and transgender. They are likely to internalize negative messages about girls and their gender roles and expectations within the culture, furthering their despair, low self-esteem, and poor opinions about females in general.

These experiences of socialized and internalized sexism intersect with racism and raise more complexities for Black girls and adolescents. Racism is an oppressive system of structuring opportunity and assigning value based on the social interpretation of skin color, or how someone looks (Jones, 2002; Sue, 2006). It disadvantages one group, while advantaging another group (Jones, 2002; Sue, 2006). Racism can lead to chronic stress reactions and disease in children and adults, now defined as racial trauma (Comas-Diaz et al., 2019). Stress that a Black mother experiences during pregnancy has been linked to high Black infant mortality (Trent et al., 2019). Intersecting with classism, Black girls raised in Black communities by single Black mothers are more likely to live in homes with higher unemployment and lower incomes with less access to adequate housing, nutrition, health care, and quality education than White children. Such disparities increase their risk of physical health and mental health problems, chronic lower-class status, poorer educational outcomes, lower job status, and less-resourced communities (Trent et al., 2019; McCarthy, 2020).

For Black girls, the educational system can be a dangerous and perplexing place. Their race and gender render their educational needs invisible and marginalized. They deserve specialized educational services similar to My Brothers' Keeper, which targets Black boys (Ricks, 2014). Black girls experience higher rates of sexual harassment and racial slurs in school settings than White girls. When these experiences of marginalization and microaggressions cause an activation of the trauma survival response of "fight or flight," Black girls face greater risks of punitive and violent oppressive responses when they choose to "fight" or speak up about injustices. Black girls are twice as likely to receive multiple suspensions and they are expelled at rates six times higher than White girls (Crenshaw et al., 2015; Morris, 2016). These responses by the educational system are based on racist and sexist stereotypes that characterize Black girls as "aggressive, angry, hypersexual, and promiscuous," which justify punitive measures (Tucker & Chaudhry, 2017; Ricks, 2014; Morris, 2016).

Black girls also experience higher rates of sexual abuse and assault than boys and this rate continues throughout their lives, making them more vulnerable to trauma. More than 1 in 5 girls in general have reported sexual violence, but for Black girls that rate is 1 in 4 (Barlow, 2020). Black girls who identify as lesbian or queer have even higher rates; almost 1 in 3 girls reported experiencing either sexual assault or other violence (Tucker & Chaudhry, 2017). Sexual violence is just one type of violence that Black girls and women experience at higher rates than their White counterparts. Black girls are at greater risk of experiencing violence in their teen dating relationships. Acts of intimate partner violence are 35% higher for Black women than for White women. Black women are three times more likely to die from domestic violence than other ethnicities and this is the leading cause of death of Black women aged 18 to 35 (Petrosky et al., 2017).

The Sentencing Project (2018) reports that Black girls are detained in juvenile facilities at higher rates than White girls and receive harsher punishments than their male counterparts for similar offenses. This trend continues into adulthood, where Black women are incarcerated at a rate that is 1.7 times greater than White women. Black lesbians and transgender youth are at a higher disproportionate rate of juvenile and adult criminal incarceration (Robinson, 2017; Movement Advancement Project, 2016). Nearly half of all Black transgender people have been imprisoned (Grant et al., 2011).

Intersectional Complex Trauma

Complex trauma is a condition where an individual experiences multiple traumatic events or adversities starting in childhood that impact psychosocial development, neurodevelopment, and physical health. It generally refers to traumatic stressors that are interpersonal—premeditated, planned, and caused by other humans, such as violation or exploitation of another person; repetitive, prolonged, or cumulative, involving direct harm; and maltreatment and neglect/abandonment/antipathy (Herman, 1992).

Complex trauma is more complicated for Black women due to intersectionality. They have a form of complex trauma that can be referred to as *intersectional complex trauma*. This type of trauma involves both interpersonal and structural violence. Black women are victims of various types of interpersonal violence, such as sexual violence, intimate partner violence, child abuse and neglect, acts of discrimination and hate crimes, and so on. Black lesbians and gender nonconforming people have experienced homophobic violence and abuse from their own family members and peers, starting at young ages. For example, Black transgender girls are often detected early in childhood as gender nonconforming boys, which stigmatizes them as a "defective" boy unworthy of being valued, making them vulnerable to verbal and physical harassment as children and victims to murder as they become older (Toomey et al., 2018; Truong et al., 2020). Lesbian and transgender young women suffer at similar and sometimes higher rates of dating and intimate partner violence (Gillum, 2017). They are concurrently victims of structural violence from discriminatory policies and practices such as housing discrimination, welfare regulations, limited access to quality medical care, and so on. These traumatic experiences intersect with historical and intergenerational trauma (trauma memories passed down through generations in DNA coding) and racial trauma. Additionally, these experiences occur in the context of systemic powerlessness and oppression. *Intersectional complex trauma* can be described as multidimensional and multilayered.

Intersectional complex trauma creates vulnerabilities that contribute to social disparities, poor mental and physical health, and consequently a reduction in positive well-being for Black women and girls. For example, experiencing sexual abuse, community violence, poverty, poor educational practices, racial discrimination, and sexist ideology can negatively impact a young Black girl's self-esteem, which influences decision-making that contributes to adulthood disparities. The outcomes of these negative childhood experiences on physical health are well-documented in the Adverse Childhood Experiences Study, which found a solid correlation between negative adult health outcomes, such as heart disease, cancer, smoking, obesity, drug use, mental illness, diabetes, and high blood pressure, and chronic traumatic experiences starting in childhood (Felitti et al., 1998). Such experiences occur within an oppressive system of structural violence that intentionally limits access to supportive systems and services, increasing these vulnerabilities.

Judith Herman (1992) asserts that recovery from trauma happens in three phases. The first phase focuses on building stability and safety. Clinicians working with Black women need to understand that their recovery occurs in the context of societal oppression and structural violence and work to create "safe spaces" for healing that have both physical and emotional safety. The second phase happens when survivors tell their stories and they are believed, validated, and supported. Clinicians need to have addressed their own implicit biases that could interfere with listening and validating Black women's lived experiences of oppression and discrimination. The third phase is when the clinician works on personal and cultural connections within the self, family, and community. Helping survivors reconnect with their bodies through self-care and healthy practices can contribute to recovery, as well as building racial identity and pride through activities focusing on sociohistorical stories, cultural traditions, spirituality, religious practices, and so on. Assisting Black women with connecting to resources such as peer support groups is in line with best practices.

Black Women and Resilience

Resilience is the ability to "bounce" back after experiencing adversity and trauma. Resilience is a multidimensional dynamic process and not a static state, trait, or characteristic. It is an interaction of risk and protective factors, which are internal and external to the person. These factors include individual traits, family influences, and community variables (Powell et al., 2020). The internal protective factors include the individual's ability to self-regulate, positive outlook/optimism, problem-solving skills, self-efficacy, sense of purpose, positive self-image, positive physical health, and so on. The external factors include supportive adults (parents), safe neighborhoods, fair rules and structures, adequate living resources, healthy peer relationships, positive activities, supportive schools, and so on (Powell et al., 2020). Cultural factors, such as spirituality, religious affiliation, ethnic/cultural practices, and ties to a community are integral components of resilience. It is a process of integrating internal and external protective factors, both individual and collective, that support well-being. It is an active process that is radically intentional. It requires that the individual "take action" using both innate and newly discovered skills to disrupt the negative impacts of multiple adversity and trauma.

Black women's resilience derives from multiple levels of protective factors that include the individual, family, peers, community, and societal and institutional influences. For example, individual characteristics of "inner strength" include optimism and positivity, spirituality/religious beliefs, self-care, and perseverance. The influences of these levels are bidirectional, and the Black woman has the power to impact these levels as they impact her existence (Qiao et al., 2019; Banyard et al., 2002; Felix et al., 2019; Powell et al., 2020). As protective factors buffer them from adverse experiences, Black women are likely to achieve and sustain healthy well-being. Strengthening these factors is essential for the recovery process from intersectional complex trauma (Conway-Phillips et al., 2020). Simultaneous dismantling of oppressive systems must occur in order to strengthen resiliencies for Black women. Black women with inner strength, optimal family support, and dependable social connections will still experience distress from racism, sexism, gendered racism, classism, heterosexism, homophobia, transphobia, and so on. Therefore, it is important to build resilience but also engage in political and social activism to change systemic oppressions (De La Rue & Ortega, 2019).

Trauma Informed Recovery Builds Resilience and Resistance

Trauma-informed care approaches are strongly recommended as best practices for facilitating recovery from complex trauma in Black women. According to the Substance Abuse and Mental Health Services Administration (SAMHSA), trauma-informed care makes four assumptions about services: realization of the pervasiveness of trauma, recognition of trauma symptoms, integration of understanding about trauma in policies and practices, and resistance to retraumatization. Also, SAMHSA lists the six key principles of trauma-informed care:

- safety
- trustworthiness and transparency
- peer support
- collaboration and mutuality
- empowerment, strength-focused
- cultural, historical, and gender issues

These principles offer tools to address the psychological effects of intersectional complex trauma such as powerlessness; social disconnection; and the lack of social justice.

Trauma-informed care for Black women should integrate liberation psychology, Black psychology, womanist models, and LGBT-affirming approaches to broaden positive aspects of recovery. They underscore the sociopolitical structures negatively impacting the lives of oppressed communities. For example, liberation psychology draws upon the need for communities to (a) recover their [rich] historical memory which revives and employs methods used by their ancestors to survive, resist, and organize, and (b) strengthen cultural pride and tradition. Healing entails an explicit focus on active resistance rather than solely reactionary resilience (Chavez-Dueñas et al., 2019). Liberation psychology uses four ways to build resistance: first, members of oppressed groups view their oppression as a collective assault requiring a unified response (e.g., social organizing). Secondly, that clinicians conceptualize problems and interventions within a social-historical context. Thirdly, that clinicians promote self-determination and self-efficacy. And finally, action toward change explicitly targets institutions and systems that create and maintain oppression (Chavez-Dueñas et al., 2019).

An illustration of liberation psychology is the power of Black lesbian resilience and radical coping strategies for withstanding oppressive forces and managing their own self-care (Clark, 1981; Follins et al., 2014; Lassiter,

2017; Meyer, 2010; Walker & Longmire-Avital, 2013). Most well-functioning Black lesbians have shown great endurance and persistence through hardships over the decades and have participated in Black and LGBT activism as leaders. In fact, Black women queer activists founded the Black Lives Matter movement (Green, 2019). To place them in an historical context, Black lesbians inherited a legacy of triumph against those who target them and have found ways to resist systems of oppression and thrive despite the struggles (Lassiter, 2017), providing useful roadmaps of activism.

Finally, liberation psychology in the recovery process integrates the awareness of being a member of an oppressed group with how to "take action" through a collectivist approach. Research suggests that social action is associated with positive mental health and well-being (Chavez-Dueñas et al., 2019). All four phases can overlap, occur simultaneously, and/or be cyclical. In addition to liberation psychology are Black psychology, LGBT-affirming, and womanist models of psychotherapy, which are also in alignment with the intersectional traumatic experiences of Black women and girls (for more details see Belgrave, 2019; Ginicola et al., 2017; Myers, 2013).

Conclusions

Black women are at great risk for developing health and social disparities that impact their well-being, due to various interpersonal and societal forces that are trauma-inducing and that combine to create a type of complex trauma that is more insidious and complicated in nature. It is intersectional and includes interpersonal, structural, societal, and historical/intergenerational impacts. To support Black women's recovery from *intersectional complex trauma*, it is recommended that clinicians use a trauma-informed approach that incorporates the strengthening of resilience and the building of resistant behaviors. This approach utilizes empowerment and strength-based interventions, prioritizing client choice, creating safety, trust, and respect within the therapeutic relationship, and minimizing potential retraumatization. When working with Black women who are heteroattractional, cisgender lesbians, and transgender, a clinician must be mindful of Black cultural nuances, language, microaggressions, misgendering, nonvalidating statements, denial of societal oppressions, and other triggering behaviors that can disrupt the therapeutic alliance. For example, using a client's preferred name and asking what pronouns they use are standard best practices.

Recommendations and Call for Action

Clinicians must practice "humility" while listening and learning about Black women's lived experiences and partner with the families and communities of Black female clients. However, beyond the micro level of therapy is the work to be done on the macro level. Mental health providers must realize how trauma reflects broader oppressive forces that need to be addressed. Strategies include dismantling power differentials that disempower their clients; policies; regulations; and practices. Organizations that wish to provide a trauma-informed environment for their Black women clients need to be mindful of institutional practices that can trigger trauma reactions, for example, so-called conversion therapies used on LGBT clients. Professional development trainings that are comprehensive and inclusive of women across the entire span of variation can be beneficial when conducted frequently. Clinicians can build upon a client's resilience by helping them to make meaning of the traumatic events as an opportunity for growth, while acknowledging the impact. The need to support the development of activism and resistance cannot be stressed enough as it is the antidote to powerlessness.

More research is needed to further document and define intersectional complex trauma along with culturally appropriate trauma-informed interventions at both the micro and macro levels of well-being. All research needs to include the independent and intersectional effects of multiple forms of oppression on the health of Black lesbians and transgender women as well (Wilson et al., 2011).

Notes

1. LGBT+ are individuals who identify as lesbian, gay, biattractional, transgender, and other attractional orientations, gender identities, gender expressions, and nonbinary identities.

2. Cisgender is being used to distinguish between lesbians that are cisgender and lesbians that are transgender women, realizing that transgender women also have attractional orientations just as cisgender women do. Cisgender is a term to describe individuals whose sex assigned at birth aligns with their internal sense of gender. This further affirms the distinction between attraction and gender identity.

Resources

Association of Black Psychologists. https://abpsi.site-ym.com
black girls breathing. https://www.blackgirlsbreathing.com

Black Lesbians United. www.blacklesbiansunited.org
National Association of Black Social Workers. www.nabsw.org
National Black Justice Coalition. http://nbjc.org
Ruth Ellis Center. www.ruthelliscenter.org
Safe Black Space. www.safeblackspace.org/resources/
The Safe Place. www.facebook.com/TheSafePlaceTSP/
Taraji P. Henson's foundation [which is offering free virtual therapy]. www.borishensonfoundation.org
Therapy for Black Girls. https://www.therapyforblackgirls.com
U.S. transgender study/Black respondents report 2015. https://www.transequality.org/sites/default/files/docs/usts/USTSBlackRespondentsReport-Nov17.pdf
Zami Nobla. www.zaminobla.org

References

Angelou, M. (1978). Still I rise. In *And still I rise: A book of poems*. Random House.
Banyard, V. L., Williams, L. M., Siegel, J. A., & West, C. M. (2002). Childhood sexual abuse in the lives of Black women. *Women and Therapy, 25*(3–4), 45–58. https://doi.org/10.1300/J015v25n03_04
Barlow, J. N. (2020). Black women, the forgotten survivors of sexual assault. *In the Public Interest* [Newsletter]. https://www.apa.org/pi/about/newsletter/2020/02/black-women-sexual-assault
Belgrave, F. (2019). Womanism and African-centered psychology: Converging perspectives. *Psych Discourse, 53*(1). http://psychdiscourse.com/2013-08-20-02-30-17/version-53-2019/spring-2019-v53-1?view=article&id=748:featured-5&catid=331
Bowleg, L., Huang, J., Brooks, K., Black, A., & Burkholder, G. (2003). Triple jeopardy and beyond: Multiple minority stress and resilience among Black lesbians. *Journal of Lesbian Studies, 7*(4), 87–108. https://doi.org/10.1300/J155v07n04_06
Charles, K. K., Guryan, J., & Pan, J. (2018). The effects of sexism on American women: The role of norms versus discrimination [Working paper]. Becker Friedman Institute, University of Chicago.
Chavez-Dueñas, N. Y., Adames, H. Y., Perez-Chavez, J. G., and Salas, S. P. (2019). Healing ethno-racial trauma in Latinx immigrant communities: Cultivating hope, resistance, and action. *American Psychologist, 74*(1), 49–62. https://doi.org/10.1037/amp0000289
Comas-Diaz, L., Hall, G. N., & Neville, H.A. (2019). Racial trauma: Theory, research, and healing. *American Psychologist, 74*(1), 1–5. https://doi.org/10.1037/amp0000442
Conway-Phillips, R., Dagadu, H., Motley, D., Shawahin, L., Janusek, L. W., Klonowski, L., & Saban, K. L. (2020). Qualitative evidence for resilience,

stress, and ethnicity (RiSE): A program to address race-based stress among Black women at risk for cardiovascular disease. *Complementary Therapies in Medicine, 48,* Article 102277. https://doi.org/10.1016/j.ctim.2019.102277

Crenshaw, K. (1994) Mapping the Margins: Intersectionality, identity politics, and violence against women of color. In M. A. Fineman, R. Mykitiuk (Eds.), *The public nature of private violence* (pp. 93–118). Routledge.

Crenshaw, K. W., Ocen, P., & Nanda, J. (2015). *Black girls matter: Pushed out, overpoliced and underprotected.* African American Policy Forum & Columbia Law School Center for Intersectionality and Social Policy Studies.

Davis, T. (2019, January 2). What is well-being? Definition, types, and well-being skills. *Psychology Today.* https://www.psychologytoday.com/us/blog/click-here-happiness/201901/what-is-well-being-definition-types-and-well-being-skills

De La Rue, L., and Ortega, L. (2019). Intersectional trauma-responsive care: A framework for humanizing care for justice involved girls and women of color. *Journal of Aggression, Maltreatment and Trauma, 28*(4), 502–517. https://doi.org/10.1080/10926771.2019.1572403

Dentato, M. P. (Ed.). (2017). *Social work practice with the LGBTQ community: The intersection of history, health, mental health, and policy factors.* Oxford University Press.

Dragowski, E. A., Halkitis, P. N., Grossman, A. H., D'Augelli, A. R. (2011). Sexual orientation victimization and posttraumatic stress symptoms among lesbian, gay, and bisexual youth. *Journal of Gay and Lesbian Social Services, 23*(2), 226–249. https://doi.org/10.1080/10538720.2010.541028

Felitti, V. J., Anda, R. F., Nordenberg, D., Williamson, D. F., Spitz, A. M., Edwards, V., Koss, M. P., & Marks, J. S. (1998). Relationship of childhood abuse and household dysfunction to many of the leading causes of death in adults: The Adverse Childhood Experiences (ACE) Study. *American Journal of Preventive Medicine, 14*(4), 245–258. https://doi.org/10.1016/S0749-3797(98)00017-8

Felix, A. S., Lehman, A., Nolan, T. S., Sealy-Jefferson, S., Breathett, K., Hood, D. B., Addison, D., Anderson, C. M., Cené, C. W., Warren, B. J., Jackson, R. D., & Williams, K. P. (2019). Stress, resilience, and cardiovascular disease among Black women. *Circulation: Cardiovascular Quality and Outcomes, 12*(4), 1–14. https://doi.org/10.1161/CIRCOUTCOMES.118.005284

Follins, L. D., Garrett-Walker, J. J., & Lewis, M. K. (2014). Resilience in Black lesbian, gay, bisexual, and transgender individuals: A critical review of the literature. *Journal of Gay and Lesbian Mental Health, 18*(2), 190–212. https://doi.org/10.1080/19359705.2013.828343

Full Frame Initiative. (2020). *The five domains of wellbeing.* https://fullframeinitiative.org/wp-content/uploads/2019/09/Five-Domains-of-Wellbeing-Overview.pdf

Gillum, T. (2017). Adolescent dating violence experiences among sexual minority youth and implications for subsequent relationship quality. *Journal of Child and Adolescent Social Work, 34*(2), 137–145. https://doi.org/10.1007/s10560-016-0451-7

Ginicola, M. M., Smith, C., & Filmore, J. M. (Eds.). (2017). *Affirmative counseling with LGBTQI+ people*. Wiley.

Grant, J. M., Mottet, L. A., Tanis, J., Harrison, J., Herman, J. L., & Keisling, M. (2011). *Injustice at every turn: A report of the National Transgender Discrimination Survey*. National Center for Transgender Equality and National Gay and Lesbian Task Force.

Green, D. B. (2019, February 6). Hearing the queer roots of Black Lives Matter. National Center for Institutional Diversity. https://medium.com/national-center-for-institutional-diversity/hearing-the-queer-roots-of-black-lives-matter-2e69834a65cd

Greene, B. (1996). Lesbian women of color: Triple jeopardy. *Journal of Lesbian Studies, 1*(1), 109–147. https://doi.org/10.1300/J155v01n01_09

Herman, J. L. (1992). Complex PTSD: A syndrome in survivors of prolonged and repeated trauma. *Journal of Traumatic Stress, 5*(3), 377–391. https://doi.org/10.1002/jts.2490050305

Jones, C. P. (2002). Confronting Institutionalized Racism. *Phylon, 50*(1–2), 7–22. https://stacks.cdc.gov/view/cdc/104986

Lassiter, J. M. (2017). Black bisexual women's health in the United States: A systematic literature review. In L. D. Follins & J. M. Lassiter (Eds.), *Black LGBT health in the United States: The intersection of race, gender, and sexual orientation* (pp. 25–38). Lexington Books.

Lewis, J., Mendenhall, R., Harwood, S. A., & Browne Huntt, M. (2013). Coping with gendered racial microaggressions among Black women college students. *Journal of African American Studies, 17*(1), 51–73. https://doi.org/10.1007/s12111-012-9219-0

McCarthy, C. (2020, January 8). How racism harms children. *Harvard Health Blog*. https://www.health.harvard.edu/blog/how-racism-harms-children-2019091417788

Meyer, I. H. (2010). Identity, stress, and resilience in lesbians, gay men, and bisexuals of color. *Counseling Psychology, 38*(3), 442–454. https://doi.org/10.1177/0011000009351601

Moore, M. R. (2011). *Invisible families: Gay identities, relationships, and motherhood among Black women*. University of California Press.

Morris, M. W. (2016). *Pushout: The criminalization of Black girls in schools*. New Press.

Movement Advancement Project. (2016, June). *Infographic: LGBT and GNC girls face criminalization*. http://www.lgbtmap.org/infographic-lgbt-girls-face-criminalization

Myers, L. J. (2013). Healing, coping, & transcending the Legacy of racism, sexism, & lassism. In H. Lowman-Jackson (Ed.), *Afrikan American women: Living at the crossroads of race, gender, class, and culture* (pp. 387–396). Cognella.

National Center on Violence against Women in the Black Community. (2018). *Black women and sexual assault.* https://ujimacommunity.org/wp-content/uploads/2018/12/Ujima-Womens-Violence-Stats-v7.4-1.pdf

Petrosky, E., Blair, J. M., Betz, C. J., Fowler, K. A., Jack, S. P., & Lyons, B. H. (2017). Racial and ethnic differences in homicides of adult women and the role of intimate partner violence—United States, 2003-2014. *Morbidity and Mortality Weekly Report, 66*(28), 741-746. https://doi.org/10.15585%2Fmmwr.mm6628a1

Powell, K. M., Rahm-Knigge, R. L., & Conner, B. T. (2020) Resilience protective factors checklist (RPFC): Buffering childhood adversity and promoting positive outcomes. *Psychological Reports, 124*(4), 1-25. https://doi.org/10.1177/0033294120950288

Qiao, S., Ingram, L., Deal, M. L., Li, X., & Weissman, S. B. (2019). Resilience resources among African American women living with HIV in southern United States. *AIDS, 33,* 35-44. https://doi.org/10.1097/QAD.0000000000002179

Ricks, S. A. (2014). Falling through the cracks: Black girls and education. *Interdisciplinary Journal of Teaching and Learning, 4*(1), 10-21.

Robinson, A. (2010). Living for the city: Voices of Black lesbian youth in Detroit. *Journal of Lesbian Studies, 14*(1), 61-70. https://doi.org/10.1080/10894160903058899

Robinson, A. (2017). The Forgotten Intersection: Black LGBTQ and Gender Nonconforming Youth in Juvenile Detention in the United States. In L. Follins & J. Lassiter (Eds.), *Black LGBT health in the United States: The intersection of race, gender, and sexual orientation* (pp. 11-23). Lexington Books.

The Sentencing Project. (2018). *Incarcerated women and girls.* https://www.sentencingproject.org/publications/incarcerated-women-and-girls/

Stansbury, K., Harley, D. A., Allen, S., Nelson, N. J., & Christensen, K. (2010). African American lesbians: A selective review of the literature. *African American Research Perspectives, 11*(1), 99-108.

Sue, D. W. (2006). The invisible Whiteness of being: Whiteness, White supremacy, White privilege, and racism. In M. G. Constantine & D. W. Sue (Eds.), *Addressing racism: Facilitating cultural competence in mental health and educational settings* (pp. 15-30). Wiley.

Toomey, R. B., Syvertsen, A. K., & Shramko, M. (2018). Transgender adolescent suicide behavior. *Pediatrics, 142*(4), Article e20174218. https://doi.org/10.1542/peds.2017-4218

Trent, M., Dooley, G., Douge, J. (2019) The impact of racism on child and adolescent health. *Pediatrics, 144*(2), 3-14. https://doi.org/10.1542/peds.2019-1765

Truong, N. L., Zongrone, A. D., & Kosciw, J. G. (2020). *Erasure and resilience: The experiences of LGBTQ students of color, Black LGBTQ youth in U.S. schools.* Gay, Lesbian and Straight Education Network (GLSEN).

Tucker, J., &Chaudhry, N. (2017). Overview and key findings. In *Let her learn: Stopping school pushout*. National Women's Law Center.

Walker, J. J., & Longmire-Avital, B. (2013). The impact of religious faith and internalized homonegativity on resiliency for Black lesbian, gay, and bisexual emerging adults. *Developmental Psychology, 49*(9), 1723–1731. https://psycnet.apa.org/doi/10.1037/a0031059

Wilson, B. D., Okwu, C., & Mills, S. A. (2011). Brief report: The relationship between multiple forms of oppression and subjective health among Black lesbian and bisexual women. *Journal of Lesbian Studies, 15*(1), 15–24. https://doi.org/10.1080/10894160.2010.508393

Chapter 15

"I Feel Some Type of Way"
Experiences of Relationship Violence, Resilience, and Resistance among Urban Black Girls

LeConté J. Dill, Bianca D. Rivera, Shavaun S. Sutton, and Elizabeth O. Ige

Introduction

The concept of resilience describes the dynamic process of individuals and communities to adapt positively and successfully despite adversities (Luthar et al., 2000). Resilience acknowledges exposure to risk factors with which populations must contend, and these risk factors tend to be significant and ongoing during adolescence (Fergus & Zimmerman, 2005). The last nearly 70 years of resilience research has called for a shift in our analysis and our interventions toward the mechanisms and strategies that individuals and communities activate in the pursuit of wellness and healthy living (Benard, 1991; Dill, 2011; Fergus & Zimmerman, 2005; Garmezy, 1991; Luthar et al., 2000; Masten et al., 1999; Rutter, 1985; Werner et al., 1971; Werner & Smith, 1977). Nevertheless, much of resilience research has been criticized for (1) focusing too much attention on the individual and family levels of influence, and not giving enough attention to the community and political level contexts, (2) not attending to youth's agency and their active participation in the self-actualization process, and (3) only considering nationally representative or White middle-class samples (Wright & Masten, 2015; Fergus & Zimmerman, 2005; Ungar et al., 2007; Zimmerman & Arunkumar, 1994).

Importantly, research by Spencer (1995; Spencer et al., 1997) and Jarrett (1995, 1997) contribute to our fields' understanding of the concept of adolescent resilience for Black youth. Their research highlights families and other supportive adults as protective factors and identifies the salience of developing positive racial identity for successful adaptation among Black youth. However, the larger risk and resilience research discourse still has much to learn and explore in terms of the role of gender in the lives of young people. The under-theorization of gender and gender-based inequities in resilience research has major implications for the ways that structural oppressions, violence, and health outcomes manifest and the ways in which programs, policies, and funding are subsequently doled out and restricted in communities. In fact, Black girls experience intersecting forms of oppressions and exhibit multiple forms of agency based on their race, gender, class, sexuality, age, and ability status (Crenshaw, 1991; Jones, 2000; Ford & Airhihenbuwa, 2010).

"Feel some type of way" is a colloquial term used to both define one's complex emotions and the inability to fully articulate such complexity. In our weekly interactions with African American, Caribbean American, and West African high school girls participating in a violence prevention program, to be detailed later in the chapter, they frequently used the phrase "feel some type of way" regarding a myriad of issues. In particular, one girl said, "I feel some type of way" when discussing her experiences with dating violence. Unhealthy, abusive, or violent relationships can have severe consequences and short- and long-term negative effects across the life course. Teen dating violence is specifically defined as the infliction, or threat of infliction, of physical, sexual, psychological, or emotional violence within a dating relationship to establish control over a romantic partner (Hays et al., 2009). Nationally, 21% of young women and 10% of young men report experiencing physical violence or sexual dating violence annually (Vagi et al., 2015). Notably, the 2013 Youth Risk Behavior Surveillance System (YRBS), administered by the Centers for Disease Control and Prevention (CDC), was the first time that a national survey began to assess both physical teen dating violence and sexual teen dating violence (Vagi et al., 2015). Additionally, much of the research on teen dating violence has focused on White, middle-class college students, while communities of color, younger populations, and low-income youth remain underexamined (Jackson, 1999; Sugarman & Hotaling, 1989; West & Rose, 2000). This oversight is glaring, because communities of color, due to their marginalized status, are actually at increased risk for dating violence victimization. In particular, Black and Latinx high school youth generally experience more teen dating violence than White high school youth (Alleyne-Green et al., 2012; Catalano et al., 2009; East & Hokoda, 2015).

As Black girls seek out safe spaces in, around, and for themselves in their dating relationships, as well as in their families, neighborhoods, and schools, our chapter illuminates mechanisms of Black girls' resilience and resistance. Through this chapter, we show how high school–aged Black girls enact multiple socio-ecological and biocultural strategies in order navigate safety and healing amid relationship violence.

Methods

Research Setting

Our study is focused on a violence prevention program for high school girls based in two small schools in Central Brooklyn—the Women's Program of the Kings against Violence Initiative (KAVI). Four small high schools occupy the educational campus in Central Brooklyn in which KAVI's programs for high school–aged youth take place. At the time of data collection, KAVI programming engaged a sample of students from two of these small schools, reaching an average of 15 high school girls each year. KAVI uses a combination of multiple approaches and strategies, as recommended by the Centers for Disease Control and Prevention (CDC), to prevent youth violence by utilizing local resources, mentorship, and a social skill-building curriculum. The curriculum is comprised of one-hour, 30-session interactive interventions categorized into 5 modules: (1) Gender Pride/Self Worth, (2) Healthy Relationships, (3) Sexual Health, (4) Conflict Management, and (5) Dream and Goal Setting. The KAVI Women's Program engaged approximately 40 high school–aged African American, Caribbean American, West African, and Latinx young women in its programming from 2011 to 2016. The 2015–2016 cohort of KAVI Women's Program participants (with whom individual interviews took place) consisted of 18 girls. KAVI's programming, reach, and visibility has grown exponentially since the time of our study.

Data Collection and Analysis

To inform our analyses of our participants' experiences with dating, we use multiple and innovative methodological approaches that are culturally, politically, and epistemologically suited for working with this population (Emerson et al., 2011; Lindsay-Dennis, 2015). In particular, the coauthors, all women of color, spent three and a half years conducting direct and participant observation at weekly KAVI sessions. After gaining approval from the Institutional Review Board of the State University of New York Downstate Medical Center, we conducted one-hour semistructured interviews with 15 young women of African American, Caribbean American, and West African descent, ages 16–21, who attend or have attended the focal high schools and have participated in KAVI. This was a purposive, nonproportional quota sample of current and alumnae KAVI Women's Program participants, reflecting similarly small, but rich and representative, sample sizes as other studies of adolescent development among urban youth of color (Ruglis, 2011; Wun, 2016). Interviews were audiotaped and then transcribed by the third author.

Analysis was guided by a thematic approach (Emerson et al., 2011). Interview text was read first to identify emergent themes. The first author reread interview text to develop detailed codes and subcodes (Saldaña, 2015). Next, the second author reread the transcripts and developed codes and subcodes separately. To establish inter-rater reliability, all authors met and discussed the results of their separate analyses, reconciled any inconsistencies, and agreed upon final themes, codes, subcodes, and related definitions for our codebook (Merriam & Tisdell, 2015). A total of 22 codes and 166 subcodes were developed. Codes and subcodes included: "dating," "relationships," "boyfriends," "girlfriends," "sex," "emotions," "fighting," "safe," "respect," "trust," and "understanding." Next, the Dedoose web-based analytical program was used to aid in sorting and management of the qualitative data. Analytic memos were developed that addressed the themes, analytic points, and interpretation of the analytic points (Emerson et al., 2011).

Emergent themes were initially member checked in discussions with the staff from KAVI. We also conducted a total of five poetry workshops with the young women in KAVI, incorporating the method of "participatory narrative analysis" (Dill, 2015), which provided additional member checks of the data, themes, and preliminary analyses, as a way of increasing validity (Furman et al., 2007). Through the participatory narrative analysis workshops, girls in KAVI were introduced to poetic techniques, poetic forms, and published works of Black women writers, such as Nikki Giovanni, Remica L. Bingham, Mahogany Browne, Angel Nafis, and t'ai freedom ford, which helped us engage in a deeper discussion of interpersonal relationships, romantic relationships, dating violence, trauma, and resistance in their lives. KAVI participants then created "interpretive poems" (Langer & Furman, 2004), detailed in a previous manuscript (Dill et al., 2018), which revealed their own lived experiences with relationship violence and dating violence in poetic form.

The interview excerpts below contextually illustrate and are representative of the key thematic points that emerged during analysis. These excerpts reveal the KAVI young women's experiences with navigating emotional, physical, and sexual violence and activating resilience in their dating and romantic relationships.

Results

> For women, the body, the home, and the street have all been areas of conflict.
>
> —Dolores Hayden, *The Power of Place* (1997)

THE STREET

Our participants live in environments where they have learned to expect and accept street harassment. Rihanna (all names used are pseudonyms, selected by the participants), an 18-year-old college freshman, shares:

> But it's just like the way that teens in my neighborhood acts. It's like they don't really seem to have respect for females. It's like once I step out of my house, it's like someone calling me either out my name or trying to talk to me or like walking behind me, tryna talk to me. It's just too much going on, even though I love the amount of personalities that surround me, sometimes it can become too much. . . . I have to walk past my building because I don't want anyone to know where I live.

Similarly, Tayla, a 21-year-old college sophomore shares: "If they don't get no attention, they think it's disrespectful. I try not to ignore. I would greet them and then say I am not interested. Our participants are constantly negotiating how to move through spaces and places in their neighborhoods and how to respond to others in those same spaces in ways that make them feel comfortable and that keep them safe and, quite frankly, keep them alive."

The Home

As our participants move from public spaces in their neighborhoods to private spaces around or in their homes, they realize that they still are confronted with gender-based harassment. Tayla also shares: "Like when my mom used to be with a guy, he had friends. He was very well-known in the area. He always had friends, and the friends like offered to give me a ride or—I would think of it as 'that's his friends,' but they always had a different intent." Tayla must contend with protecting herself from sexual advances from friends of her family. Some of our participants reveal that unfortunately these sexual advances shift to actual sexual assault, and not just from family friends, but also from blood relatives. Jay, an 18-year-old college freshman shares:

> I would say seven to nine, I felt like I was in a very inappropriate relationship with my brother. And I was unaware—like I knew it was wrong but I wasn't aware of the extent that like it would make me feel eventually. It was just like—he used to do things. He would touch me and do inappropriate things with me. And I didn't—I knew it was wrong, but I didn't know it was a crime. I didn't know there was a name for it. Like a word for it at that time. So I expressed it to my fifth grade teacher. I wrote it in my journal we had to write every morning. I thought that she never used to read the journals and then she actually used to read them. And she was like crying one day. I was like "What's wrong?" She was like "Do you really go through this?" I said "Yeah, you know, it just happens." She brought it to the principal's attention. They called my mom. My mom didn't believe it. And it was really hurtful for me that she felt like her son was incapable of that and I was just a liar. But like as time passed by, he joined the

Marines, came back home. He wasn't doing that to me no more, but it was just uncomfortable to be around him. . . . She [my mom] said never bring it up again. "This stays in this house and nowhere else."

Our participants share that girls of color, particularly girls from Caribbean American families, are expected to be silent after experiencing sexual violence in the home.

The Body

In addition to experiencing gender-based and sexual violence in public and private spaces from strangers and family members, our participants also experience physical abuse in their romantic relationships. Jay also shares:

> It took me a long time to accept his apology cuz like I just hated him so much. He had too much control over me at that time. I just—I forgave. I was still upset. . . . Cuz he used to like ask me for money. And he used to like—if he wanted to have sex and I didn't want to have sex, he would become very forceful and it was just like—it was not comfortable all the time and I jus—I felt like I was doing the right thing because I felt "oh he loves me so I have to this and I have to do that." But then like now, it's not what I thought it was. I'm happy to be out of it. And I'm happy to know better.

Similarly, Tayla comments: "But then, he tries so hard to be a really good person or whatever, so whenever he would try hard, I feel like I have to repay him with sex."

Our participants experience controlling and manipulative romantic relationships and justify intimacy as the right thing for someone who might love them and whom they love.

Some of our participants identify as lesbian, bisexual, and/or "I just like who I like." Lesbian, bisexual, and sexually fluid adolescents also experience dating violence. Fleeky, a 17-year-old high school senior, shares:

> It was a girl. I still speak to her. Like almost every other day. But it was just hard because we would get into an argument and she's like thicker than me. She would push me and I would

push her back. It was just—I remember one time she had my phone cuz she didn't want me to go to school that day. She was a bad influence too. She didn't want me to go to school but I wanted to go. . . . So yeah. It was like—I feel like nobody should have to go through that. Especially for education like. I could understand if I was going to like a party or something where you don't want me to go. But I was going to school. For you not to want me to go to school that was—that was big. . . . It was like, I really can't do this anymore, because like not even—I can't even explain it. She was just so horrible. Like she had trust issues with everything. And it was like how much am I supposed to tolerate? Like everything I want to do she's sucking her teeth. Like "oh you about to go do this, oh you about to go do that," when in reality I wasn't. It was just so horrible, because I knew she didn't trust me. And there was no reason for her not to trust me.

THE MIND

Our participants understand that there are multiple forms of dating violence, including psychological and emotional abuse. Jay shares: "And people don't think emotional abuse is real. It's really frustrating to see that in my generation, cuz they don't believe emotional abuse is real, because it is. It really does hurt. Sometimes people say things that are so hurtful and they think like 'Oh'—like they just apologize five minutes and think it's ok. But it's like words really do sting and they really do hurt." Similarly, Anti, a 16-year-old high school sophomore comments: "She just has a way to get, like to get me like real emotional. You know, like in public. So I just—I don't know. She knows like—she knows what gets to me. So when she's mad at me, she uses those stuff to get—to kind of keep me. She knows like all those things." In this case, Anti knows that her girlfriend is being manipulative and that this too is a form of relationship violence.

THE SOUL

In addition to navigating and experiencing these different forms of gender-based, sexual, and dating violence, our participants are actively coping with their traumas and developing various strategies of resistance. Our participants explicitly cite the KAVI program as a part of their coping and resistance strategies. Tayla and several of her peers in KAVI and in her school in general regularly meet with the school social worker. She shares that these sessions actually led her to KAVI: "Then we started talking about things and then girls started talking about how they were raped, just—she [school social worker] just realized that there was so much things going on that it [KAVI] would probably help us more." Jay has bravely shared her experiences with incest and romantic emotional, physical, sexual, and even cyber violence, as detailed in some of the excerpts above. In reflecting on how she processed these experiences in the KAVI workshops, she shares: "And then like coming to KAVI—I think that was the first time, I cried about it. It was just like I just finally got to release and be comfortable. It was just like so intense. Like they could've been like 'you were wrong for that [making a sex tape with her then-boyfriend] you know better.' But they were actually very supportive like 'you made a mistake and life is gonna go on.'" She goes on to share: "But I feel like everybody around me—like my support system, I got through it better than had I had that happen to me like before everything—like before I was in KAVI, before I started getting that kind of help."

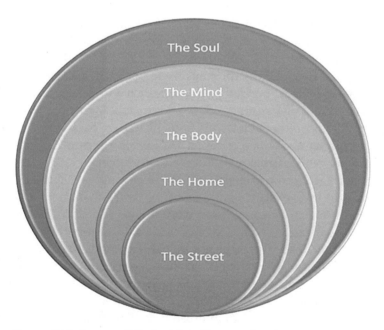

Figure 15.1. Spaces of Black girl resilience and resistance enactment.

Discussion

Our findings reveal our participants' experiences as survivors of verbal, emotional, physical, and sexual abuse from acquaintances and strangers on the street, as well as from family members, peers, and romantic partners. Our findings elucidate the macro- to microexperiences of gender-based, sexual, and dating violence, resilience, and resistance among urban Black girls. We offer such a model, informed by Black girls' own narratives, depicting the spaces where and how Black girl resilience and resistance are enacted. This visual model (figure 15.1) inverts the socio-ecological model (Golden et al., 2015) used frequently in public health, and instead centers Black girls' engagement with their environments (i.e., "the street," "the home"), then conceptualizes ways in which their physical, mental, and socio-emotional contexts (i.e., "the body," "the mind," "the soul") are shaped by risk and protective factors.

Black girls experience street harassment most saliently in their lives. Street harassment involves gender-based language and/or actions that are explicitly or implicitly sexual in nature and that are forced on a person in a public place without their consent (Davis, 1994). Our participants are often overwhelmed by the comments, gestures, and actions that they must contend with while walking in their home and school neighborhoods. They enlist what McCurn (2017) calls multiple "strategies of resistance" in order to ease uncomfortable situations with the aim of avoiding aggressive conflict on the street. Our participants try to normalize the behavior as a part of the urban daily round, they try to create physical distance between themselves and the harassers, or they work to appear friendly, so as not to come off as confrontational. We posit that street harassment creates the societal-level conditions of sexual violence in which other forms of interpersonal gender-based and sexual violence occur.

Next, Black girls encounter sexual advances and sexual abuse from loved ones in their extended and immediate families. We note a gap in the research and in evidence-based interventions related to dating violence that does not take into account victims' histories of child sexual abuse. We argue that dating violence should not and must not be siloed, but it should be considered under this broader frame of sexual violence and community violence and should be analyzed from a life-course perspective. Additionally, we were able to document experiences of sexual violence and dating violence from urban girls from the African diaspora. This is a contribution to the extant literature, which notes that there is a dearth of comprehensive studies on domestic violence among first- and second-generation immigrants (Pinnock, 2016). The few studies that do exist focusing on domestic violence among immigrants tend to focus on adult women and the domestic violence that they may experience tied to manipulation and coercion from their partners who threaten to reveal their undocumented immigrant status (Menjívar & Salcido, 2002; Reina et al., 2014). However, there are even fewer studies that focus on first- or second-generation immigrant adolescents experiencing dating violence (Herman, 2004). Our participants also reveal that when they experience sexual advances and sexual assault from extended family members and blood relatives, they are instructed to stay silent about it or keep the news "in the house." This is akin to the "culture of dissemblance" (Hine, 1989) among Black women in particular who shield their inner lives or are encouraged to shield their inner lives as a means of self-protection. This culture of dissemblance often leads to secrecy, shame, and stigma, which often manifest in other areas of one's life and which often are not met with healthy and holistic intervention.

Third, Black girls experience multiple forms of dating violence. We suggest that "relationship violence" is a more useful term for these experiences, as there is a wide spectrum of the types and levels of intimacy, roles, and duration of romantic partnerships and vast conceptions of "dating." Our participants experience what Chávez (2002) notes as a "paradox of love and violence" in which they are met with the emotions and actions of both love and violence from their partners. Our participants realize that in addition to experiencing joy in their romantic relationships, at times their love makes them vulnerable to physical and emotional abuse (Chávez, 2002; Jones, 2009).

Fourth, Black girls not only experience physical and sexual relationship violence, but also and often psychological violence. Experiences of coercion and manipulation from their partners creates the aforementioned confluence of love and violence and often results in our participants expressing self-blame and "feeling stuck" in their relationships as they want to navigate out of them. This psychological conundrum and the need to meet the psychological needs of Black girls extends the work of French (2013), who notes that many prevention programs fall short of holding abusers accountable and therefore can further victimize Black girls.

Last, but certainly not least, Black girls reveal strategies that they enlist to cope, resist, and heal from the traumas of gender-based, sexual, and relationship violence. The KAVI program serves as a safer space for them—geographically located inside their school, meeting during the school day once a week—but it also serves as a psychosocial safer space for them as they form supportive networks among their peers and with adult women workshop facilitators. Our participants also seek our professional social workers, both school social workers and social workers who are part of the KAVI staff, on a regular basis. Furthermore, our participants also use artwork in order to express and cope with their complex and multiple traumas and begin to engage in safety planning and healing for themselves and their peers.

Creary (2018) terms "biocultural citizenship" the complex interplay of biological, cultural, and societal factors among individuals who strive to gain full citizenship. As our participants "feel some type of way," they are embodying their biocultural citizenship of both trauma and healing, of risk and resilience and resistance. As the "citizenship" of urban Black girls is far too often constrained, the resistance strategies of participants illuminate the inverted socio-ecological approach (Golden et al., 2015) to violence prevention and intervention which advocates, practitioners, and researchers must be vigilant about pursuing. As such, an epistemological focus on Black feminist thought (Hill Collins, 1990) and Black girlhood studies (Brown, 2013) has been critical in our understanding of urban Black girls' experiences and in our attention to making needed revisions and enhancements to KAVI's curriculum, programming, and volunteer and staff training in order to meet the needs of current and future KAVI participants. Relatedly, as queer youth experience dating violence at rates equal to or higher than their heterosexual peers (Gillum & DiFulvio, 2014), KAVI is being more intentional about making their program more culturally humble and inclusive to meet the needs of queer, questioning, and gender-expansive participants.

Recommendations and Call for Action

We assert that youth development and violence intervention programs must consider curricular and psychosocial components specifically related to teen dating violence and relationship violence in order to be responsive and equitable to the holistic social, physical, psychological, emotional, and spiritual needs of their participants. Black girls demonstrate strategies of resilience on a regular basis. May we urgently shift our metrics, recognizing their resistance and supporting their healing.

Resources

Justice for Black Girls. https://www.justiceforblackgirls.com/
Kings against Violence Initiative. https://kavibrooklyn.org/
A Long Walk Home. http://www.alongwalkhome.org/
Saving Our Lives, Hear Our Truths (SOLHOT). https://www.solhot.com/
Stop Telling Women to Smile. http://stoptellingwomentosmile.com/

References

Alleyne-Green, B., Coleman-Cowger, V. H., & Henry, D. B. (2012). Dating violence perpetration and/or victimization and associated sexual risk behaviors among a sample of inner-city African American and Hispanic adolescent females. *Journal of Interpersonal Violence, 27*(8), 1457–1473. https://doi.org/10.1177/0886260511425788

Benard, B. (1991). *Fostering resiliency in kids: Protective factors in the family, school, and community.* Western Center for Drug-Free Schools and Communities.

Brown, R. N. (2013). *Hear our truths: The creative potential of Black girlhood.* University of Illinois Press.

Catalano, S., Smith, E., Snyder, H., & Rand, M. (2009). *Female victims of violence.* US Department of Justice, Office of Justice Programs.

Chávez, V. (2002). Language, gender and violence in qualitative research. *International Quarterly of Community Health Education, 21*(1), 3–18. https://doi.org/10.2190/URHT-A2KX-GK95-AAA0

Creary, M. S. (2018). Biocultural citizenship and embodying exceptionalism: Biopolitics for sickle cell disease in Brazil. *Social Science and Medicine, 199,* 123–131. https://doi.org/10.1016/j.socscimed.2017.04.035

Crenshaw, K. (1991). Mapping the margins: Intersectionality, identity politics, and violence against women of color. *Stanford Law Review, 43*(6), 1241–1299. https://doi.org/10.2307/1229039

Davis, D. (1994). The harm that has no name: Street harassment, embodiment, and African American women. *UCLA Women's Law Journal, 4*(2), 133–178.

Dill, L. J. (2011). *Routes to resilience: Mechanisms of healthy development in minority adolescents from high-risk urban neighborhoods* [Doctoral dissertation]. University of California, Berkeley.

Dill, L. J. (2015). Poetic justice: Engaging in participatory narrative analysis to find solace in the "killer corridor." *American Journal of Community Psychology, 55*(1–2), 128–135. https://doi.org/10.1007/s10464-014-9694-7

Dill, L. J., Rivera, B., & Sutton, S. (2018). Don't let nobody bring you down: How urban Black girls write and learn from ethnographically-based poetry to understand and heal from relationship violence. *Ethnographic Edge*, *2*(1), 57–65. https://doi.org/10.15663/tee.v2i1.30

East, P. L., & Hokoda, A. (2015). Risk and protective factors for sexual and dating violence victimization: A longitudinal, prospective study of Latino and African American adolescents. *Journal of Youth and Adolescence*, *44*(6), 1288–1300. https://doi.org/10.1007/s10964-015-0273-5

Emerson, R. M., Fretz, R. I., & Shaw, L. L. (2011). *Writing ethnographic fieldnotes*. University of Chicago Press.

Fergus, S., & Zimmerman, M. A. (2005). Adolescent resilience: A framework for understanding healthy development in the face of risk. *Annual Review of Public Health*, *26*, 399–419.

Ford, C. L., & Airhihenbuwa, C. O. (2010). The public health critical race methodology: Praxis for antiracism research. *Social science and medicine*, *71*(8), 1390–1398. https://doi.org/10.1016/j.socscimed.2010.07.030

French, B. H. (2013). More than Jezebels and freaks: Exploring how Black girls navigate sexual coercion and sexual scripts. *Journal of African American Studies*, *17*(1), 35–50. https://doi.org/10.1007/s12111-012-9218-1

Furman, R., Langer, C. L., Davis, C. S., Gallardo, H. P., & Kulkarni, S. (2007). Expressive, research and reflective poetry as qualitative inquiry: A study of adolescent identity. *Qualitative Research*, *7*(3), 301–315. https://doi.org/10.1177/1468794107078511

Garmezy, N. (1991). Resilience in children's adaptation to negative life events and stressed environments. *Pediatrics*, *20*(9), 459–466. https://doi.org/10.3928/0090-4481-19910901-05

Gillum, T. L., & DiFulvio, G. T. (2014). Examining dating violence and its mental health consequences among sexual minority youth. In D. Peterson & V. R. Panfil (Eds.), *Handbook of LGBT Communities, Crime, and Justice* (pp. 431–448). Springer.

Golden, S. D., McLeroy, K. R., Green, L. W., Earp, J. A. L., & Lieberman, L. D. (2015). Upending the social ecological model to guide health promotion efforts toward policy and environmental change. *Health Education and Behavior*, *42*(1 Suppl.), 8–14. https://doi.org/10.1177/1090198115575098

Hayden, D. (1997). *The power of place: Urban landscapes as public history*. MIT Press.

Hays, D. G., Forman, J., & Sikes, A. (2009). Using artwork and photography to explore adolescent females' perceptions of dating relationships. *Journal of Creativity in Mental Health*, *4*(4), 295–307. https://doi.org/10.1080/15401380903385960

Herman, K. A. (2004). Developing a model intervention to prevent abuse in relationships among Caribbean and Caribbean-American youth by partnering with schools. *Journal of Immigrant and Refugee Services*, *2*(3–4), 103–116. https://doi.org/10.1300/J191v02n03_07

Hill Collins, P. (1990). *Black feminist thought: Knowledge, consciousness, and the politics of Empowerment*. Routledge.

Hine, D. C. (1989). Rape and the inner lives of Black women in the Middle West. *Signs, 14*(4), 912–920. https://doi.org/10.1086/494552

Jackson, S. M. (1999). Issues in the dating violence research: A review of the literature. *Aggression and Violent Behavior, 4*(2), 233–247. https://doi.org/10.1016/S1359-1789(97)00049-9

Jarrett, R. L. (1995). Growing up poor: The family experiences of socially mobile youth in low-income African American neighborhoods. *Journal of Adolescent Research, 10*(1), 111–135. https://doi.org/10.1177/0743554895101007

Jarrett, R. L. (1997). Resilience among low-income African American youth: An ethnographic perspective. *Ethos, 25*(2), 218–229. https://doi.org/10.1525/eth.1997.25.2.218

Jones, C. P. (2000). Levels of racism: A theoretic framework and a gardener's tale. *American Journal of Public Health, 90*(8), 1212. https://doi.org/10.2105%2Fajph.90.8.1212

Jones, N. (2009). *Between good and ghetto: African American girls and inner-city violence.* Rutgers University Press.

Langer, C. L., & Furman, R. (2004). Exploring identity and assimilation: Research and interpretive poems. *Forum: Qualitative Social Research, 5*(2). https://doi.org/10.17169/fqs-5.2.609

Lindsay-Dennis, L. (2015). Black feminist-womanist research paradigm: Toward a culturally relevant research model focused on African American girls. *Journal of Black Studies, 46*(5), 506–520. https://doi.org/10.1177/0021934715583664

Luthar, S. S., Cicchetti, D., & Becker, B. (2000). The construct of resilience: A critical evaluation and guidelines for future work. *Child Development, 71*(3), 543–562. https://doi.org/10.1111/1467-8624.00164

Masten, A. S., Hubbard, J. J., Gest, S. D., Tellegen, A., Garmezy, N., & Ramirez, M. (1999). Competence in the context of adversity: Pathways to resilience and maladaptation from childhood to late adolescence. *Development and Psychopathology, 11*(1), 143–169. https://doi.org/10.1017/S0954579499001996

McCurn, A. S. (2017) "I am not a prostitute": How young Black women challenge street-based micro-interactional assaults. *Sociological Focus, 50*(1), 52–65. https://doi.org/10.1080/00380237.2016.1218216

Menjívar, C., & Salcido, O. (2002). Immigrant women and domestic violence: Common experiences in different countries. *Gender and society, 16*(6), 898–920. https://doi.org/10.1177/089124302237894

Merriam, S. B., & Tisdell, E. J. (2015). *Qualitative research: A guide to design and implementation* (4th ed.). Wiley.

Pinnock, C. (2016). *A means to an end: Articulations of diasporic Blackness, class and survival among female Afro-Caribbean service workers in New York City* [Doctoral dissertation]. City University of New York.

Reina, A. S., Lohman, B. J., & Maldonado, M. M. (2014). "He said they'd deport me": Factors influencing domestic violence help-seeking practices among Latina immigrants. *Journal of Interpersonal Violence, 29*(4), 593–615. https://doi.org/10.1177/0886260513505214

Ruglis, J. (2011). Mapping the biopolitics of school dropout and youth resistance. *International Journal of Qualitative Studies in Education, 24*(5), 627–637. https://doi.org/10.1080/09518398.2011.600268

Rutter, M. (1985). Resilience in the face of adversity: Protective factors and resistance to psychiatric disorder. British Journal of Psychiatry, *147*(6), 598–611. https://doi.org/10.1192/bjp.147.6.598

Saldaña, J. (2015). *The coding manual for qualitative researchers* (3rd ed.). Sage.

Spencer, M. B. (1995). Old issues and new theorizing about African-American youth: A phenomenological variant of ecological systems theory. In R. L. Taylor (Ed.), *Black youth: Perspectives on their status in the United States* (pp. 37–69). Praeger.

Spencer, M. B., Dupree, D., & Hartmann, T. (1997). A phenomenological variant of ecological systems theory (PVEST): A self-organization perspective in context. *Development and Psychopathology, 9*(4), 817–833. https://doi.org/10.1017/S0954579497001454

Sugarman, D. B., & Hotaling, G. T. (1989). Dating violence: Prevalence, context and risk markers. In M. A. Pirog-Good & J. E. Stets (Eds.), *Violence in dating relationships: Emerging social issues* (pp. 3–32). Praeger.

Ungar, M., Brown, M. Liebenberg, L., Othman, R., Kwong, W. M., Armstrong, M., & Gilgun, J. (2007). Unique pathways to resilience across cultures. *Adolescence, 42*(166), 287–310.

Vagi, K. J., Olsen, E. O., Basile, K. C., & Vivolo-Kantor, A. M. (2015). Teen dating violence (physical and sexual) among US high school students: Findings from the 2013 National Youth Risk Behavior Survey. *JAMA Pediatrics, 169*(5), 474–482. https://doi.org/10.1001/jamapediatrics.2014.3577

Werner, E. E., Bierman, J. M., & French, F. E. (1971). *The children of Kauai*. University of Hawaii Press.

Werner, E. E., & Smith, R. (1977). *Kauai's children come of age*. University of Hawaii Press.

West, C. M., & Rose, S. (2000). Dating aggression among low income African American youth: An examination of gender differences and antagonistic beliefs. *Violence against Women, 6*(5), 470–494. https://doi.org/10.1177/10778010022181985

Wright, M. O., & Masten, A. S. (2015). Pathways to resilience in context. In L. C. Theron, L. Liebenberg, & M. Ungar (Eds.), *Youth resilience and culture* (pp. 3–22). Springer.

Wun, C. (2016). Against captivity: Black girls and school discipline policies in the afterlife of slavery. *Educational Policy, 30*(1), 171–196. https://doi.org/10.1177/0895904815615439

Zimmerman, M. A., & Arunkumar, R. (1994). Resiliency research: Implications for schools and policy. *Social Policy Report*, *8*(4), 1–20. https://doi.org/10.1002/j.2379-3988.1994.tb00032.x

Chapter 16

Womanist Theological Bioethics
A Healing and Culturally Responsive Approach to Death and Dying in Black Communities

NICOLE TAYLOR MORRIS

In the midst of a global pandemic, various health disparities affecting lifetime morbidity and mortality persist for Black people in the United States due to systemic inequity and injustice. As the coronavirus (COVID-19) continues to devastate families and communities across the US and globally, its particular impact on Black communities is pronounced, as is the lack of access to quality health care to reduce the likelihood of death due to this virus (Fortuna et al., 2020). Aside from death directly related to COVID-19, the impact of the stress and grief accompanying this season of profound loss of life and of means for living will have lasting effects on the health of Black communities; particularly, on the Black women that often act as primary caregivers for loved ones while facing disparities themselves.

In addition to the unjust familial, communal, and socioeconomic losses that have resulted and continued from COVID-19, many Black communities have also been forced to further confront the racism that pervades daily life in the form of live videos of murder-by-police, police and communal racialized violence, and mob riots in the name of White supremacy. Considering these factors, the way that the field of bioethics approaches both the implications of these experiences on health and health care for Black communities and the morality of different health-care policies and interventions is critical. It is important to use an equity-centered lens to explore diverse approaches to death and dying. Bioethics, particularly when informed by a womanist theological approach, may provide vital insights as we shape a more justice-oriented future transformed by our current realities and intent on providing opportunities for wellness and vitality for all.

Standardized Bioethical Approaches to Death and Dying

The four main principles of bioethics are beneficence, nonmaleficence, autonomy, and justice; these principles must be balanced when considering death and dying, with justice elevated to inform an equity-centered lens. Porter et al. (2005) provided an overview of the major dilemmas regarding death and dying in the field of bioethics in their article, "Bioethical Issues Concerning Death: Death, Dying, and End-of-Life Rights"; these include physician-assisted suicide (PAS), advance directives, and other forms of "death with dignity" centered on the bioethical principles of patient self-determination and autonomy. These topics have been the primary focus of bioethical approaches to practices and policies regarding death, as demonstrated by several other bioethicists including Robert Veatch (2000), Lisa Cahill (2005), and Susan Wolf (1996).

Though these are conversations surrounding "death with dignity" and Porter et al.'s imperative that individuals provide detailed instructions of what they want dying and death to look like for themselves, these popularized notions do not consider how cultural and historical relationships with health care may inform end-of-life care decisions and the interest in medical interventions. Bioethical practices and policies must also be culturally relevant when approaching death and dying. Due to the disproportionate impacts of structural violence, disparities in health outcomes, and the legacy of mistreatment in health care on Black communities, it is important to consider bioethics in this context. This is especially pertinent as the urgency of conversations surrounding health-care proxies, advance directives, and other end-of-life care interventions has increased in the time of COVID-19, yet these issues remain harder to address in a culturally competent manner within Black communities (Janwadkar & Bibler, 2020).

Limitations of Standardized Approaches

In direct opposition to Porter et al.'s suggested approaches to "death with dignity," Wojtasiewicz cited several studies suggesting that not only do African Americans seek more "aggressive end-of-life interventions," but also that advance directives may be perceived as "a death warrant; a license to kill to avoid the cost of maintaining a patient on life support" (Wojtasiewicz, 2006; Tucker, 1994). According to Wojtasiewicz and other researchers, such as Prograis and Pellegrino (2007) in their book *African American Bioethics: Culture, Race, and Identity*, it is necessary to consider the ways in which culture, race, ethnicity, and other aspects of identity inform approaches to care and considerations at end of life (Levin & Sprung, 2003; Koenig & Williams-Gates,1995).

As bioethical approaches and suggestions continue to be valued in defining practices and policies for the medical and health-care fields, especially those that pertain to racial and ethnic disparities in health, in access to care, and in causes of death, a critical look at the application of "standardized" bioethical approaches to these issues must be taken. Aside from determining culturally relevant interventions regarding what kinds of end-of-life care plans and treatments may be acceptable and accessible for these marginalized groups, bioethics as a field must be transformed to be more inclusive of principles that are applicable to the diverse identities who all ultimately face death.

Danis et al. (2016) have noted the limitations of traditional practices in this field and criticized that "bioethicists have not contributed substantially to addressing [issues related to racism]. Concern for justice has been one of the core commitments of bioethics. For this and other reasons, bioethicists should contribute to addressing these problems." As end-of-life technology and care continue to innovate, it is important and urgent for the field of bioethics to acknowledge communal experience and practice and to be intentional about inclusion, as "standardized" approaches have varied implications for members of marginalized groups.

Death and Dying in Black Communities

When examining death and dying within African American communities, Levin and Sprung (2003) found that Black Americans were least likely to accept life-sustaining treatment because of factors such as costs and distrust in doctors, though they were the most likely to desire life-sustaining treatment. They also indicated that African Americans often urged for resuscitation efforts as they feared physicians may be unwilling to do so without being urged—these findings are noteworthy as this study also examined end-of-life decisions for White Americans and found that they were both less likely to seek life-sustaining treatment and to urge for resuscitation. This study demonstrates how bioethical approaches to death, which focus on individuals attempting to "control death" rather than sustain life, may be more relevant to dying within White communities than in Black communities (Levin & Sprung, 2003). Degenholtz et al. (2003) conducted a literature review to examine racial differences in both end-of-life care and ICU care and found that Black patients, particularly with their family members as proxies, are more likely to seek life-sustaining treatment but less likely to complete a living will or prepare an advanced directive.

The authors of this study note that some of the reasons for differences in approaches to end-of-life care include mistrust of the medical system, historical mistreatment and medical disenfranchisement, the role of family in making decisions at end-of-life, and reluctance toward planning ahead for death and dying. Additionally, they found that increased costs for care for Black patients is often due to increased use of costly, emergency life-saving care because of less engagement with preventative care over individuals' lifetimes (Degenholtz et al., 2003). The aforementioned factors, in addition to ongoing intergenerational trauma due to historical medical maltreatment, can be heavily attributed to the ongoing roles that racism and discrimination play in the lives of members of Black communities.

Another important consideration is the role that spirituality plays in end-of-life care decisions for many Black individuals. Johnson et al. (2005) cite a significant body of research suggesting that desiring aggressive life-sustaining treatment once hospitalized but lack of seeking preventative medical intervention earlier on may be related to beliefs about death and God as the ultimate decision-maker for mortality for those that practice Christianity (Pew Research Center, 2013). Spirituality and religion not only influence end-of-life care, but also play a role in the ways that Black community members may address health concerns throughout their lifetimes and how some may view death as a spiritual passage to a divine afterlife, therefore accepting dying and death as God's will rather than engaging with preventative or life-sustaining health care (Phillips, 2011).

CONSIDERATIONS FOR VIOLENT DEATH AND DEATH ANXIETY IN BLACK COMMUNITIES

Bioethical conversations surrounding death and dying for African Americans must be culturally relevant and consider how racism, discrimination, and marginalization have affected approaches to end-of-life care for those who are dying. They must also consider the effects of violence on communal experiences with death. Bioethics plays a key role in shaping the health-care systems at large that are still often not equipped to manage the familial, communal, and sociopolitical implications of violent death and injury that occur in many African American communities due to layered systemic oppression (Liebschutz et al., 2010; Alang et al., 2017; Gire, 2014).

Several authors demonstrated that Black youth have a disproportionately higher risk for facing death due to violence in the United States compared to their White counterparts; these disparities directly result from ongoing experiences of structural racism and discrimination (Sheats et al., 2018; Najem et al., 2004). Researchers also indicated that structural violence and interactions with law enforcement not only impact absolute death for individuals, but also prompt communal trauma and death anxiety, which greatly reduces quality of life for these community members (Bailey et al., 2013; Kwate & Threadcraft, 2017).

This death anxiety due to violence is important to note for its impacts on African Americans across age groups and gender; however. it is also connected with fears of aging and, subsequently, seeking preventative health care and long-term health-care planning (Thorson et al., 1998). Luth and Prigerson (2018) and Tucker (1994) described how advanced care planning, including living wills, advance directives, and healthcare proxies, for Black individuals can actually cause psychological distress and sadness for both dying individuals and their caretakers as compared to White counterparts; this may be related to greater experiences with personal and communal loss as well as both violent and nonviolent trauma due to factors related to racism. For many Black people in the United States, there are constant risks and anxieties surrounding death and dying, particularly in medicalized settings, due to structural and interpersonal racism and maltreatment. Communal care, and especially the Black women who often lead in alternatives to traditional bioethical and health-care approaches, must be acknowledged.

Bioethical Implications for Black Women

When examining death and dying, violent or nonviolent, within African American communities, it is important to consider how Black women are particularly impacted. African American women disproportionately face many disparities in health and health care due to the combined effects of racism and sexism, which influence quality of life and causes of death, including less publicly recognized instances of police violence causing death, as well as extreme disparities in maternal mortality related to racism in pregnancy care (Jacobs, 2017; Owens & Fett, 2019). Despite these alarming trends in mortality, Black women are often delegated as end-of-life caregivers for spouses, parents, and other family members (Anderson & Turner, 2010).

Black populations, regardless of age and gender, are more likely to die from all-cause mortality including chronic illnesses like cancer, kidney disease, cardiovascular disease, and stroke, among others, than White counterparts (Marron et al., 2018; Cunningham et al., 2017). Due to these disparities and because of cultural and gender pressures, African American women often take on the role of end-of-life caregivers within their families despite the plethora of disparities and illnesses that they face themselves; this role is in addition to the other social and childrearing labor expectations for Black women (Jones et al., 2018; Anderson & Turner, 2010).

Jones et al. (2018) demonstrated that stress from these roles often contributes to chronic conditions, such as hypertension, which in turn shorten the lives of Black women. Despite the physical and social tolls these types of roles can have for Black women, Anderson & Turner (2010) demonstrated that some Black women who are caregivers do not expect generational reciprocity and do not want to "burden" their own children with the stressors of caregiving. The women in this study also mentioned that they would be willing to be placed in nursing homes, but they insisted that their family would be essential as constant visitors and as advocates for their care. They did not mention anything related to autonomy in the right-to-die as potential methods for not "burdening" their families (Anderson & Turner, 2010). Black women's roles as end-of-life caregivers serve as an intervention beyond care in medical settings, which reasserts the importance of family in end-of-life care in many Black communities.

In addition to caregiving roles, Black women are also often invisibilized in police-related death and are often most impacted by death anxiety and PTSD related to familial loss due to violence (Jacobs, 2017; Bailey et al., 2013). Though Black women's experiences of police violence resulting in death, disability, and various forms of trauma are often underreported in popular media, these experiences persist and have sparked the social media movement #SayHerName to direct specific attention to Black women who face this violence in addition to the boys and men whose names have been popularized by the Black Lives Matter movement (Crenshaw et al., 2015; Jacobs, 2017). Black women are also often most impacted by grief due to violent death within communities, and this can have long-term effects on life meaning-making and subsequently health and willingness to engage with care (Bailey et al., 2013).

In addition to these experiences of institutionalized violence related to overpolicing and environments shaped by structural racism, Black women also face racialized violence leading to death in hospitals; a popularized example of this is the crisis of perinatal mortality (Owens & Fett, 2019). Black women are most likely to face pregnancy-related death than counterparts nationally in America; this disproportionate rate is overwhelmingly influenced by experiences of ongoing racism in perinatal health care (Owens & Fett, 2019). These experiences of death must also be acknowledged in bioethical conversations as the intersections of gender and race inform both violent death and experiences of loss for Black women, which can impact both willingness to engage with and trust in medicalized institutions and interventions. These settings, which are theoretically meant to be life-saving, are simultaneously perpetuators of unjust death and racialized violence for Black women.

A Justice-Oriented Approach to Death and Dying in Black Communities

Approaches to death and dying within the field of bioethics have focused on patient autonomy and self-determination regarding end-of-life care decisions—these concentrations are not considerate of the ways that conceptions of death, life experience, historical relationships to healthcare, and identity may have varied impacts for different groups of people, particularly those who are already sociopolitically marginalized. Approaching death and dying from an equity-oriented perspective both values the experiences of life and death within Black communities and accounts for the complex dynamics of family, spirituality, and structural oppression as they impact both health and healthcare. Womanist theological bioethics is an applicable and culturally relevant framework for shaping bioethical conversations that are inclusive and prioritize experiences within Black communities, and particularly those of Black women.

A womanist perspective centers the experiences of Black women as a lens for approaching justice that emphasizes the humanity of all and seeks to magnify the voices of those most marginalized in a heterosexist, White-supremacist, and capitalism-based society. A womanist approach, as defined by Alice Walker and other critical womanist scholars, is rooted in both theory and praxis, so it is a lens toward tangible actions, practices, and policies that move toward justice (Townes, 2011). Theological bioethics centers the role of spirituality in informing decisions regarding health and health care (Cahill, 2005). A womanist theological bioethics lens, as informed by the work of womanist bioethicist Wylin Wilson, prioritizes "justice" in terms of how we might improve health and health care models by grounding our understanding in Black women's health and experiences—as Black women are both often at risk for poorest health outcomes and tasked with the socio-emotional labor of caring for others (Wilson, 2019).

Emilie Townes wrote, "The challenge for a womanist ethicist is to create and then articulate a positive moral standard that critiques the elitism of dominant ethics at its oppressive core and is relevant for the African-American community and the larger society" (Townes, 2011, p. 37). This statement summarizes how womanist theological bioethics not only recognizes and decenters "dominant" notions of ethics that focus on experiences rooted in Whiteness, but also how it emphasizes creating and acknowledging ethics that are applicable within Black communities. Womanist theological bioethics is also deeply informed by the major influences on both life and death in Black communities and emphasizes the role of familial and communal relationships, spirituality, and how structural and interpersonal experiences of violence inform interactions with health and health care.

The significance of understanding these relationships to health care through this lens and its implications for policies and end-of-life care have been magnified by the impact of COVID-19 and increased publicity of police violence in Black communities in the United States. A womanist theological bioethical lens is useful in shaping policies and practices that are mindful of the role of support persons and spirituality, among other sociocultural factors that influence death both in medical settings and due to racialized violence, even during unprecedented and emergency situations. These factors and this lens need to be regularly incorporated into health-care settings and decisions for treatment, as they can reduce the disproportionately negative experiences that Black community members face.

The Need for Change

Institutionally, bioethics informs the decisions made by policymakers, public health practitioners, health-care providers, researchers, and law enforcement (Kwate & Threadcraft, 2017; Alang, 2017). These decisions play a large role in shaping health determinants, life experience, and the end-of-life care that many Black people in America experience. A womanist theological bioethics lens not only informs policies and practices that guide practitioners in these various fields toward equitable and justice-oriented strategies for addressing care, but it also centers healing and recognizing one another's humanity as guides to moral treatment and practice. The prioritization of autonomy and self-determination at end of life in mainstream bioethics is rooted in White supremacist constructs that focus on power and control, even to the point of attempting to "control death." Womanist theological bioethics allows for justice and communal experiences to be at the core of approaches and moves toward indigenous ways of communal knowledge, trust, and a deep sense of humanity that allows for gentle end-of-life care and opportunities for death, dying, and grieving; to also allow for healing, rather than further trauma.

Advocating for Black voices to be emphasized both within the field of bioethics and within daily life are challenges, as those that benefit from these conversations and those who have the power to shape these conversations tend to not be marginalized themselves. The moral issue within approaching solutions for reshaping the field of bioethics and addressing unjust causes of death in Black communities—is whether those with power are willing to recognize and value the humanity of Black people enough to advocate for change. Factors that shape inequity in health and health care, and subsequently in death and dying, in Black communities have existed in America for over 400 years with the enslavement of Africans and continued forms of oppression. It is time that the field of bioethics is not only critiqued for its lack of inclusivity, but that tangible changes are made for improving the field and shifting its lens toward justice and equity.

Recommendations and Call for Action: The Ongoing Necessity of Bioethics

In Lucille Clifton's poem "won't you celebrate with me," she wrote, "come celebrate / with me that everyday / something has tried to kill me / and failed" (Clifton et al., 2012, p. 427). This poem reiterates the necessity of a womanist theological bioethical perspective for death and dying within Black communities. Survival is not guaranteed by the forces that shape life experiences, especially for Black people in the United States, and sometimes those forces that "try to kill" do not fail and end life for many too soon. The field of bioethics needs to both take seriously and to emphasize varied causes for death and dying and how they are approached in the context of care for Black communities; this often requires a focus on justice more than on autonomy. There is an opportunity, with the mass and disproportionate loss of life in Black communities and other communities of color during the COVID-19 pandemic and the continued racialized police violence, for the field of bioethics to not only offer guidance toward humane and justice-oriented practices and policies, but also to support and emphasize the importance of acknowledging persistent grief and the necessity of opportunities and resources for healing in these communities. There is much work to do in shaping and hopefully someday mitigating the forces that constantly try to diminish and destroy Black life, but the field of bioethics, particularly when using a womanist theological lens, is at a vantage point in sparking change and must be transformed itself in order to do so.

Resources

Going with Grace [Alua Arthur, Death Doula]. https://goingwithgrace.com

Moore, S. E., Jones-Eversley, S. D., Tolliver, W. F., Wilson, B., & Harmon, D. K. Cultural responses to loss and grief among Black Americans: Theory and practice implications for clinicians. *Death Studies*, 46, no. 1 (2020):1–11. https://doi.org/10.1080/07481187.2020.1725930

Wilson, W. D. (2021). Womanist bioethics [Unpublished manuscript]. Theological Ethics, Duke Divinity School.

References

Alang, S., McAlpine, D., McCreedy, E., & Hardeman, R. (2017). Police brutality and black health: Setting the agenda for public health scholars. *American Journal of Public Health*, 107(5), 662–665. https://doi.org/10.2105/ajph.2017.303691

Anderson, J. R., & Turner, W. L. (2010). When caregivers are in need of care: African-American caregivers' preferences for their own later life care. *Journal of Aging Studies*, 24(1), 65–73. https://doi.org/10.1016/j.jaging.2008.06.002

Bailey, A., Hannays-King, C., Clarke, J., Lester, E., & Velasco, D. (2013). Black mothers' cognitive process of finding meaning and building resilience after loss of a child to gun violence. *British Journal of Social Work, 43*(2), 336–354. https://doi.org/10.1093/bjsw/bct027

Cahill, L. S. (2005). *Theological bioethics: Participation, justice, and change.* Georgetown University Press.

Crenshaw, K. W., Ritche, A. J., & Harris, L. (2015, May 20). *Say her name: Resisting police brutality against Black women.* https://www.aapf.org/_files/ugd/62e126_9223ee35c2694ac3bd3f2171504ca3f7.pdf

Cunningham, T. J., Croft, J. B., Liu, Y., Lu, H., Eke, P. I., & Giles, W. H. (2017). Vital signs: Racial disparities in age-specific mortality among Blacks or African Americans—United States, 1999–2015. *Morbidity and Mortality Weekly Report, 66*(17), 444–456. https://doi.org/10.15585/mmwr.mm6617e1

Clifton, L. (2012). *The Collected Poems of Lucille Clifton, 1965–2010* (K. Young & M. S. Glaser, Eds.). BOA.

Danis, M., Wilson, Y., & White, A. (2016). Bioethicists can and should contribute to addressing racism. *American Journal of Bioethics, 16*(4), 3–12. https://doi.org/10.1080/15265161.2016.1145283

Degenholtz, H. B., Thomas, S. B., & Miller, M. J. (2003). Race and the intensive care unit: Disparities and preferences for end-of-life care. *Critical Care Medicine, 31*(5), S373–S378. https://doi.org/10.1097/01.ccm.0000065121.62144.0d

Fortuna, L. R., Tolou-Shams, M., Robles-Ramamurthy, B., & Porche, M. V. (2020). Inequity and the disproportionate impact of COVID-19 on communities of color in the United States: The need for a trauma-informed social justice response. *Psychological Trauma, 12*(5), 443–445. https://doi.org/10.1037/tra0000889

Gire, J. (2014). How death imitates life: Cultural influences on conceptions of death and dying. *Online Readings in Psychology and Culture, 6*(2), Article 3. https://doi.org/10.9707/2307-0919.1120

Jacobs, M. S. (2017). The violent state: Black women's invisible struggle against police violence. *William & Mary Journal of Women and the Law, 24*(1), 39–100. https://scholarship.law.wm.edu/wmjowl/vol24/iss1/4

Janwadkar, A. S., & Bibler, T. M. (2020). Ethical challenges in advance care planning during the COVID-19 pandemic. *American Journal of Bioethics, 20*(7), 202–204. https://doi.org/10.1080/15265161.2020.1779855

Johnson, K. S., Elbert-Avila, K. I., & Tulsky, J. A. (2005). The influence of spiritual beliefs and practices on the treatment preferences of African Americans: A review of the literature. *Journal of the American Geriatrics Society, 53*(4), 711–719. https://doi.org/10.1111/j.1532-5415.2005.53224.x

Jones, L. M., Moss, K. O., Wright, K. D., Rosemberg, M.-A., & Killion, C. (2018). "Maybe this generation here could help the next generation": Older African American women's perceptions on information sharing to improve health in younger generations. *Research in Gerontological Nursing, 11*(1), 39–47. https://doi.org/10.3928/19404921-20171129-01

Koenig, B. A., & Williams-Gates, J. (1995). Understanding cultural differences in caring for dying Patients. *Western Journal of Medicine, 163*(3), 244–249.

Kwate, N. O., & Threadcraft, S. (2017). Dying fast and dying slow in Black space: Stop and Frisk's public health threat and a comprehensive necropolitics. *Du Bois Review, 14*(2), 535–556. https://doi.org/10.1017/s1742058x17000169

Levin, P. D., & Sprung, C. L. (2003). Cultural differences at the end of life. *Critical Care Medicine, 31*(5), S354–S357. https://doi.org/10.1097/01.ccm.0000065275.30220.d2

Liebschutz, J., Schwartz, S., Hoyte, J., Conoscenti, L., Christian, A. B., Muhammad, L., Harper, D., & James, T. (2010). A chasm between injury and care: Experiences of Black male victims of violence. *Journal of Trauma, 69*(6), 1372–1378. https://doi.org/10.1097/ta.0b013e3181e74fcf

Luth, E. A., & Prigerson, H. G. (2018). Unintended harm? Race differences in the relationship between advance care planning and psychological distress at the end of life. *Journal of Pain and Symptom Management, 56*(5), 752–759. https://doi.org/10.1016/j.jpainsymman.2018.08.001

Marron, M. M., Ives, D. G., Boudreau, R. M., Harris, T. B., & Newman, A. B. (2018). Racial differences in cause-specific mortality between community-dwelling older Black and White adults. *Journal of the American Geriatrics Society, 66*(10), 1980–1986. https://doi.org/10.1111/jgs.15534

Najem, G. R., Aslam, S., Davidow, A. L., & Elliot, N. (2004). Youth homicide racial disparities: Gender, years, and cause. *Journal of the National Medical Association, 96*(4), 558–566.

Owens, D. C., & Fett, S. M. (2019). Black maternal and infant health: Historical legacies of slavery. *American Journal of Public Health, 109*(10), 1342–1345. https://doi.org/10.2105/ajph.2019.305243

Pew Research Center. (2013). *Views on end-of-life medical treatments.* http://www.pewforum.org/2013/11/21/views-on-end-of-life-medical-treatments/

Phillips, N. R. (2011). Death unto life: The power of the incarnation. *Pastoral Psychology, 60*(3), 339–354. https://doi.org/10.1007/s11089-011-0333-z

Porter, T., Johnson, P., & Warren, N. A. (2005). Bioethical issues concerning death: Death, dying, and end-of-life rights. *Critical Care Nursing Quarterly, 28*(1), 85–92. https://doi.org/10.1097/00002727-200501000-00009

Prograis, L., & Pellegrino, E. D. (Eds.). (2007). *African American bioethics: Culture, race, and identity.* Georgetown University Press.

Sheats, K. J., Irving, S. M., Mercy, J. A., Simon, T. R., Crosby, A. E., Ford, D. C., Merrick, M. T., Annor, F. B., & Morgan, R. E. (2018). Violence-related disparities experienced by Black youth and young adults: Opportunities for prevention. *American Journal of Preventive Medicine, 55*(4), 462–469. https://doi.org/10.1016/j.amepre.2018.05.017

Thorson, J. A., Powell, F. C., & Samuel, V. T. (1998). Age differences in death anxiety among African-American women. *Psychological Reports, 83*(3 Suppl.), 1173–1174. https://doi.org/10.2466/pr0.1998.83.3f.1173

Townes, Emilie M. (2011). Ethics as an art of doing the work our souls must have. In K. G. Cannon, E. M. Townes, & A. D. Sims (Eds.), *Womanist theological ethics: A reader* (pp. 35–50). Westminster John Knox Press.

Tucker, R. T. (1994). Patient Self-Determination Act: An African American perspective. *Cambridge Quarterly of Healthcare Ethics, 3*(3), 417–419.

Veatch, R. M. (2000). *The Basics of Bioethics*. Prentice Hall.

Wilson, W. D. (2019, February). Bioethics on the margins: Vulnerable populations and health outcomes [Lecture]. Harvard Divinity School.

Wojtasiewicz, M. E. (2006). Damage compounded: Disparities, distrust, and disparate impact in end-of-life conflict resolution policies. *American Journal of Bioethics, 6*(5), 8–12. https://doi.org/10.1080/15265160600856801

Wolf, S. M. (1996). *Feminism and bioethics: Beyond reproduction*. Oxford University Press.

Chapter 17

Blissful Balance

Spirituality, Healing, and Restoration

IMANI MA'AT AND CHERYL TAYLOR

Caring for myself is not self-indulgence—it is self-preservation.

—Audre Lorde

Introduction

Soul Sister, Sister love, Queen Mother, Sister girl, and Beloved are terms commonly used in reference to Black women. The importance of how we address ourselves is directly connected to our spiritual beliefs and the belief in ourselves. Through the lens of Black women, this chapter focuses on Black women's spirituality, faith, and healing practices from ancient times through current day. According to Musgrave et al. (2002) the meaning of spirituality is fluid and difficult to define. On one hand, it may mean an inner quality that facilitates connectedness with the self, other people, and nature, and, on the other hand, the traditional definition involves one's acknowledgment of and relationship with a higher power. For many women of color, it appears that the traditional definition is more often embraced (Musgrave et al., 2002).

Spirituality, however, can be described as the soul force of Black women and is a foundational and ancestral core value in Black culture.

Spirituality and faith serve as core constructs that are nonquantifiable, while their processes and outcomes concerning healing among individuals and communities have measurable and immeasurable dimensions. Practices such as meditation, prayer, yoga, music, dance, drumming, and singing are observable healthy lifestyle expressions of spirituality. While health outcomes of spiritual practices including those listed above are designed to progress to blissful balanced lives, think of spirituality as a required course, and not as extracurricular activities. Think of spirituality as a progressive flow of positive energy that sustains itself based on beliefs, ritual ceremonies, and practices. Faith consists of belief patterns that ground and guide authentic living and give meaning to one's world (Dyess, 2011). Faith and spirituality are connected with each other and integral to experiencing the fullness of joy, peace, and love—the fuel that drives the ability to be resilient.

Table 17.1 summarizes nine research studies from an integrated review of the literature on the intersectionality of Black women's spirituality and health. Of the studies reviewed, the majority used qualitative methods, which limits the generalizability of findings to the larger population. However, the studies found religion, spirituality, and social support to be important indicators of Black women's health. Two research studies investigated the use of sister circles as culturally specific public health interventions to reduce anxiety (Neal-Barnett et al., 2011) and reduce cardiovascular risk factors (Taylor & Tilton, 2004). Included in some of the research studies is the womanist theory perspective (Smith 2015), which involves Black women honoring their unique experiences, cultural heritage, and contributions historically made to religious discourse and society. African American women's sense of confidence, power, creativity, and leadership are highlighted in the womanist framework. Several research studies reviewed in table 17.1 used the womanist framework as their conceptual framework.

Absent from the literature reviewed was research assessing the impact on Black women's own health and well-being as a result of working in the public health arena. Black women have a visible presence in the public health arena, contributing to public health research, policies, and programs. From personal and shared experience, we are aware of the racism, misogyny, and discrimination in general experienced by Black women in top public health institutions, as well as amazing stories of resilience. Some have not been so resilient and have succumbed while working or shortly after retirement. One may argue that people of all races and genders have

Table 17.1 Black Women's Resilience: Spirituality Research Review of Literature

Authors (year) and topic time frame	Theoretical framework, research design/purpose, and study participants sample size	Major findings or conclusions	Limitations and recommendations
Lynn, Yoo, and Levine, "Religious and Spiritual Practices of African-American Breast Cancer Survivors" (2013).	Grounded theory; qualitative. 47 African American women ages 34–82, Muslim and Christian.	Spiritual community provided emotional, tangible, social and spiritual support. Comfort via prayers by others and encouragement through reading scriptures was achieved. Women who participated in both individual and communal spiritual practices coped successfully from breast cancer diagnosis through breast cancer survivorship.	Religious and spiritual practice language labels were used interchangeably.
Taylor and Chatters, "Spirituality in the Lives of African American Caribbean Blacks and Whites" (2010).	No theoretical framework. Secondary data analysis. Quantitative design. 5,000 African Americans including Caribbean Blacks. Data collected 2001–2003.	90% of African Americans and Caribbean Blacks found religion and spirituality to be very important in their daily life.	Public health practitioners should incorporate practice principles and guidelines that include religion and spirituality in their professional work with clients and centered care.
Yolanda Smith, "Empowering Black Women: Womanist and Womanist Theology" (2008).	Womanist theology framework. Quantitative historical. Annual womanist consultation meeting at the American Academy of Religion for the Society of Biblical Literature.	Christian education issues revealed racism, ignored contributions or devaluing them. Sexism and lack of equalitarian leadership. Womanist theology can play significant roles in shaping the content, method, and process of African American Christian education.	The study lacked differentiation between spirituality and religion focused concepts and focused denominations.

continued on next page

Authors (year) and topic time frame	Theoretical framework, research design/purpose, and study participants sample size	Major findings or conclusions	Limitations and recommendations
Denham, Holt, Clark et al., "Religious Relationship Social Support with Health Behaviors in African Americans" (2010).	Health behavior and social network theory. Secondary data analysis from the National RHIAA study. 2,300 African Americans National sample from telephone interviews.	Religious support served as a predictor for fruit and vegetable consumption and physical activity and decreased alcohol use.	There is a lack of generalizability of the findings to African Americans who do not attend churches. Participants self-reported data.
Musgrave, Allen, and Allen, "Spirituality and Health for Women of Color" (2002).	Review of the literature culture.	Spirituality enhances some public health interventions among women of color. Spiritual well-being and social support improve coping and health promotion behaviors.	A review of literature emphasizing the multilayered integration of spirituality and health. Further study comparing rural and urban women of color is necessary.
Michele Mahon, "Sisters with Voices: Black Women in London Baptist Association" (2015).	Liberation theology-Black theology. Womanist? Feminist framework. Mixed methods design. 9 women ministers, African and Caribbean descent. Online survey.	Women ministers serve multiple roles in multiethnic communities undergirded by a love for God and their neighbors.	More gender focused, limited sample size. Methodological confusion and lack of generalizability.

Neal-Barnett, Stadulis, et al., "Sister Circles as Culturally Relevant Interventions for Anxious African American Women" (2011).	Social support Intervention Research Pilot Study testing the efficacy of sister circles as a public health intervention for anxiety. Investigate the utility of sister circles.	Sister circles are culturally relevant and may exist in communities and organizations where Black women live. Black women need each other's support.	Further research is needed.
Mary Abrums, "How African American Women from a Storefront Church Resist Oppression in Healthcare" (2004).	Black family theory, Black feminist theory. Ethnography, qualitative design. Secondary analysis of data. 35 participants. Life history interviews. In-church storytelling. Thematic analysis.	Analysis results included understanding meanings of (1) intelligence versus education, (2) the power of prayer, (3) demonstrating agency in health care encounters, and (4) trust in (higher power) Jesus.	
Pamela Ayo Yetunde, "From Strong Black Women to Remarkably Resilient Women: Black Christian Women & Black Buddhist Lesbians in Dialogue" (2017)	Grands' "theory of sacrifice." Womanist theory and Buddhist conceptual framework. 31 African American Buddhist lesbians.	The strong Black woman mythology is grounded in oppressive beliefs and practices that foster internalized racism and oppression justified by early Christianity. Practicing mindfulness through meditation could facilitate conscious interdependence and relational resilience.	

been known to transition shortly after (or even before) retiring. However, to what extent do job stressors on Black female public health professionals contribute to increased mortality and early morbidity? How might spiritual beliefs and faith practices enhance the effectiveness and resilience of Black female public health workers and officials? Even the tough issues like the extent to which internalized racism can turn African Americans public health professionals against each other needs examination. How is internalized racism experienced in this arena and how is it resolved? The research questions need to be asked, and the data need to be examined. These research questions may require qualitative studies initially, in order to formulate the questions for further research. Examples of Black women's lived experiences leading and navigating with resilience and progressively navigating societal racism and injustices are described herein.

In addition to daily trials and tribulations in the form of racial and sexist insults and violations, Black women carry centuries of atrocities that are imprinted in our DNA and our very souls (Heinzelmann and Gill, 2013; Sipahi et al., 2014). Systemic, societal, and interpersonal racism combined with misogyny wear heavily on the Black woman, and our defense mechanisms are many. Without a place to deposit the hurt, the pain, the rage, these feelings can fester and rot and may transform into bitterness, illnesses, and diseases. Our spiritual and faith practices are a necessary cultural response and come in many forms. Black women have explored and used them all as individuals and in collectives as women striving to remain whole and healthy. Take our hair for example. A federal court once ruled it legal for employers to ban dreadlocks (Arefin, 2020; Allen, 2020). The fact that the right to wear our hair in natural styles is still being discussed and debated in state legislation and corporate board rooms is a sad commentary on society and a small example of what Black women experience daily (Arefin, 2020; McGregor, 2019). Moreover, New Jersey, Tennessee, Michigan, Wisconsin, Illinois, and other states have proposed legislation to explicitly ban race-based hair discrimination—tackling a remaining loophole in the law governing discrimination in workplaces, schools, and other public places. California and New York were the first to sign such legislation into law in July, and New York City issued guidelines on the issue (McGregor, 2019). There is a federal bill that now makes it illegal to discriminate based on your hairstyle entitled the Crown Act, which has passed the House but not yet the Senate (Christiani, 2021).

Our very existence as strong, smart, creative, resourceful women worthy of dignity, respect, and support is captured in the words of Sojourner

Truth in her famous speech entitled "Ain't I a Woman?": "That man over there says that women need to be helped into carriages, and lifted over ditches, and to have the best place everywhere. Nobody ever helps me into carriages, or over mud puddles, or gives me any best place. And ain't I a woman? Look at me!" (Truth, 2016).

In recognition of the unique needs of African American women stemming from historical and current injustices and the need for holistic healing, both traditional and nontraditional caregivers of African American women have incorporated spiritual activities in treatment and healing protocols. Research studies have shown that significant relationships were found between spiritual well-being and the quality of life (QOL) domains of physical, emotional, and functional well-being. These specific findings suggested that nurses should incorporate spiritual and religious support in the care of African American women during the breast cancer treatment phase (Heinzelmann & Gill, 2013).

Worship and Prayer

Typically, houses of worship are the first response to the question of what spiritual practices sustain Black women and contribute to the ability to achieve balance and wholeness—mind, body, and spirit. In Christian churches, Black women have held and still do hold leadership roles as ministers, choir directors, singers in the choirs, Sunday school teachers, and more. Honorable mention is due to the late Dr. Barbara King, founder and minister of the Hillside International Truth Center, whose new age/new thought ministry touched thousands of lives in Atlanta, Georgia, where her church was based, as well as in communities around the world where she was often invited to speak. We have also explored and participated in other faiths such as Judaisms (including but not limited to Hebrew Israelites), Bahai, Islam, Buddhism, and Chiism (a world peace and compassion-promoting religion started in Nigeria, West Africa). Studies of African Americans and faith have indicated that African Americans are "demographically (87%) the most religious group in the nation" (Withrow, 2017).

We are indeed a praying people often reinforced by our mothers, grandmothers, and great-grandmothers. Consistent with the understanding that everything is energy and everything carries a vibration, praying has been a primary way of Black women communicating with their higher power and bringing the energy of healing and survival to the focus of our prayers. Black women's prayers carry the mighty force of the ancestors—looked to for guidance and support. Often transcending time and space, our prayers guided by our beliefs have been known to work miracles that changed the course of history. Many believe that Harriet Tubman was led by her spiritual beliefs, or she could never have guided so many enslaved Africans out of slavery to freedom. Although not allowed to practice African religions and other cultural practices from Africa during slavery, it is a fact that our deep-rooted spiritual beliefs far predated the religions aforementioned and slavery in the US.

Queen Afua, a nationally renowned herbalist, natural health and nutrition expert, and healer of women's bodies practices a unique form of Afrocentric spirituality. She guides women through a process that includes meditation, affirmations, and rituals rooted in Ancient Egyptian temple teachings.

She teaches how to love and rejoice in our bodies by spiritualizing the words we speak, the food we eat, the spaces we live in, the beauty we create in our lives, the healing energy we transmit to self and others, the relationships that we nurture, the service we offer, and the divine spirit we manifest (Queen Afua, 2000).

Meditation

It is often said that when we pray, we are speaking to God, but when we meditate, God is speaking to us and we are listening. Black women have been tuning in as a way of staying balanced and healthy and to deflect the worries of the world. Meditation helps to center and take our minds off of the worries of the world and back on to ourselves. "Meditation, in its own way, is a form of self-care: another way to take time out to show yourself love, patience, and grace . . . meditation is another great form of taking care of yourself from the inside out. It also helps you increase your focus for more clarity in order to be able to tackle another day. . . . Being able to take a breath through meditation not only gives you time to mentally gear up for the day, but it also re-energizes you so that you can bring your full self to the world—a world that needs you for all that you are, Black woman" (Bedford, 2020).

As an instructor and the former manager of inmate services for the DeKalb County Sheriff's Office in Decatur, Georgia, I often started my classes with a brief but deep guided meditation session for both the male and the female classes. The purpose was to calm and relax them in a rigid, structured, and sometimes anxiety-producing environment. I took them on a journey sometimes on a beach, other times in a vehicle on a wide-open road in the country, where they encountered someone that told them about themselves and reminded them of their purpose in life. Both therapeutic and enlightening, meditation is a powerful spiritual tool that aids in healing body, mind, and spirit.

Yoga

Yoga practices are as ancient and wholesome as our breath. These practices affect us mind, body, and spirit in a way that few practices do. The stretching postures, breathing, and balancing impact us at our core—strengthening and rejuvenating simultaneously. According to Queen Afua, our ancestors used the element of air-breath (referred to as prana)—through what was called Ari Ankh Ka, now known as Hatha Yoga. The various movements and poses from those practices depicted on the walls of temples and pyramids were carved by African people thousands of years ago (Queen Afua, 2000).

Data have shown that yoga is effective for improving health-related outcomes in breast cancer survivors. While breast cancer is the most commonly diagnosed cancer among Black women, Black women were less likely to engage in yoga compared to other ethnic groups. One study of the impact of yoga on African American breast cancer survivors showed positive results for the participants, and the authors encouraged further study to document the efficacy of yoga in healing protocols for Black women recovering from breast cancer (Taylor et al., 2018).

According to Leslie Salmon Jones, creator of Afro Flow Yoga, a research-based technique for healing cultural and personal trauma: "The colonization process cut us off from our roots and our history, and these practices—the drumming, the dance, the yoga—help to heal that. . . . The memory of our lineage and history begins to awaken in the DNA and the cells, it gives us agency and freedom" (Kripalu Center for Yoga and Health, 2020).

Fasting

There are as many different types of fasting as there are clouds in the sky. From ancient times, there have been religious fasts, such as the fast of Ramadan practiced by the those in the Islamic faith. Practiced for 30 days each year from sun up to sun down, Ramadan includes daily prayers, discipline, the reading of the Koran holy book, and mass worship. There are also fasts for weight loss, balance, peace, and spiritual growth. How people fast also varies. For some it means abstaining from eating food; however, liquids including water, juices and smoothies are fine. Some only drink water. There are, for example, Black women, such as Queen Afua, who have championed and taught the discipline of fasting for cleansing and spiritual development. According to Queen Afua, fasting benefits include spiritual peace, mental clarity, weight loss, more beautiful skin, burning up of cellulite, and greater womb wellness (Afua, 2000). It is imperative that self-care behaviors demonstrate aspects of love for beauty, peace, harmony, and holistic care for ourselves.

Writing as a Spiritual Healing Outlet

Outside of and in addition to participating in established religions, contemporary Black women have sought and engaged in both traditional and nontraditional spiritual practices. We pray, meditate, practice yoga, and we write it down. Writing has been as much of a spiritual healing outlet for many of us as the other practices described above, but is not normally recognized as a spiritual healing outlet. Searching for meaning in an often senseless and unforgiving world sends me and lots of Black women from all walks of life and socioeconomic and educational backgrounds to pen and paper, and now to the computer. It is as though dissecting frivolous acts of racial hatred, self-hatred, and soul annihilation with the pen creates solutions and remedies (at least in our minds) that make this world more tolerable. As such, it serves as a healing balm. In a world that outwardly deems us as superfluous but inwardly envies the ease with which we carry ourselves and navigate through life's challenges; along the vast continuum of strategies for self-love and self-care, writing it down as poetry and prose is right up there with breathing. Writing in some cases serves to document the obvious and not so obvious atrocities while planting seeds of hope for a greater tomorrow.

The senseless murder of Sandra Bland, among other Black women who chose to challenge the system, yielded poetic justice from this public health scientist designed to soothe my soul and the souls of others who became paralyzed by the thought of hanging from a noose in a jail because of a minor traffic infraction (changing lanes without signaling while Black).

Writing by and for Black women is something we have done for centuries in this country. It is part of the resilience story that quite frankly gets overlooked. Codifying our pain and process through the written word has liberated us on one level and validated us on another in ways that only we can do for each other. This includes the lyrics of gospel songs, poetry, fiction, and nonfiction, as well as prose. The following narrative includes personal accounts of experiences.

As a young girl, I (one of the coauthors) wrote frequently for the fun of it or to fulfill a homework and later scholarly assignments. However, the desire to write turned into the need to write for the very sustenance of my mind, body, and spirit. It became a way to remember details, as details often get lost or twisted when it comes to telling our story.

I wrote it down when on a public health epidemiological investigation of the "coming" AIDS epidemic in South Africa—I saw a thin, weak, very young sister on a gurney outside a crowded health clinic whose lifeless body spoke to me. It spoke to me in a way that colleagues in my group missed, telling me (and I wished this for her) that she had already returned to spirit—because that was no way to operate and optimally function otherwise (Ma'at, 2008)!

African American female writers over the past century—literary giants such as Zora Neal Hurston, Toni Morrison, Alice Walker, and Sonia Sanchez—have through their stories chronicled the passion and pain experienced by African Americans and Black women in particular. *Beloved*, by Toni Morrison, the story of Seth who is haunted by her baby (referred to as Beloved), is a painful tale. However, it is painful in a way that allows us to experience and then release it—the tragedies and choices that African American women have had to make while enslaved and as indentured servants concerning their bodies and their children. Difficult decisions are made to this day. Many Black women have turned to other sisters for support and healing. Sisters circles have offered such support.

Sister Circles

When I (one of the coauthors) first moved to Atlanta from New York, I knew very few people outside of the CDC and felt very much like a fish out of water—or like I had moved to a different country. Everything seemed so strange and unfamiliar. While I loved my new job, I was also experiencing personal issues at home. I stumbled upon sister circles held by the National Black Women's Health Initiative (NBWHI) at a time when in many ways my inner world, my personal world was falling apart. While attending a public health conference of the NBWHI in Washington, DC, I attended a break-out session devoted to sister circles.

Sister circles are support groups that build upon existing friendships, fictive kin networks, and the sense of community found among African American females (Neal-Barnett et al., 2011). Giddings (1984) credits the Black club movement with launching sister circles. Originally known as Black women's self-help groups, sister circles have been a vital part of Black female life for the last 150 years. Sister circles were designed to provide support, encouragement, spiritual guidance, and love among women that were on a mission to make changes in themselves and the world. Sister circles exist directly in the community and within organizations that are components of women's lives. Many women have ties to these organizations that go back generations. Members often refer to one another as Sister X or Sister Y, building on a sense of collectivism and existing kinship networks (Black Women's Health Imperative, 2016; Boyd, 1993). Inherently, sister circles provide Black women with help, support, knowledge, and encouragement (Boyd, 1993; Giddings, 1984; Neal-Barnett et al., 2011).

One organization that facilitated sister circles was the National Black Women's Health Project. In 1983, Byllye Y. Avery, founder of the Black Women's Health Imperative (formerly the National Black Women's Health Project) and the Avery Institute for Social Change, has been a health-care activist for over 30 years, focusing on the specific needs of African American women. The National Black Women's Health Project was committed to defining, promoting, and maintaining the physical, mental, and emotional well-being of Black women and their families. Ms. Avery combined activism and social responsibility to develop a national forum for the exploration of the health issues of Black women (PrEp, 2021).

Within the sister circle that I helped to launch were seven powerful African American women from different walks of life—several of whom were working in public health. We often started our weekly sessions with open-eye meditation—taught by one of the participants. It was for focus, grounding, and getting centered prior to our discussion. We shared our dreams and plans and provided a spiritual bond of sisterhood that lasted for decades. Dazon Dixon Diallo is the creator and executive director of Sister Love, Inc., an HIV prevention women's organization which had its roots in our sister circle and proved to be very instrumental in actualizing our goals. Ms. Dixon Diallo went on to become a prominent voice in public health, starting an international arm of her program in South Africa.

Her programs incorporated the culture of the women served, including, among other practices, the music. With music being known for its healing value as the universal language, music and dance serve as transformative ways of simultaneously being with self and community. "Lift every voice and sing, till earth and heaven ring. Ring with the harmonies of Liberty" (Johnson & Johnson, 1899).

Music

From African drumming to jazz to rhythm and blues to soul music— music indeed stirs our soul, both soothing and inspiring Black women. Music ignites us to hum and dance for reasons and no reasons, both of which have their place in the restoration process and keeping us whole. Our presence as musicians, as instrumentalists, singers, and writers, is part of the American story. Nina Simone, Leontyne Price, Billie Holiday, Alice Coltrane, Aretha Franklin, Bessie Smith, Ella Fitzgerald, Etta James,

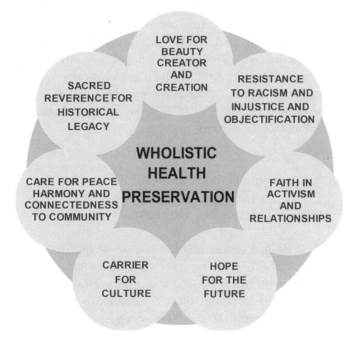

Figure 17.1. Spiritual dimensions of Black women's resilience. *Source*: Author.

to name a few of the great Black female singers and musicians over the past century. The resilience of Black women is intricately connected to and compelled by music of all genres!

Considering the magnitude of Black women's' spiritual and faith practices related to health and wellness, the need for more dialogue, support, and practical application is evident.

Summary

This chapter has presented a broad overview of issues and practices related to Black women's spiritual and faith practices that impact our health, well-being, and ability to be resilient. Each of the topics here within must be examined in richer detail and depth. While many practices exist and have existed for decades, little empirical research exists to document the health benefits of such practices. With a focus on improved health outcomes, further study would highlight the benefits of the practices discussed. It will also facilitate enhanced visibility and possibilities for integrating these practices into the workplaces, places of worship, and wellness centers serving Black women in their communities.

Spirituality and faith undergirds Black women's resilience and preserves their health through loving ways of being. Black women's unlimited spirituality and faith is manifested like a light beaming dignity, divinity, joy, mutual respect, self-awareness, and self-compassion. Personal, community, and global health and healing all benefit from the love, hope, faith, and activism of resilient Black women.

Recommendations and Call for Action

Public Health Practitioners and Researchers

More research is needed concerning the impact of spirituality and faith on Black women's health outcomes. For example, when collecting personal health history, include questions about behavioral practices related to spiritualty. Also inquiry about Black women's view of their spiritual and social support systems. Design and conduct research studies that specifically evaluate the impact of behavioral health interventions—for example, sister circles, meditation, and yoga groups—on the health outcomes of Black women.

As indicated above, there is a huge opportunity to closely examine the experiences of Black public health researchers and other professionals in institutions such as the Centers for Disease Control and Prevention (CDC), the National Institutes of Health (NIH), and other prominent public health institutions. Stories need to be shared of Black women's resilience in these institutions—identifying the barriers to success as well as those variables such as spiritual beliefs and faith practices that contribute to our resilience.

Public Health Policy

Consistent with the tenets of social determinants of health, consider the provision of funding to local and regional, rural and urban Black women's health resource centers that include alternative health practices and intervention. Specific measurements are needed of the intersectionality of health promotion interventions and spirituality. Include a rigorous evaluation component to document and disseminate the findings.

Also of benefit would be an annual conference held for a three–five year time period featuring exemplars/healers, public health practitioners, and other leaders who, through the exchange of ideas, workshops, and presentations, can help to define best practices for holistic and spiritual health practices. Scholarships should be provided for Black women nationwide to participate, and rigorous evaluations done that include both quantitative and qualitative variables.

Consider the Following for Forums, Discussions, and Research

Ask questions about the public health strategies to help ensure Black women's holistic health is being addressed. Ask whether institutional resources—people and funding—are being appropriately designed and deployed to support the health needs of Black women. Ensure that there is a focus on spirituality as a human dimension, and not just physicality as the basis of health resiliency. Regularly provide resources to improve Black women's resilience with support systems at personal, organizational, community, and institutional levels.

Allocate funds for further study and celebrate mental health, spiritual health, and meditation practices. An evidence-based support of Black women's resilience is a critical component to promote. Include time on agendas to discuss institutional and public policy issues of Black women's health.

Resources

Black Women's Health Imperative. https://bwhi.org/
Breakfast Club Power 105.1 FM. Queen Afua & SupaNova Slom on ultimate healing of the mind, body & spirit, feminine wellness + more. March 22, 2021. https://youtu.be/kGVtye47wq0
The Energy Project. https://theenergyproject.com/
From Ruby Sales' Front Porch. https://fromrubysalesfrontporch.wordpress.com/
Prayer Academy Global: Raising Elite Praying Warriors. https://prayeracademy-global.com/
Sister Love, Inc. https://www.SisterLove.org
SpiritHouse Project Public Group. Facebook. https://tinyurl.com/10blckyogateachers
SWAY'S Universe. Queen Afua celebrates sacred woman: A guide to healing the feminine body, mind and spirit on SITM. March 25, 2021. https://youtu.be/vXkSp2xC_HM
Taider, S. Black women on what the art of doing nothing means to them. *xoNecole*, January 17, 2021. https://www.xonecole.com/what-embracing-stillness-truly-means/

In memory of both Qairo "Shevevyah" Ali, who championed the funding and support for HIV prevention faith-based initiatives at the Centers for Disease Control and Prevention (CDC), and the phenomenal actress Cicely Tyson, whose talent, grace, and power exemplified a spiritual life!

References

Afua, Q. (2000). *Sacred woman: A guide to healing the feminine body, mind and spirit*. Ballentine.
Allen, Maya. (2020, February 24). 22 Corporate women share what wearing their natural hair to work means. *Byrdie*. https://www.byrdie.com/natural-hair-in-corporate-america
Arefin, D. S. (2020, April 17). Is hair discrimination race discrimination? *Business Law Today* (American Bar Association). https://www.americanbar.org/groups/business_law/publications/blt/2020/05/hair-discrimination/
Bedford, B. A. (2020, July 15). What meditation means to Black women. *The Everygirl*. https://theeverygirl.com/what-meditation-means-to-black-women/
Black Women's Health Imperative. (2016). *IndexUS: What Healthy Black Women Can Teach Us about Health*.

Boyd, J. (1993). *In the company of my sisters: Black women and self-esteem*. Dutton.
Christiani, P. E. (2021, January/February). I am not my hair. *Essence Magazine*.
Dyess, S. M. (2011). Faith: A concept analysis. *Journal of Advanced Nursing*, 67(12), 2773–2731. https://doi.org/10.1111/j.1365-2648.2011.05734.x
Giddings, P. (1984). When and where I enter: The impact of Black women on race and sex in America. Morrow.
Heinzelmann, M., & Gill, J. (2013). Epigenetic mechanisms shape the biological response to trauma and risk for PTSD: A critical review. Nursing Research and Practice, 2013, Article 417010. https://doi.org/10.1155/2013/417010
Kripalu Center for Yoga and Health. (2020). Black yoga and meditation teachers who are changing the world. https://kripalu.org/resources/10-black-yoga-and-meditation-teachers-who-are-changing-world
Johnson, J., and Johnson, R. (1899). Lift every voice and sing. https://www.naacp.org/naacp-history-lift-evry-voice-and-sing/
Ma'at, I. (2008). *Promoting healthy knowledge, attitudes and behaviors among youth using haiku and creative expression: A training manual for mentors*. Focused Health.
McGregor, J. (2019, September 19). More states are trying to protect black employees who want to wear natural hair styles. *Washington Post*. https://www.washingtonpost.com/business/2019/09/19/more-states-are-trying-protect-black-employees-who-want-wear-natural-hairstyles-work/
Musgrave, C. F., Allen, C. E., & Allen, G. J. (2002). Spirituality and health for women of color. *American Journal of Public Health*, 92(4), 557–560. https://doi.org/10.2105/AJPH.92.4.557
Neal-Barnett, A., Stadulis, R., Payne, M. R., Crosby, L., Mitchell, M., Williams, L., & Williams-Costa C. (2011). In the company of my sisters: Sister circles as an anxiety intervention for professional African American women. *Journal of Affective Disorders*, 129(1–3), 213–218. https://doi.org/10.1016/j.jad.2010.08.024
PrEP. (2021). Board member Byllye Y. Avery. http://prep.bwhi.org/staff-and-board-members/board-member/byllye-nbsp-y.-nbsp-avery-nbsp/
Sipahi, L., Uddin, M., Hou, Z.-C., Aiello, A. E., Koenen, K. C., Galea, S., & Wildman, D. E. (2014). Ancient evolutionary origins of epigenetic regulation associated with posttraumatic stress disorder. *Frontiers in Human Neuroscience*, 8, Article 284. https://doi.org/10.3389/fnhum.2014.00284
Smith, M. J. (Ed.). (2015). *I Found God in Me: A Womanist Biblical Hermeneutics Reader*. Wipf and Stock.
Taylor, C., & Tilton, C. (2004). Community lifeguards of Black women's health. *The Women's Health Activist*, 29(6), 3.
Taylor, T. R., Barrow, J., Makambi, K., Sheppard, V., Wallington, S. F., Martin, C., Greene, D., Yeruva, S. L. H., & Horton, S. (2018). A restorative yoga

intervention for African-American breast cancer survivors: A pilot study. *Journal of Racial and Ethnic Health Disparities*, 5(1), 62–72. https://doi.org/10.1007/s40615-017-0342-4

Truth, S. (2016). *Speech entitled Ain't I a Woman* (Delivered at the 1851 Women's Convention in Akron, Ohio). https://thehermitage.com/wp-content/uploads/2016/02/Sojourner-Truth_Aint-I-a-Woman_1851.pdf

Withrow, B. (2017, September). Black atheists: A minority within a minority. *Free Thought Today*. https://ffrf.org/publications/freethought-today/item/30453-black-atheists-a-minority-within-a-minority-by-brandon-withrow

Commentary

Organized Resistance Is Necessary

Linda Rae Murray

> To be a Negro in this country and to be relatively conscious, is to be in a rage almost all of the time. So that the first problem is how to control that rage so that it won't destroy you.
>
> —James Baldwin, interview, WBAI-FM
> New York City, January 10, 1961

When I was a little girl growing up in Cleveland during the 1950's my maternal great-grandmother came to live with us. Born during reconstruction, she was one of my early teachers on what it means to be a Black woman. Each day, around noon she would call us in from play: "Come in out that sun before you turn Black." Not wanting to interrupt my play I would always complain, "But I'm already Black." Once inside we would have lunch and spend the next hour resting out of the heat. During that break she would tell us stories of her childhood, how to behave, what to watch out for, and most importantly the peculiar ways of White folks. One day after being perplexed by our inability as Negroes just to live I asked how we could possibly know what was the right thing to do. "Oh, don't worry that is easy," she assured me. "Just remember baby—White folks will always knock you down. The *only* thing you have to decide in life is how often you stand back up." A calm settled over me and has lasted until this day.

White folks did not think we Negroes were people and would always knock us to the dirt. But we were people and, at least to my young mind, it would be easy indeed to stand back up. I did not think of this as "resilience," it was simply a fact of life. After all, no matter what White folks thought—you could not cease to be human. And since I was a human being—I would choose to stand back up.

Like most of our sisters, I experienced many of the stereotypes that plague little Negro girls and young women, the demands placed on Black mothers and grandmothers. But to me there never was a choice. It is not even a question of the mythical super strong Black women . . . my great-grandmother said nothing about how long you might have to lie in the dirt gathering your strength. No, her point was simply—decide how often you will stand back up and assert your humanity.

A decade after the conversation with my great-grandmother, I had another critical lesson from my first and best teacher—my mother. She reminded me of the importance of observing events around the world and appreciating history. "The important lesson from World War II is that Black people will be the first to be exterminated if fascism ever comes to America," she warned. "Remember how you were raised—do not walk quietly into gas chambers." It was as if the pieces of a puzzle clicked into place. The White power structure would continue to deny our humanity. It is possible for fascism to come to America; and, therefore, resistance is critical.

Today I have more nuanced language to describe these two lessons. I have spent decades learning those nuances. Decades in classrooms dominated by European thought and science, decades in settings with sisters and brothers trying to decolonize the oppressive lessons of Western philosophy, decades of living and working as a Black mother in America, decades involved in struggles fighting for the humanity of all peoples.

I have learned how the very land we live on was stolen from Indigenous peoples throughout this hemisphere. The stealing of the land and colonization of the world based on the racist ideology of White supremacy allowed racial capitalism to shape today's world (Dunbar-Ortiz, 2014).

As the great W. E. B. Dubois points out, "Black labor became the foundation stone not only of the Southern social structure, but of Northern manufacture and commerce, of the English factory system, of European commerce of buying and selling on a world-wide scale; new cities were built on the results of black labor, and a new labor problem, involving all white labor, arose both in Europe and America" (DuBois, 1935).

Racism creates a false hierarchy involving all peoples and nations of the world. This oppression—murder and genocide—continues today and its historical roots are hidden by myths and lies (Immerwahr, 2019).

Dr. Maria Yellow Horse Brave Heart, a Hunkpapa, Oglala Lakota professor, developed her concept of historical trauma based on lessons of the Holocaust and the lived experience of Native communities in the United States and Canada. She argues that you cannot understand the profound health inequities faced by Native (and not by accident also Black) men without understanding historical trauma (Brave Heart, 2012).

Black women must reconnect with the 95% of Africans in the trans-Atlantic slave trade who landed *outside* of the Thirteen British Colonies. We must listen carefully to the many other stories of the transformation of the world by racism and capitalism (Carrigan & Webb, 2013; Ortiz, 2018; Seijas, 2014).

An essential role of Black women has been to educate our young, whether as mothers and grandmothers or more formally in our state controlled, racist education systems. Education (not simply formal degrees) was seen as a major tool to achieve emancipation and secure the democracy necessary for us to become and remain free:

> Black education was a fugitive project from its inception—outlawed and defined as a criminal act regarding the slave population. . . . Enslaved people learned in secret places. During Jim Crow black educators wore a mask of compliance in order to appease the white power structure, while simultaneously working to subvert it. (Givens, 2021)

> When my youngest granddaughter, TY, was about 6 years old, I asked the usual question adults ask: "What did you learn in school today?" I expected the usual—"Nothing." But one day, she surprised me and replied, "Did you know that eggs are really dead baby chickens?" I chuckled, "Yes, baby, I knew that." Her little face looked suspicious. "Then did you know that we used to be slaves?" Yes, I responded. She pointed her finger and shook it at me, saying "You are supposed to tell us the important stuff!" (Murray, 2011)

This small encounter perfectly sums up my grandmotherly responsibilities. To continue to provide the fugitive pedagogy Black women have followed for centuries—to tell the young the "important stuff."

In 73 years of life, I still do not have the answers. I have, however, gained some clues about the "important stuff."

In my over 40 years of clinical practice as a Black physician, I know I stand on a great tradition of Black healers. That tradition is not limited to interactions with individual patients. It is a tradition deeply embedded in our struggles for freedom as a people and the struggle for justice throughout the world (Byrd & Clayton, 2000, 2001; McBride, 1991).

Ours is a struggle carried on not only by healers (i.e., the health sector) alone, but encompassing every discipline, every nook and cranny of our people. We are facing crises in every arena. The maternal mortality rate of American mothers continues to climb in stark contrast to the fall of maternal mortality in other rich nations. The rate of pregnancy-related mortality is highest for Black mothers. Black men comprise a smaller percent of medical students today than when I trained as a resident almost 50 years ago (Morris et al., 2021). Our children and youth continue to be murdered in the streets, now often recorded on cell phones. Inequities continue to grow in wealth, income, incarceration, and any area we choose to measure.

I consider the ecosocial theory proposed and developed by Nancy Krieger as the major contribution to public health of our generation. Her concept of embodiment expresses in academic terms something Black women deeply understand. Our Latin American cousins have enriched public health theory by insisting that the collective health and its *social determination* must be explored and understood if we are ever to produce healthy people and a healthy world (Breilh, 2021; Krieger, 2021). With these tools and others, Black public health practitioners can make important contributions to changing the world.

I am reminded that, for each step forward, we are confronted with a wave of reaction. I have watched my son and daughter-in-law's generation join their energy and strength to my generation as we struggle to hold back the forces of reaction. They have passed on their understanding of the "important stuff" to my grandchildren.

Today we face the very real threat of fascism engulfing the nation, a worldwide increase in inequities, and the existential threat of climate change. I worry about the very survival of my grand babies, all them related to me by history, not merely DNA. The tasks they face are overwhelming. Resilience—particularly the kind that adapts to injustice and oppression—has never been enough. Resistance is required. Organized resistance that understands the profound connections between oppressions based on racism, class, and gender is a goal that Black women have passionately pursued. We, Black women, who stand at the center of this triple oppression have always fought to organize the power needed to defeat our enemies (Gore, 2011; Jones, 2020; McDuffie, 2011)

Our grandchildren must create a world where every human being is valued, patriarchy is abolished, and racism is a ghost of the past. A world where the few can no longer steal the wealth created by the many; and all have a chance to achieve their dreams. A planet that is healthy and sustainable. A world where peace and social justice is the law of the land: "I know what I'm asking is impossible. But in our time, as in every time, the impossible is the least that one can demand—and one is, after all, emboldened by the spectacle of human history in general, and the American Negro history in particular, for it testifies to nothing less than the perpetual achievement of the impossible" (James Baldwin, *The Fire Next Time*).

References

Brave Heart, M. Y. H., Elkins, J., Tafoya, G., Bird, D., & Savlador, M. (2012). Wicasa Was'aka: Restoring the traditional strength of American Indian boys and men." *American Journal of Public Health*, 102(Suppl. 2), S177–S183.

Breilh, J. (2021). *Critical epidemiology and the people's health*. Oxford University Press.

Byrd, W. M., & Clayton, L. A. (2000). *An American health dilemma: Vol. 1, Beginnings to 1900*. Routledge.

Byrd, W. M., & Clayton, L. A. (2001). *An American health dilemma: Vol. 2, Race, medicine, and health care in the United State,s 1900–2000*. Routledge.

Carrigan, W. D., and Webb, C. (2013). *Forgotten dead: Mob violence against Mexicans in the United States, 1848–1928*. Oxford University Press.

DuBois, W. E. B. (1935). *Black reconstruction in the United States*. Atheneum.

Dunbar-Ortiz, R. (2014). *An indigenous peoples' history of the United States*. Beacon.

Givens, J. R. (2021). *Fugitive pedagogy: Carter G. Woodson and the art of Black teaching*. Harvard University Press.

Gore, D. F. (2011). *Radicalism at the crossroads: African American women activists in the Cold War*. New York University Press.

Immerwahr, D. (2019). *How to hide an empire: A short history of the greater United States*. Random House.

Jones, M. S. (2020). *Vanguard: How Black women broke barriers, won the vote, and insisted on equality for all.* Hachette.

Krieger, N. (2021). *Ecosocial Theory, Embodied Truths, and the People's Health.* Oxford University Press.

McBride, D. (1991). *From TB to AIDS: Epidemics among urban Blacks since 1900.* State University of New York Press.

McDuffie, E. S. (2011). *Sojourning for freedom: Black women, American communism, and the making of black left feminism.* Duke University Press.

Morris, D. B., Gruppuso, P. A., McGee, H. A., Murillo, A. L., Grover, A., & Adashi, E. Y. (2021). Diversity of the national medical student body—Four decades of inequities. *New England Journal of Medicine, 384*(17), 1661–1668.

Murray, L. R. (2011, November/December). The important stuff: Parting words from APHA's president. *The Nation's Health.* https://www.thenationshealth.org/content/41/9/3.1

Ortiz, P. (2018). *An African American and Latinx History of the United States.* Beacon.

Seijas, Tatiana. (2011). *Asian slaves in colonial Mexico: From Chinos to Indians.* Cambridge University Press.

Conversations with Thought Leaders
Beacons of Light

JENNIFER F. KELLY, JEMEA DORSEY, AND ADDIE BRIGGS

Question: What one word describes Black women to you? Why? What does that word mean to you?

SELECTED EXCERPTED RESPONSES

- Strong. I know that whatever obstacles we [Black women] have, we can handle those situations, because we are a very resilient breed of people.

- Resilient. We [Black women] push forward regardless of personal pain and frustration that we have personally experienced. Anger that we [Black women] may feel activates us and contributes to our own healing and ability to use our power in an effective way. We propel ourselves to use our energy to heal ourselves and others.

- Resilient. We [Black women], no matter what the situation, will always rise to the occasion. Black women have been the centerpiece of keeping our race together. Not just for our families; but our entire race.

Question: Can you describe how you see Black women as a critical part in establishing cultural norms and/or trends in our society?

Selected Excerpted Responses

- We [Black women] are natural leaders and thinkers and must stop being overlooked. We started many of the popular styles and trends that are considered mainstream. "Greatness is innately in us [Black women]"

- Hair styles. More recently we [Black women] are sporting various different hairstyles and embracing the "natural hair movement." Our hair is an accessory. We are so creative and expressive.

- It is our confidence and courageous self that is at the forefront of American culture.

- Creativity and self-expression. Even if we [Black women] are having challenges, we're not going to let the world see us sweat. We're going to have on our dresses, hair done, and makeup on. We're going to be creative.

Question: What are some of the challenges that you believe Black women must overcome in navigating through our society? How do you think we demonstrate resilience?

Selected Excepted Responses

Challenges

- One major challenge is living as our authentic self in a societal structure that does not affirm us [Black women].

- Getting rid of negative stereotypes and images of us [Black women]. There are so many untold stories and contributions that we should get credited, but we don't.

Resilience

- We demonstrate resilience by the support that we offer each other—in our families and communities. It becomes a form of self-care that recharges us as women and our bonding together. "We Never Leave Anyone Behind."
- "Despite it all, we show up and show out!"

Question: What do you believe are the most significant health concerns facing Black women and families today?

Selected Excepted Responses

- Stress and mental health issues.
- Sexual health and reproductive health issues/literacy; especially for young Black women.
- Body image concerns. While many other cultures try to emulate our look, there remain many problems.
- Interpersonal violence against women and family members.

Part Four

Advocacy and Activism for Social Justice

Perseverance /pərsəˈvirəns/
Continued effort to do or achieve something despite difficulties, failure, or opposition

Me Ware Wo
West African Adinkra Symbol for Perseverance

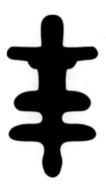

Okodee Mmowere
West African Adinkra Symbol for Bravery and Strength

308 | Part Four

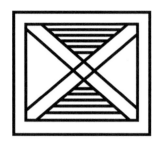

Mframadan
West African Adinkra Symbol for Fortitude

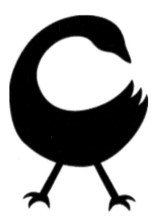

Sankofa
West African Adinkra Symbol for Learn from the Past

Sandra Bland

Imani Ma'at

I Think of you all the time
I drive daily and change lanes often without signaling.
In fact every time I do, I say your name in my head
Sandra Bland
Your name is now synonymous with
Changing lanes without permission
Sandra Bland
Synonymous with speaking your mind
Sandra Bland
Telling the truth and pissing people off
Perhaps your crime wasn't really about changing lanes at all
Sandra Bland
But refusing to stay in the lane assigned
By your birthright as a Black woman
Stay in your place.
Follow the rules.
Do as you are told
Put out your cigarette, pledge allegiance
To the flag
Shut the — up! Sandra Bland
Speaking up has never been a crime for other women
Well certainly not to the same extent.
Sandra Bland, your life was anything but Bland.

You lived in technicolor with
Explosive and powerful words for your people.
Your crime was speaking up—speaking out and
Telling the truth
While you were focused on liberating others by telling the truth,
They hung you in a jail cell and Lied about you hanging yourself.
Well, well, well,
Black woman swinging from a noose
In a cell
Not a pretty site. It's not right.
Black women's lives matter.
Say her name . . . Sandra Bland. . . . Say her name . . .
Sandra Bland. . . . Say her name. . . .

Chapter 18

#SayHerName

Honoring Black Women Victims of Violence

MAISHA STANDIFER AND SYDNEY LOVE

It is our obligation to acknowledge and honor Black women who have been victims of violence in the US due to fatal interactions with police officers. It is significant to say their names today, more than ever, due to the pervasive unjust actions and circumstances Black women have succumbed to over centuries of generational traumatic experiences in America. We must say her name because I am her—she is me. I must say her name to clear the elevated space Black women hold in America. We must say her name to rectify the innocence lost (while asleep); we must say her name to stand for righteous communication (in the midst of chaos); we must say her name to render homage to Black women's sanctity (vilified by systemic forces beyond her control).

To protect and serve is not a simple task—neither is being a Black woman in America!

Since 2015, nearly 250 women in total have been killed by police officers, of which 48—about a fifth—were Black, according to a *Washington Post* database. (Tate et al., 2020).

According to a study of 548 cases of arrests of police officers for sex related crimes between 2005 and 2007, over half were for sexual misconduct on duty (51.3%) or when acting in an official capacity (52.9%). (African American Policy Forum [AAPF], 2015)

According to a study of 548 cases of arrests of police officers for sex related crimes between 2005 and 2007, 32.2% involved forcible or statutory rape. (AAPF, 2015)

According to a study of 548 cases of arrests of police officers for sex related crimes between 2005 and 2007, 19.5% involved forcible fondling. (AAPF, 2015)

According to a study of 548 cases of arrests of police officers for sex related crimes between 2005 and 2007, 10.8% involved statutory rape. (AAPF, 2015)

Black women are disproportionately at risk for domestic violence, sexual abuse, and death at the hands of family members, partners, and people they know. *Time* magazine revealed that they are almost three times more likely to experience death as a result of domestic violence than are White women (African American Policy Forum, 2015). The CATO Institute's 2010 annual report on police misconduct found that "sexual misconduct was the second most common form of misconduct reported throughout 2010 [after excessive force] with 618 officers involved in sexual misconduct complaints during that period, 354 of which were involved in complaints that involved forcible non-consensual sexual activity such as sexual assault or sexual battery."

We say her name unapologetically as tenderly, as serenely, as sweetly, as majestically as we can. We must say her name to force others who interact with us to no longer see us as they once knew. We say their names until there are no more!

Ma'Khia Bryant

As similar to the others, on April 20, 2021, 16-year-old Ma'Khia Bryant was fatally shot and killed by a police officer outside of her foster home in Columbus, Ohio, highlighting the unfortunate police brutality and gender racism Black young women and women continue to face. Ma'Khia Bryant will be remembered as a funny, loving, and bright student, child, cousin, friend, and family member to so many.

Priscilla Slater

Priscilla Slater was arrested and taken into police custody on the morning of June 9, 2020, and found unresponsive over 24 hours later. Today, her loved ones, family members, and activists are still requesting closure and demanding justice, as her death marks another case where a Black American has been found harmed or dead after an encounter with an officer of the law.

Breonna Taylor

On March 12, 2020, a Jefferson County Court Judge approved search warrants for Breonna Taylor's home for her boyfriend suspected of illegal drug activity. Shortly after midnight, three officers/detectives used a battering ram to break down the door of her home and fatally shot the 26-year-old.

Atatiana Jefferson

On the morning of October 12, 2019, officers responded to a welfare check at the home where 28-year-old Atatiana Jefferson was babysitting her 8-year-old nephew. Bodycam footage shows officer Aaron Dean firing a shot through the window of her home and fatally killing Atatiana, sparking yet another outcry for racial justice and accountability in the judicial and policing system.

Dominque Clayton

African-American woman Dominique Clayton was fatally shot in the head and killed while sleeping in her home on Sunday morning, May 19, 2019. It is presumed she had a relationship with her killer, office Matthew Kinne, who has since been indicted and pled not guilty to the murder of 32-year-old Dominque Clayton.

Pamela Turner

On May 13, 2019, the death of Pamela Turner was recorded on video. Officer Delacruz of the Baytown Police Department fatally shot Pamela Turner after approaching her under false pretenses.

Jasmine McBride

Young and beautiful Jasmine McBride was 30 years old when she passed away on February 12, 2019 from one of the most prominent public health disasters in America, Legionnaires' disease from the water source and treatment crisis in Flint, Michigan. Her death marks an unjust political issue, where officials have spent years neglecting its social and physical infrastructures, exposing communities to poisoned circumstances that still exist today.

Aleah Jenkins

Aleah Jenkins was arrested November 27, 2018 after a traffic stop due to an expired tag. While in police custody, Aleah went into medical distress, suffering from an overdose and lack of oxygen that would later result in her death on December 6, 2018.

Charleena Lyles

Charleena Lyles called 911 on the date of June 18, 2017 to report a burglary. The Seattle police officers who responded to her north Seattle apartment fatally shot her in her home where her children were present, representing a continuous pattern of excessive force against Black American women.

Alteria Woods

Alteria Woods was a young and bright honors student at the Indian River State College in Florida. On the day before her death, she spent time with her mother and later retired for the night with her boyfriend, a young man whose father was the focus of the Indian River Shores County Sheriff's Department for possession of a stimulant drug, cocaine. On the early morning of March 19, 2017, Alteria Woods was fatally shot multiple times while lying in the bed. The officers involved in the raid were later exonerated from the murder of the young Alteria Woods.

Deborah Danner

Deborah Danner was fatally shot by sergeant Hugh Barry in her Bronx, New York, apartment on the date of October 18, 2016. Since then, the family and loved ones of Deborah have had to mourn her death knowing the New York Police Department (NYPD) has been acquitted of both murder and manslaughter.

> We say their names—delicate, defiant, gentle, resilient souls.
> May their souls continue to blossom.

References

African American Policy Forum. (2015). *Say her name: Resisting police brutality against women.* https://44bbdc6e-01a4-4a9a-88bc-731c6524888e.filesusr.com/ugd/62e126_9223ee35c2694ac3bd3f2171504ca3f7.pdf

Tate, J., Jenkins, J., & Rich, S. (2020, January 22). Fatal force: Police shootings database. *The Washington Post.* https://www.washingtonpost.com/graphics/investigations/police-shootings-database/

Chapter 19

Black Women, Public Health, and Resilience
Political Power

BRIAN MCGREGOR AND ANANA JOHARI HARRIS PARRIS

> I'm thinking about my mother, Shyamala Gopalan Harris, and the generations of Black women who came before me who believed so deeply in an America where a moment like this is possible.
>
> —Vice President Kamala Harris (Harris, 2019)

Introduction

Black women in the United States have long endured attacks on their physical, emotional, spiritual, and psychological well-being and have been forced to access deep and wide reservoirs of knowledge, skill, courage, creativity, and power to mitigate harms arising from individuals and systems that sought to devalue and destroy them. Historically, institutionalized racism and sexist oppression have served to limit the power of Black women to control the decisions and resources needed to protect their opportunities to achieve optimal health. As a result, they have had to cultivate individual and community resilience in various forms to withstand attacks on their lives and, in many cases, the lives of their children, families, communities, and indeed the nation. This chapter will examine how Black women have demonstrated that resilience since the beginning of their journey in the United States, and how it has been leveraged to create political power used to withstand harms to their well-being and promote advancements in public health.

It is critically important to examine Black women's resilience at the intersection of political power and the public-health arena for several reasons. First, we are not aware of any other published work that examines the role of individual and community resilience in developing political power, broadly defined, used by Black women to thwart public-health threats and achieve important public-health outcomes. Second, Black women experience some of the most significant and pervasive health disparities, including incidence rates of breast cancer, maternal mortality, and infertility, to name a few (Petersen et al., 2019; Krieger et al., 2018; Chandra et al., 2013). Third, there has been a recent awakening of the importance of Black women's influence and significance in the political arena, particularly within electoral politics. Black women have long been engaged in the political process, and have been elected or appointed to local, state, and national offices, with examples such as Crystal Bird Fauset (Pennsylvania), Stacey Abrams (Georgia), Carol Moseley Braun (Illinois), Barbara Jordan (Texas), Lelia Foley (Oklahoma), Shirley Chisolm (New York), and Madame Vice President Kamala Harris (California). Finally, and perhaps mostly importantly, while Black women are thriving in many areas of public life, there continue to be numerous examples of systematic and institutionalized disregard, disrespect, and attempted depreciation of the worth and value of the lives of Black girls and women in this country.

It is important to describe how this chapter frames political power. It is not only the kind that is born out of the thoughts and actions of Black women in elected office who leveraged their position to impact public health. It also refers to the visible and invisible power, cultivated from the effective collaboration of individuals working together to achieve sustainable goals, that may intersect with the machinery of government but often emerges outside of the political apparatus. Thus, political power can be developed and nurtured outside of spaces where it is born and exercised, such as the halls of Congress, corporate board rooms, or at exclusive country clubs. Indeed, Black women have inhabited these spaces and used those resources to achieve health benefits; however, there are many examples of grassroots efforts, that is, community born and bred, that Black women led that created considerable political power to effect change.

While it is recognized that resilience is a powerful tool that Black women must possess and cultivate, it can only aid their survival if their health and safety are not compromised in the process of developing political power. What does it profit a Black woman to gain political power yet forfeit the quality of her life? It is important to examine the physical, emotional, and psychological sacrifices that too many Black women experience along the journey to protect and promote the health of their counterparts, a bitter irony. The injuries are often numerous, debilitating, and obstinate, making for a challenging recovery process, and all of which may occur away from the public eye.

This chapter will explore the development of individual and community resilience of Black women and how both aided in the cultivation of political power leveraged to impact public health. We will conclude by reviewing lessons learned and consider how those lessons can contribute to increasing the political power of Black women and how best to leverage it to increase health equity among Black women and improve the nation's public health.

Black Women's Political Power: Developed and Sustained through Individual, Familial, and Community Resilience

Resilience has been a requirement for the survival of Black women on American soil for hundreds of years. One of the many gifts Black women throughout the diaspora have received from their African ancestors is the skill of using resilience as fuel for achieving political power. This resilience can be found in their recovery from damage and injury and in the way they search for resources and support to heal and create safe environments to learn, network, and strategize. There are various forms of resilience; however, Black women have used them all to creatively connect, recover from repeating injuries, and face trials and tribulations, which has been necessary for the pursuit and attainment of political power.

Family, community member, Black, and being a woman are a few of the social and political identities Black women carry on their intersectional walk, without reprieve from the institutionalized burdens that accompany those identities. Moreover, they are expected to do so with grace and aplomb while successfully addressing a multitude of micro- and macro-level challenges. Black women's efforts to respond to these challenges have been collaborative and organized, assuring their existence beyond mere survival for centuries.

Black women have organized strategic responses to a myriad of threats in above- and underground spaces that have saved countless lives and shifted political landscapes. Some churches, school systems, and community organizations have provided respite for Black women to nurture resilience and craft political strategies for use in local, regional, and national arenas. These institutions have been protected educational and training spaces for leadership development, mentorship, and fundraising for Black women. Unfortunately, black women could not completely shield themselves from the harsh consequences of sexism, which tends to lead to limited access to resources.

Resilience has fed every aspect of Black women's political power dating back thousands of years. John Henrik Clarke, a pioneer of Pan African studies, details an example from antiquity in *Black/White Alliances* (Clarke, 1976). The complexities of battling multiple challenges while holding a position of political power plagued the Egyptian Queen Hatshepsut, fifth pharaoh of the Eighteenth Dynasty. She faced the disgruntled people of her kingdom while simultaneously fighting off invaders. This is an example of the rich and storied tradition of Black women leaders mastering the skill of resilience to navigate treacherous political landscapes to garner and maintain political power. Harriet Tubman conquered the mental, emotional, and physical brutality of slavery and created familial and community leadership to make the Underground Railroad a success. Her courage and unwavering resilience can be identified in the organizing efforts of key Black women in the civil rights movement like Ella Baker, Shirley Chisolm, and Fannie Lou Hammer, as well as present day leaders like Vice President Kamala Harris and Stacey Abrams (Harris, 2019). Examples of challenges Black women have overcome include voter fraud, medical apartheid, poor access to social determinants of health such as transportation and safe housing, employment insecurity, economic/wage gaps, corporate glass ceilings, maternal and infant mortality, and the criminalization of Black girls in the school system, to name a few (Morris, 2016; National Partnership For Women and Families, 2020; Noonan et al., 2016; Marsh et al., 2014). Black women have also faced internal challenges through generationally learned behaviors including self-neglect and poor self-care practices (Parris, 2016).

Tobin and Dobard (1999) present historical evidence of the innovative and collective resilience of Black women in the stories of quilters who created secret codes embedded in the fabric of quilts. Their research reveals that certain quilt patterns, including a prominent one called the Charleston Code, were in fact, essential tools for escape along the Underground Railroad. Additionally, they chronicled the oral testimony of Ozella McDaniel, a descendant of enslaved Africans. McDaniel claims that her ancestors passed down the secret of the quilt code from one generation to the next. The code facilitated communication to another person without others discovering what was being said. The quilts would hang in plain sight in windows helping enslaved Africans navigate their escape through the Underground Railroad and ultimately to freedom (Tobin & Dobard, 1999). Charles Payne (1990) described the engagement of women who canvassed, demonstrated, and registered to vote more often than men during the civil rights movement. They were also involved in voter registration, led meetings in town halls, participated in church groups, and held political rallies. The movement would allow for different leaders to develop and allowed women to be participants as well as organizers. Women's influence in the movement was more pronounced than that of many other leaders, making their roles irreplaceable (Payne, 1990). Further, many Black women also navigated gender inequality during the Black Power movement. "The racial solidarity for which women hoped, the community they imagined, was weakened by male dominance and sexism. The movement empowered women while simultaneously angering and disappointing them" (Breines, 2006, p. 51).

Many of the same threats to the health and quality of life of Black women that need to be addressed, serve as the barriers keeping them from power. They are present in the environments where aspiring Black women leaders live, work, play, age, and worship and often show up when they are extremely vulnerable.

Politics is often a misused term, because the true goal of politics is not equanimity. The true goal of politics rests in one word, power. Power to protect, power to decide, and power to direct is typically seen to be left in the hands of those in public office; however, for Black women who have fought to contribute to and lead in the strengthening of the Black community to remain safe, the road to acquiring power has had to be hidden, finagled, developed, and sustained over time.

To discuss the political power of Black women, we must first discuss the danger and repercussions of exposing power. How can Black women expect to develop and sustain power in their own homes and communities when the country they reside in has never consistently protected them while doing so? If it has been consistently demonstrated that Black women are unsafe in the quiet of their own bedrooms at night, like Breonna Taylor, who was killed by law enforcement in her own home a few steps from her bed, how can Black women be guaranteed protection?

While unbridled resilience is a hallmark of their achievements, it does not come without a cost. There are told and untold stories of the trauma experienced by Black women who have sought and achieved political power. These injuries include threats and attempts to kill them, or to undermine and infiltrate their organizations; neglect of their health and safety; and attempted defeat of their legislative agendas. Additionally, many of these leader's experiences could be described as misogynoir, a term coined by Moya Bailey, that addresses anti-Black sexism that is uniquely experienced by Black women. This was on full display during Michelle Obama's time as First Lady and will no doubt characterize the vitriol aimed at Vice President Harris. Marilyn Mosby, the city of Baltimore's state attorney, one of 45 women of color who are elected prosecutors in the US, faced threats against her and her families' lives after she charged six police officers in the murder of Freddie Gray (Carrega, 2020). Suffice it to say, the evils of misogynoir did not begin with the popular use of the term and will only get worse as the country becomes more politically and racially polarized. However, in our examination of the resilience of Black women building political power, what is our collective responsibility to disrupt systems that compel these leaders to suffer in silence, particularly those at the local and state level, where the spotlight is dimmer? Are we to say to them and their sons, daughters, mothers, and fathers that this is an unavoidable by-product of Black women's political engagement that they should endure because they are pillars of resilience? If we understand that Black women political leaders' resilience may be our best chance at enhancing a movement that prioritizes the needs of individuals described as poor and working-class in policy making, improves family and community quality of life, and embraces a public health equity lens in its challenge to the status quo, the answer must be a resounding "No!". Yes, resilience is necessary, but it is not sufficient when it comes to resources Black women need to continue the fight for health equity and social justice in America.

Black women can be found vulnerable in the hospitals giving birth, walking their children to school, and navigating sexual advances in the workplace. This is where Black women are left vulnerable on a regular basis. Many Black women begin the journey toward political power without a list of specific needs being met and quickly learn that they need more than the spirit of resilience to cultivate sustainable leadership.

Political power has been described as activities associated with the governance of a country or other area, and is often exercised during debate or conflict among individuals or parties that have or hope to achieve power. Mistakenly, many only attribute political power to the images of and decisions made in the White House and governmental agencies. The definition of power and political power for Black women is multidimensional. Through the drafting and research of this chapter, we have identified seven different internal and external categories of support and impact that strengthen the resilience of Black women's rise to political power.

The seven categories of support to develop political power for Black women include:

1. familial and personal resources (external)
2. social network, mentorship, and safe environments (external)
3. mindset resilience and mental toughness training (internal)
4. strategic self-care planning and needs assessment (internal)
5. educational development and exposure to political strategies (internal)
6. knowledge of local, national, and global community dynamics (internal/external)
7. access to other social determinants of health (external)

Each of these influential factors helped to establish and nurture leadership that has helped Black women achieve success in politics, including key Black women leaders in Georgia during the 2018 and 2020 election seasons, where they had a significant impact on voter turnout.

Both Stacey Abrams and Kamala Harris have had a groundswell of support in all of these categories of support throughout their leadership development. Stacey Abrams's 2018 gubernatorial loss created an opportunity to expose and respond to inequities. In an interview with TIME.com, the CEO of the New Georgia Project, Nsé Ufot, outlined how determinedly Stacey Abrams worked to garner this historical election-shifting impact. Ufot explained how Abrams' years of organizing and strategizing efforts put a spotlight on Georgia, created political leverage for Georgia voters, and gave them a voice (Waxman, 2021). Ms. Abrams was able to benefit from the "seven categories of support" to develop political power for Black women. Abrams' journey to political power included creating a safe space in launching Fair Fight Action.

In the face of adversity, Abrams did not give up. She instituted a mindset of staunch resilience in order to adjust her political strategy. "Because I suddenly saw opportunity where I had never been brave enough to look before, and I found that failure wasn't fatal, that otherness held an extraordinary power for clarity and invention" (Waxman, 2021).

As Black women have increased their involvement in the political process, their political power has increased, which they have used to design and promote health policy legislation aimed at increasing health equity, a benefit for the entire society. Atlanta Mayor Keisha Lance Bottoms appointed the city's first Chief Health Officer in 2019, Dr. Angelica Geter, a public health expert who played a central role in the strategy to mitigate the spread of COVID-19, which disproportionately impacts Black men, women, and children (Williams, 2019). Sandra Barnhill earned her BA in political science at Georgia State University (1982), and her JD at the University of Texas (1984) (Foreverfamily, n.d.). From 1983 to 1987, she served as a staff attorney for the Southern Prisoners' Defense Committee. In this role, she represented indigent prisoners in class action challenges to prison conditions and in post-conviction challenges on capital convictions. During this time, Barnhill became frustrated by the lack of support given to imprisoned mothers and their families. In 1987, she founded Foreverfamily (originally named Aid to Imprisoned Mothers (AIM)), which is a nonprofit Atlanta-based organization advocating for inmate parents and their children. She was also instrumental in getting child visiting centers placed at Pulaski State Women's Prison and Lee Arrendale Women's Prison, both in the state of Georgia.

Also, consider the rise and legacy of Shirley Anita Chisholm, the first Black woman elected to Congress and the first Black candidate to seek the Democratic Party's nomination for president of the United States. Chisholm was a strong advocate for increased participation of women in public affairs through her work with organizations such as the League of Women Voters and the Brooklyn Democratic Clubs in the 1960s, early in her political career (Chisholm, 2010). She also challenged the leadership in these and other organizations to increase their engagement of women of color, often encountering strong opposition (Chisholm, 2010). Despite sexism, racism, and threats to her physical and psychological safety, Chisholm committed to building her political power with an agenda that centered underserved women's issues and needs, including increased support for childcare, better housing, and increased access to employment (Chisholm, 2010). This proved to be effective, given her success in being elected as a New York State senator and a US congresswoman from the same state.

After considering the wide range of examples of Black women's political power through the works of Stacey Abrams, Harriet Tubman, Ella Baker, Sandra Barnhill, Barbara Jordan, Shirley Chisolm, Able Mable Thomas, Njere Akosua Aminah Alghanee, Fannie Lou Hammer, Charlotta Bass, Loretta Lynch, Ida B. Wells, Ameena Matthews, Sojourner Truth, and Vice President Kamala Harris, we must conclude that resilience was paired with above- and underground political strategies as a way of protecting black women, warding off foreseen challenges to the movement and especially in the area of voting and voters' rights.

Black Women Utilizing Political Power to Achieve Public-Health Goals

Black women's health and quality of life have been neglected and abused in the United States since their captivity and enslavement centuries ago (Owens & Fett, 2019). Through the years, protecting themselves and their families meant understanding the power in their individual and collective agency and having the courage to act on it. Some of their power grew out of tragic events that harmed them. Some of it came from recognition and awareness of an increasing health burden on Black women that the public-health mainstream was ignoring, for example, maternal and child health. In many cases, the positive health outcomes experienced by Black women extend to other communities and thus have broader societal impact. In this section, we address two essential questions. First, how has Black women's political power been used to improve the health of Black women and, in some cases, the health of the nation? Though initial objectives may specifically identify Black women as the population of interest, initiatives often result in impacts to other groups. Second, how has the resilience of Black women contributed to the achievement and sustainability of these goals? Threats to the health and quality of life of Black women challenging the status quo is unquestionable and their resilience is fundamental to the positive outcomes that result from their efforts.

An essential example of how Black women have used their resilience and a special integration of above- and underground political strategies to empower themselves and strengthen their communities is in motherhood. Midwives, doulas, neighborhood aunties, and elder Black women in communities coordinated interventions during the many critical moments in a woman's life. Maternal mortality and severe maternal morbidity are critical health issues in the United States, with unacceptably high rates and racial, ethnic, and geographic disparities (Owens & Fett, 2019). Various Black women–led organizations are raising awareness about racial and ethnic disparities in maternal health and poor access to public health resources. A partnership between the Center for Reproductive Rights and the Black Mamas Matter Alliance developed a toolkit that includes a policy framework to address disparities, talking points for advocates, and research and informational resources about maternal mortality (Center for Reproductive Rights & Black Mamas Matter Alliance, 2018). The Black Mamas Matter Alliance also implemented its first-ever Black Maternal Health Week in April 2018, and this continues to be observed on an annual basis.

The United States has been promoting standardization in the reporting of maternal mortality data across 50 states—an important first step toward identifying ways to reduce pregnancy-related deaths across the country. The data, released in January 2020 by the National Center for Health Statistics, show that the national maternal mortality rate—deaths caused or aggravated by pregnancy—was an estimated 17.4 maternal deaths per 100,000 live births in 2018 (Hoyert et al., 2020). Using the new coding method, researchers found that of the 658 women who died of maternal causes in 2018, Black women fared the worst, dying 2.5 times more often than White women (37.1 vs. 14.7 deaths per 100,000 live births), while Hispanic women had the lowest rate of maternal mortality, 11.8 deaths per 100,000 live births. Advocates for Black women hailed these new data as an important step to empower themselves and strengthen their communities. Advocates assert that it is the government's responsibility to promote and advance maternal health care that is safe and respectful, which cannot be achieved without lasting political will and continued investments in the health and well-being of Black girls and women in particular (Center for Reproductive Rights & Black Mamas Matter Alliance, 2018).

The rapid response often initiated to support and educate a young Black girl in a community who has just begun her menstrual cycle is a micro-level example of Black women organizing to respond to a health need (Cooper & Koch, 2007). That young girl will need protection, safe spaces to learn more about her body, products, discretion, and most importantly strategies on how to navigate her new responsibilities of becoming a woman. In this example, Black women collectively have historically moved in a well-organized fashion not only to offer safety and education but also to encourage this new young woman not to feel ashamed. This cultural practice can be an informative experience in the development of a young girl's understanding of power and self-care cultivated by Black women. If they had not come together to provide the needed support and education, from where else would it have come? The collective agency demonstrated by these women serves as a model to girls of how to leverage skills, knowledge, and material resources at the community level to potentially prevent the harm of a neglected developmental need.

Taboos, secrecy, fear, shame, and embarrassment associated with discussing menstruation hinder young Black girls from seeking advice from parents and teachers on appropriate menstrual hygiene management (MHM) practices. Positive social norming of menstruation would help destigmatize discussions about it in public spaces large and small. This work would go a long way in supporting MHM improvements in the Black community and similar communities situated in low- and middle-income settings (Shah et al., 2019).

Marsh et al. (2014) found that the proportion of heavy menstrual bleeding among participants was higher than the nationwide prevalence. However, a gap existed in knowledge of heavy menstrual bleeding among the women surveyed. Their findings indicate an opportunity for community-based education to raise awareness of heavy menstrual bleeding, its associated clinical presentations, and available treatment modalities.

In 2020, the Black Women's Health Imperative (BWHI) released the second edition of its *Black Women Vote: National Health Policy Agenda for 2020–2021*. The national health policy agenda for Black women was created to help inform and support partnerships with policymakers and other stakeholders on the critical health policy issues that impact and improve the well-being of Black women. This agenda also provides an opportunity for voters to engage in substantive policy discussions—particularly around key health policy issues impacting Black women and girls—and to seek meaningful solutions (BWHI, 2020).

Byllye Yvonne Avery, founder of the National Black Women's Health Project (NBWHP), led transformational work through this organization, now named Black Women's Health Imperative (BWHI), that illustrates the unique journey that black women must travel to improve the health of their communities, and how political power shapes those outcomes (a detailed case example was made available at http://sistercarealliance.org).

Black women's leadership and use of their individual and collective political power has improved the landscape of public health for Black women and society in general. Their impact ranges from legislative victories such as the Crown Act, which protects against natural hair discrimination, to exposing Johnson & Johnson for talc-based products that have been linked to ovarian cancer (O'Donnell, 2020), to ensuring voters' rights protections. Their contributions to improving the nation's health is profound and undeniable.

Black women have used their political power to support investigations into threats and safety concerns that Black women have experienced and used the findings to justify funding they can use for their protection and outreach efforts. Funding allows organizations and individuals to increase the outreach to more Black women in need of an increase in support. An increase in funding can create better access to the social determinants of health, more family and personal resources (e.g., childcare and emergency funds), political strategy education, entrepreneurial network development, safe environments to learn in, increased trainings around self-care planning, mindset resilience, and mental toughness. Other benefits to the political power of Black women improving the quality of public health includes governmental agencies being pressured to be more accountable for better monitoring and action on the inequalities that exist for Black women. The prevalence of inequalities is about more than closing a gap. These disparities in health equity also highlight the origins of the ripple effect created, which causes a cascading of additional health issues for Black women.

There are several takeaway lessons to note that we hope are instructive for continued growth and development of Black women's public health and political power.

When Black women use their political power to improve their own health, everyone benefits from the fruits of their labor. Much of the impact of the work of Black women benefits more than just Black women, like the election changing work of Stacy Abrams and all the other Black women who fought to improve voters' rights that extended to military personal, elderly citizens challenged with transportation, and citizens completing absentee ballots. Improving the quality and accuracy of the national voting system has had a lasting impact on the future of our country and our children.

Black women experience unique challenges on their journey to political power and thus require support and protection if they are to thrive. Black women political and community leaders like former Georgia State representative "Able" Mable Thomas, member of the Atlanta Reproductive Justice Commission who convened the first group of women that coined the term "reproductive justice," and Monica Simpson, executive director of Sister Song, did not elevate to their political positions easily. The scope of access to political power for Black women like Thomas and Simpson must be expanded to include more opportunities and funding that can be used to support and protect emerging Black women leaders, allowing candidates for elected office, for example, to compete with their opponents on equal footing and with the inalienable rights that all citizens of the United States are supposed to receive.

Recommendations and Call for Action

Movement work to promote a higher quality of care for Black women should include a strategic self-care and needs assessment. An example of this can be found in the work of the SisterCARE Alliance, a network of Black women who promote self-care as a form of social justice. They have developed such an assessment which is outlined in the book *Self Care Matters: A Revolutionary's Approach* (Parris, 2016). The program described therein can help communities and organizations craft an accurate assessment of the needs of Black women while simultaneously empowering them to craft and follow their own Strategic Self Care Plan.

Another powerful step toward improving support for Black women in political leadership positions should include training in the seven categories of impact and support in their preparation to develop political power. This training will offer a safe environment for Black women to study political strategies, organizing, and activism, as well as leadership styles.

The expensive cost to the bodies, bank accounts, emotional health, communal support systems, and mindset of Black women who choose to lead cannot be fueled or sustained by unflinching resilience alone. Moving forward to the continued liberation of the Black community from health inequities and societal injustices will require more financial investment in the support of Black women leaders and community members holistically. There must be an immediate increase in the investment in emerging and existing Black women political leaders and the programs that support them.

Resources

Self-Agency. https://www.SelfCareAgency.com
SisterCARE Alliance. https://SisterCareAlliance.org

References

Avery, B. (2002). Who does the work of public health? *American Journal of Public Health, 92*(4), 570–575. https://doi.org/10.2105/AJPH.92.4.570

Black Women's Health Imperative. (2020). Black women vote: National health policy agenda, 2020–2021. https://3hqwxl1mqiah5r73r2q7zll1-wpengine.netdna-ssl.com/wp-content/uploads/2020/10/BWHI_Black-Women-Vote_2020.pdf

Black Women's Health Imperative. (n.d.). Our story. Retrieved January 4, 2021, from bwhi.org/our story/

Breines, W. (2006). *The trouble between us: An uneasy history of White and Black women in the feminist movement.* Oxford University Press.

Carrega, C. (2020, March 21). For the few black women prosecutors, hate and "misogynoir" are part of life. *ABC News.* https://abcnews.go.com/US/black-women-prosecutors-hate misogynoir-part-life/story?id=68961291

Center for Reproductive Rights & Black Mamas Matter Alliance. (2018). *Black Mamas Matter: Advancing the human right to safe and respectful maternal health care.* www.reproductiverights.org/sites/crr.civicactions.net/files/documents/USPA_BMMA_Toolkit_Booklet-Final-Update_Web-Pages.pdf

Chandra, A., Copen, C. E., & Stephen, E. H. (2013). *Infertility and impaired fecundity in the United States, 1982–2010: Data from the national survey of family growth* (National Health Statistics Reports No. 67). National Center for Health Statistics

Chisholm, S. (2010). *Unbought and Unbossed* (Expanded 40th anniv. ed.). Take Root Media.

Clarke, J. H. (1976). *Black/white alliances: A historical perspective.* Institute of Positive Education.

Cooper S. C., & Koch, P. B. "Nobody told me nothin": Communication about menstruation among low-income African-American women. *Women and Health, 46*(1), 57–78. https://doi.org/10.1300/J013v46n01_05

Foreverfamily. (n.d.). Fulfilling a vitale role—Foreverfamily. Retrieved on January 20, 2021, from https://www.foreverfam.org/our-work-2/

Hoyert, D. L., Uddin, S. F. G., & Miniño, A. M. (2020, January 30). *Evaluation of the pregnancy status checkbox on the identification of maternal deaths* (National Vital Statistics Reports, Vol. 6, No. 1). National Center for Health Statistics, Division of Vital Statistics.

Krieger, N., Jahn, J. L., Waterman, P. D., & Chen, J. T. (2018). Breast cancer estrogen receptor status according to biological generation: US Black and White women born 1915–1979. *American Journal of Epidemiology, 187*(5), 960–970. https://doi.org/10.1093/aje/kwx312

Marsh, E. E., Brocks, M. E., Ghant, M. S., Recht, H. S., & Simon, M. (2014). Prevalence and knowledge of heavy menstrual bleeding among African American women. *International Journal of Gynaecology and Obstetrics, 125*(1), 56–59. https://doi.org/10.1016/j.ijgo.2013.09.027

Morris, M. W. (2016). *Pushout: The criminalization of Black girls in schools*. New Press.

National Partnership for Women and Families. (2020). *Black women and the wage gap*. https://www.nationalpartnership.org/our-work/resources/economic-justice/fair-pay/african-american-women-wage-gap.pdf

Noonan, A. S., Velasco-Mondragon, H. E., & Wagner, F. A. (2016). Improving the health of African Americans in the USA: An overdue opportunity for social justice. *Public Health Review, 37*(12), Article 12. https://doi.org/10.1186/s40985-016-0025-4

O'Donnell, C. (2020, July 8). Nonprofits urge Johnson & Johnson to halt sales of baby powder globally. Reuters. https://www.reuters.com/article/idUSL1N2EF2E3

Owens, D. C., & Fett, S. M. (2019). Black maternal and infant health: Historical legacies of slavery. *American Journal of Public Health, 109*(10), 1342–1345. https://doi.org/10.2105/AJPH.2019.305243

Parris, A. J. H. (2016). *Self care matters: A revolutionary's approach*. YBF Publishing.

Payne, C. (1990). "Men Led, But Women Organized: Movement Participation of Women in the Mississippi Delta." In V. L. Crawford, J. A. Rouse, & B. Woods, *Women in the Civil Rights Movement: Trailblazers and Torchbearers, 1941–1965*. Carlson.

Petersen, E. E., Davis, N. L., Goodman, D., Cox, S., Syverson, C., Seed, K., Shapiro-Mendoza, C., Callaghan, W. M., & Barfield, W. (2019). Racial/ethnic disparities in pregnancy-related deaths-united states, 2007–2016. *Morbidity and Mortality Weekly Report, 68*(35), 762–765. http://dx.doi.org/10.15585/mmwr.mm6835a3

Shah, V., Nabwera, H. M., Sosseh, F., Jallow, Y., Comma, E., Keita, O., & Torondel, B. (2019). A rite of passage: a mixed methodology study about knowledge, perceptions and practices of menstrual hygiene management in rural Gambia. *BMC Public Health, 19*(1), Article 277. https://doi.org/10.1186/s12889-019-6599-2

Tobin, J., & Dobard, R. G. (1999). *Hidden in plain view: The secret story of quilts and the underground railroad*. Doubleday.

Waxman, O. B. (2021, January 8). Stacey Abrams and other Georgia organizers are part of a long—but often overlooked—tradition of Black women working for the vote. *Time*. https://time.com/5909556/stacey-abrams-history-black-women-voting/

Williams, D. (2019, July 25). City of Atlanta gets its first chief health officer. *Atlanta Business Chronicle*. https://www.bizjournals.com/atlanta/news/2019/07/25/city-of-atlanta-gets-first-chief-health-officer.html

Chapter 20

Standing on the Shoulders of Those Before Us

Allyson S. Belton, Ashley Kennedy Mitchell, and Katrina M. Brantley

Introduction

Leadership can be defined in numerous ways. *Merriam-Webster.com Dictionary* (Merriam-Webster, n.d.) notes that leadership is "the act or an instance of leading." Others state that it is a process of influence over others to accomplish an objective. Though there are many definitions, leadership has a subjective nature defined by who we are as leaders and by those who see us in those roles. Current public health leaders encounter increasingly complex barriers and challenges while serving as leaders in the communities in which they live, work, and serve (Carlton et al., 2015).

Leaders develop over time and continue developing as they grow in experience. Early leaders learn to find their voice, whereas more seasoned leaders are continuously refining their leadership traits. Having a professional title, a certain level of education, and access to a specific type of audience does not make a great leader, nor does it make a poor leader. Yet identifying one's personal leadership style helps create an understanding of how to best lead and be effective as a leader. One hallmark of a leader is the ability to learn as he or she leads others. Dr. David Satcher, 16th US Surgeon General, once stated that "leaders must be good learners, continually learning more about themselves, those they lead, and the cause or missions for which they work." As leaders grow in their respective careers and personal lives, they have experiences that serve as learning tools, ultimately developing, shaping, and molding their leadership skills and abilities. These experiences may be positive or negative in nature; but ultimately any experience serves as a growth marker as one matures into an effective leader. As public health practitioners, identifying and leaning into one's leadership style harnesses the leadership skills needed to effect change in the public health landscape.

Experiencing and Navigating Personal Conflict and Navigating the Growing Pains

By its very definition, the term "growing pain" assumes you must go through a challenging circumstance and grow from it. The longer we live, we will all go through something challenging in life. Whether it is physical pain, mental illness, disappointments, or failures, we learn something from every opportunity. A *Berkeley News* article described the "strong black woman" as merely a stereotype that women feel pressured to act like a Superwoman (Manke, 2019). Delving further, researchers have coined the phrase "Superwoman Schema" to describe when Black women feel an obligation to present an image of strength while suppressing their emotions and rejecting offers of help (Woods-Giscombé, 2011). This has been reported as a protective factor for health and diminishes the effects of chronic racial discrimination (Allen et al., 2019). Though this does not change the fact that discrimination exists, African American women have a learned skill of refocusing on success while suppressing the stressful parts of their lives. The field of public health is no different than any other obligations in women's lives. Women must overcome growing pains to succeed. Women of all racial/ethnic backgrounds will need to remember their past, thrive in their present, and stay focused on their future to overcome life challenges.

Why would Black women need to focus on the past? We have a better appreciation for our current opportunities when we focus on how far women have come; as we reflect on days when women did not have the right to vote, compared to 2020 when the first African American woman was voted in as the vice president of the United States of America. The ancestor's journeys have been fought hard to provide the opportunities women have today. Examples of formidable great women from the past include Sojourner Truth and Harriet Tubman. These women faced death to provide for so many. More recent women such as Coretta Scott King and Betty Shabazz stood behind strong political, outspoken men, despite the fact that both men were assassinated primarily because of their focus of work. One thing that all these women have in common is that they overcame major obstacles. Some of them raised children during their struggle. They helped people in the midst of their own personal struggles. Many Black women today look up to these ladies due to the strength they showed in the middle of their struggle. Black women embody the struggles from our ancestors as proof that we too can overcome our current situation and succeed in life. Anything worth having is worth fighting for.

Black women thrive in current situations mainly because of their support structures that assist them in all situations. Women's support systems could consist of coworkers, family, or friends whom they confide in to help support decision making, calm them down from despair, or encourage them to keep moving. All women need to identify a confidante who will help them through life's growing pains. A professional confidante can help guide a career ladder, provide support for a difficult work situation, or simply read a resume. A family or friend confidante can help to take one's mind off work, celebrate the important milestones in a woman's life, and provide that shoulder to lean on when things do not go as planned. African American women keep thriving in current situations with their support systems while they keep their eyes on future goals and aspirations.

For women, the future gives them hope for what could be. Every day is a new opportunity to turn a fantasy into reality. Some women use a check-off list of their accomplishments. They may follow in the footsteps of a mentor or create a new path never considered as a possibility. Women must do a better job of telling their story. For every woman who has succeeded in life, a mentee may be watching them learning from the obstacles and successes set before them. Currently, we need to tell others our stories. How did we overcome? What lessons did we learn? This information can help a few women to not make the same mistakes or at least learn how they may overcome life challenges. So, as we celebrate every milestone, we can inspire a new group of women behind us to take on those superwomen personas and "push through" various situations.

Dealing with Imposter Syndrome and Tokenism

Imposter syndrome, also called the imposter phenomenon, is a persistent doubt of one's capabilities or accomplishments, often despite external proof of competence (Sanford et al., 2015; Harvey & Katz, 1985). The terminology was first used in the 1970s by psychologists Pauline Rose Clance and Suzanna Imes in their study of high-achieving women (1978). They state that, unlike men, who tend to own success as attributable to a quality inherent in themselves, women are more likely either to project the cause of success outward to an external cause (luck) or to a temporary internal quality (effort) that they do not equate with inherent ability (p. 2). Imposter syndrome is prevalent among minority populations who may be predisposed to psychological distress due to low minority representation and heightened expectations (Bravata et al., 2020). In organizational culture, minority employees can often represent their societal group; therefore, success and challenges take on greater meaning than if they were just representing themselves. Therein lies imposter syndrome's intersectionality with tokenism.

Tokenism describes when companies hire a token member into the company, often as a gesture, that differs in some way from the majority or dominant workforce (Lewis, 2016; Yoder et al., 1996). Negative outcomes associated with tokenism often include stress from heightened visibility, social isolation from other workers, and the performance pressures. Therefore, tokenism and imposter syndrome can work in tandem to create a stressful and demoralizing work environment for minorities and women. Since Black women belong to two marginalized groups (Black people and women), the intersectionality of racism and sexism can lead to heightened effects of both phenomena. As an academician of color, Mikkaka Overstreet writes, "I ingested tokenism and bled racial battle fatigue. I breathed in microaggressions and exhaled service." Imposter syndrome often stems from burdensome societal pressures and stereotypes. This is true for Black women who are impacted by several negative stereotypes, including characterizations of heightened aggression, overbearingness, and ignorance (Ashley, 2014). Though not entirely derogatory, the idea of the "strong Black woman"—a perception that Black women are inherently resilient, strong, self-contained, and self-sacrificing—can affect imposter syndrome and make it more pronounced (Donovan & West, 2015). The pressures, both external and often internal, to fit the ideal of a "strong Black woman" or "Superwoman" translate into feeling unprepared for or unworthy of career milestones.

Apart from the individual concerns, imposter syndrome has a larger sociological implication: Why do so many Black women feel like they do not belong or that they are not accepted in the spaces in which they exist? The larger sociological answer is a simple one: in the past, they were not accepted in these spaces. Historically, many jobs and jobs sectors were not open for or heavily guarded against both women and minority members. Even today, Black women are disproportionately represented in lower earning positions, often only making minimum wage (Tucker & Vogtman, 2020). Black women are often less likely to be promoted and supported within their organizations (Coury et al., 2020). There are systemic and righteous reasons for this unease felt by Black women in the workplace. As more Black women enter these spaces, both the internal and external reasons for imposter syndrome can be assessed and challenged.

As with its concerns, imposter syndrome should be understood and tackled on two levels. For individuals, there are several methods to combat imposter syndrome. Knowing the signs of the imposter phenomenon can help in the identification of unwanted feelings. These signs include attributing success to external factors such as luck, difficulty accepting praise, setting unreasonably high standards, and self-doubt (Persky, 2018). Mentorship and peer group discussions encourage self-reflection and the adoption of strategies to address the imposter phenomenon when it arises. These conversations can also induce a sense of solidarity, especially when engaging "comrades in similar adversity," as Pedler (2011) termed it. Another strategy is developing a healthy relationship with perfection. Striving toward a goal can be a great motivator, but self-oriented perfectionism, or required perfection from oneself, can decrease productivity (Sherry et al., 2010).

Often imposter syndrome is treated as a personal issue, but when its scale becomes larger, organizations must engage with their constituents and enact cultural and policy changes (Mullangi & Jagsi, 2019). Work cultures can value perfectionism and certainty, leading to increases in feelings of inadequacy (LaDonna et al., 2018). Work cultures can also be mired in systemic racism and discriminatory practices that actively pressure conformity and detract from the well-being of minority employees (Ashe & Nazroo, 2017). As imposter syndrome can lead to burnout and loss of productivity in employees, institutions, especially those with less diverse worker populations, must evaluate and adjust organizational policies that can lead to the imposter phenomenon.

Overcoming Stereotypes

Navigating leadership amid the intersectionality of being Black and being a woman is complicated. For Black women, embracing certain leadership styles may lead to unfortunate stereotyping of behaviors and characteristics. The perceptions brought on by stereotyping can be detrimental to one's professional growth, even stifling in the pursuit of opportunities. Age and career stage also play into these stereotypes, unfairly labeling one as inexperienced or not qualified to take on specific leadership roles. Already positioned in some professional spaces to execute double the effort for half the recognition, simultaneously tackling and disproving stereotypes presents a significant challenge to the professional Black woman.

Certain stereotypes are associated with certain leadership styles. As noted previously, the intersectionality of race and gender make the leadership journey even more complex for Black women leaders. To persistently be labeled "too ___" while trying to lead effectively becomes discouraging at some times and motivational at others. For example, if a Black woman leader embraces the traits of a servant leader, then she may be labeled as too accommodating and not firm enough in her approach. Conversely, if she embraces more authoritarian traits, then she may be labeled as too aggressive or "angry."

Overcoming these stereotypes, while going along in the leadership journey and also maintaining one's personal sanity, requires strong effort. In some instances, it requires self-advocacy to avoid mislabeling, while in other cases, relenting and silently managing is the only solution. Many Black women leaders have had to "dim their lights" on occasion to fit into certain professional cultures. Others have had to practice "code switching" to create relatability and be heard in the workplace (Cheeks, 2018). One means of handling stereotypes is by seeking the guidance and advice of others, especially those who have had personal experiences of being unjustly labeled or perceived in uncomfortable lights. Learning from others' experiences pours into the bucket of lessons learned throughout the stages of growth. Additionally, part of developing resilience is practicing self-care, especially with one's emotional health. Managing stereotypes can take a great toll on one's emotional health, ushering in feelings of confusion, disenchantment, frustration, and underappreciation. To better deal with the negative emotions that stir up from battling stereotypes, professional counseling with a mental health practitioner or spiritual counseling provides another outlet for working through these challenges.

BUILDING YOUR DREAM TEAM

The leadership journey is not meant to be taken alone. One crucial step in career growth is identifying and engaging professionals who can provide useful advice, resources, and opportunities along the journey. Although one may develop leadership skills by one's own efforts, creating a dream team of mentors, coaches, and sponsors to guide and encourage the journey enhances those efforts, cultivating a more effective leader with a supportive ecosystem in place. When building a dream team, special consideration should be given to the team's roles and functions. There are many types of team members, including mentors, coaches, sponsors, and supporters. Each role functions in different capacities; however, a member of the dream team may serve in multiple roles, thereby not requiring a sole person for each role. Just as there is no requirement for a sole person to serve in one role only, there is no requirement to how many members comprise a dream team or for how long in the career trajectory one must engage with the dream team. Black women especially face a myriad of barriers and challenges along the leadership journey, so having additional support in place to help navigate the changing tides can help one in the journey. To understand how these roles contribute to the development of effective leaders, each role must be defined.

Mentors provide guidance and insight into your career path planning and navigation. The focus of the mentor is the conversational navigation of career spaces. A mentor is defined in numerous ways by multiple sources. For the purposes of this text, a mentor is defined as an individual experienced in a particular area or discipline supporting a less experienced individual ("mentee") with professional development and socialization into the profession (Hernandez et al., 2017). A mentor may be one who has experienced similar personal and/or professional encounters and brings a set of knowledge and lessons learned that can be applied in the leader's current situation. Sorkness et al. (2017) note that robust mentoring enhances mentee productivity, while also encouraging "self-efficacy and career satisfaction." Mentors provide "professional and psychological assistance and support to help mentees achieve career and personal achievements through long-term professional relationships that develop and deepen over time" (Hansman, 2016; Schunk & Mullen, 2013). Mentoring is often a less structured agreement that focuses on professional development through relationship building and expertise sharing without adherence to the professional's current job.

Similarly, coaches can also offer dialogue and resources to professionals. The coach's role is often interchanged with the mentor's role, due to the similar nature of engagement. Coaching involves a more structured process and focuses heavily on performance and performance metrics. Coaches are positioned to address certain areas of professional development or gaps in one's skillset (Helms et al., 2016). However, what differentiates the coach from the mentor is that there may not be a deeper relationship that develops over time, as a coach may only be needed for a specific period of time or for a more specific reason. Coaches are present to "help individuals confront and overcome obstacles to success," "encourage perseverance and resilience," and refine goals or refine the methods by which the goal may be achieved (MacLennan, 2017).

Unlike mentoring and coaching, which focus on advice and training between two individuals, sponsor and supporter roles are defined by what these individuals provide for the professional's career externally. Sponsors are those who advocate for another individual's career advancement (Helms et al., 2016). They are those who have evidence of a professional's work and work ethic and willingly communicate those positives in the presence of leadership and career growth prospects. Sponsors are persons of influence, individuals with the ability and willingness to offer tangible opportunities for career growth. According to Ibarra et al. (2010), they may advocate for specific assignments, promotions, or be a shield against negative publicity. Sponsors may also be mentors; yet mentors in the role of the sponsor go beyond just providing advice and are prepared to wield their influence as needed to promote their mentee's professional growth (Helms et al., 2016).

Supporters are members of your social circles who participate in your career development through engagement. These individuals often reshare social media postings and attend events. They are a valuable component of the team that can provide useful feedback, like audience preferences and real-time performance evaluations.

Though many individuals in a professional's life can fulfill one or more roles, an effective dream team requires diversity. This includes a diversity of experience, thought, and personality types. The successful collaboration of the different voices allows the professional to grow in their own self-reflection and career navigation. In essence, diverse and effective dream teams make dreams come true.

Conclusion: Resilience in the Growth Process

Thriving as a leader requires ongoing development personally and professionally. As one grows into an effective leader, the journey is shaped by wins and losses, good and bad experiences, and interpersonal conflict. This journey can take a toll on one's mental/emotional—and even physical—well-being. It brings about challenges that are not easy to overcome and some that may not appear to have a resolution. Yet, how one thrives and grows as a leader is by way of the resilience that she holds within. There is no singular strategy toward becoming a resilient leader, as it is an individual journey. However, there are some strategies that can be implemented to help along the way. As previously mentioned, developing a dream team is one strategy for growth; and engaging with an executive coach is another approach. Below are other suggested strategies.

To successfully navigate their careers, Black women must know the direction in which they want to go. One way to assure career cohesiveness is to develop an individual development plan, or IDP. An IDP is a template to assist professionals in their career and personal development. There are several benefits. It allows tracking of career development and progress over periods of time. An IDP also provides a visual representation of goals, objectives, and steps toward achievement. Professionals can utilize their IDPs to align their personal career goals with institutional needs and missions. This alignment creates an opportunity to convincingly argue for promotions, raises, or new job titles and descriptions.

Another strategy for becoming a resilient leader is to step out of the shadows of others and blaze your own pathway. Realize that your journey is unique to you and others' respective journeys are unique to who they are. So often young leaders strive to emulate those they revere and attempt to model or replicate the pathway of others to become like said person. What goes unrecognized are the nuances of that other person's journey and how they impacted that person along the way. Also, following along someone else's pathway can result in intensified pressure to succeed and achieve outcomes similar to those of another. It is great to have role models—there are many great leaders from whom we draw inspiration; however, the respect and reverence that we have for these leaders should serve as a guiding light rather than a concrete roadmap.

Becoming a resilient leader commences at any stage in life and is an ongoing growth process. It is a marathon, not a sprint. As Black women in public health, there are trailblazers such as Dr. Dorothy Boulding Ferebee, Dr. Donna Christensen, Ms. Mary Eliza Mahoney, Dr. Marilyn Hughes Gaston, and far too many more to name, who have set the stage for future public health leaders—leaders who are Black women and influential in their own right—to thrive and serve as champions of public health and health equity. We honor those who ventured before us and proudly stand on their shoulders.

Recommendations and Call for Action

1. Build a dream team: Identify and engage a support system consisting of peers and professionals who can provide useful advice, resources, and opportunities along the journey. Team members may consist of a mentor, coach, sponsor, or general supporter. Special consideration should be paid to everyone's role and function on the team.

2. Create an individual development plan (IDP): IDPs can help with tracking career development and progress over periods of time, as well as align an individual's career goals with institutional needs. An IDP also provides a visual representation of goals, objectives, and steps towards achievement, including arguing for promotions, raises, new job titles, or new roles.

3. Blaze your own trail: Step out of the shadows of others and blaze your own pathway. Realize that your journey is unique to you and others' respective journeys are unique to who they are. Recognize the strength and talent within yourself!

Resources

Black Ladies in Public Health. https://bliph.org/ and https://www.linkedin.com/company/bliph/

The National African-American Women's Leadership Institute. https://www.naawli.org/

References

Allen, A. M., Wang, Y., Chae, D. H., Price, M. M., Powell, W., Steed, T. C., Black, A. R., Dhabhar, F. S., Marquez-Magana, L., & Woods-Giscombe, C. L. (2019). Racial discrimination, the superwoman schema, and allostatic load: Exploring an integrative stress-coping model among African American Women. *Annals of the New York Academy of Sciences, 1457*(1), 104–127. https://doi.org/10.1111/nyas.14188

Ashe, S., & Nazroo, J. (2017). *Equality, diversity and racism in the workplace: A qualitative analysis of the 2015 Race at Work Survey*. https://hummedia.manchester.ac.uk/institutes/code/research/raceatwork/Equality-Diversity-and-Racism-in-the-Workplace-Full-Report.pdf

Ashley, W. (2014). The angry Black woman: The impact of pejorative stereotypes on psychotherapy with Black women. *Social Work in Public Health*, 29(1), 27–34. https://doi.org/10.1080/19371918.2011.619449

Carlton, E. L., Holsinger, J. W., Jr., Riddell, M., & Bush, H. (2015) Full-range public health leadership, Part 1: Quantitative analysis. *Frontiers in Public Health*, 3, Article 73. https://doi.org/10.3389/fpubh.2015.00073

Cheeks, M. (2018, March 26). How Black women describe navigating race and gender in the workplace. *Harvard Business Review*. https://hbr.org/2018/03/how-black-women-describe-navigating-race-and-gender-in-the-workplace#

Clance, P. R., & Imes, S. A. (1978). The imposter phenomenon in high achieving women: Dynamics and therapeutic intervention. *Psychotherapy*, 15(3), 241–247. https://psycnet.apa.org/doi/10.1037/h0086006

Coury, S., Huang, J., Kumar, A., Prince, S., Krivkovich, A., & Yee, L. (2020). *Women in the Workplace 2020*. McKinsey and Co. and LeanIn.org. https://wiw-report.s3.amazonaws.com/Women_in_the_Workplace_2020.pdf

Donovan, R. A., & West, L. M. (2015). Stress and mental health: Moderating role of the strong Black woman stereotype. *Journal of Black Psychology*, 41(4), 384–396. https://doi.org/10.1177/0095798414543014

Hansman, C. A. (2016), Mentoring and informal learning as continuing professional education. *New Directions for Adult and Continuing Education*, 2016(151), 31–41. https://doi.org/10.1002/ace.20193

Harvey, J. C., & Katz, C. (1985). *If I'm so successful, why do I feel like a fake? The impostor phenomenon*. St. Martin's Press.

Helms, M. M., Arfken, D. E., & Bellar, S. (2016). The importance of mentoring and sponsorship in women's career development. *SAM Advanced Management Journal*, 81(3), 4–16.

Hernandez, P. R., Bloodhart, B., Barnes, R. T., Adams, A. S., Clinton, S. M., Pollack, I., Godfrey, E., Burt, M., & Fischer, E. V. (2017). Promoting professional identity, motivation, and persistence: Benefits of an informal mentoring program for female undergraduate students. *PLoS One*, 12(11), Article e0187531. https://doi.org/10.1371/journal.pone.0187531

Ibarra, H., Carter, N. M., & Silva, C. (2010, September). Why men still get more promotions than women. *Harvard Business Review*. https://hbr.org/2010/09/why-men-still-get-more-promotions-than-women

LaDonna, K. A., Ginsburg, S., & Watling, C. (2018). "Rising to the level of your incompetence": what physicians' self-assessment of their performance reveals about the imposter syndrome in medicine. *Academic Medicine*, 93(5), 763–768. https://doi.org/10.1097/ACM.0000000000002046

Lewis, C. (2016). Gender, race, and career advancement: When do we have enough cultural capital? *Negro Educational Review, 67*(1–4), 106–132,169.

MacLennan, N. (2017). *Coaching and mentoring*. Taylor and Francis.

Manke, K. (2019, September 30). Does being a "superwoman" protect African American women's health? *Berkeley News*. https://news.berkeley.edu/2019/09/30/does-being-a-superwoman-protect-african-american-womens-health/

Merriam-Webster. (n.d.). Leadership. In *Merriam-Webster.com Dictionary*. https://www.merriam-webster.com/dictionary/leadership

Mullangi, S., & Jagsi, R. (2019). Imposter syndrome: Treat the cause, not the symptom. *JAMA, 322*(5), 403–404. https://doi.org/10.1001/jama.2019.9788

Pedler, M. (2011). Leadership, risk and the imposter syndrome. Action Learning, 8(2), 89–91. https://doi.org/10.1080/14767333.2011.581016

Persky, A. M. (2018). Intellectual self-doubt and how to get out of it. *American Journal of Pharmaceutical Education, 82*(2), Article 6990. https://doi.org/10.5688/ajpe6990

Sanford, A. A., Ross, E. M., Blake, S. J., & Cambiano, R. L. (2015). Finding courage and confirmation: Resisting impostor feelings through relationships with mentors, romantic partners, and other women in leadership. *Advancing Women in Leadership Journal, 35*, 31–41.

Schunk, D., & Mullen, C. (2013). Toward a conceptual model of mentoring research: Integration with self-regulated learning. *Educational Psychology Review, 25*, 361–389. https://doi.org/10.1007/s10648-013-9233-3

Sherry, S. B., Hewitt, P. L., Sherry, D. L., Flett, G. L., & Graham, A. R. (2010). Perfectionism dimensions and research productivity in psychology professors: Implications for understanding the (mal) adaptiveness of perfectionism. *Canadian Journal of Behavioural Science/Revue canadienne des sciences du comportement, 42*(4), 273–283. https://psycnet.apa.org/doi/10.1037/a0020466

Sorkness, C.A., Pfund, C., Ofili, E.O. Okuyemi, K. S., Vishwanatha, J. K., Zavala, M. E., Pesavento, T., Fernandez, M., Tissera, A., Deveci, A., Javier, D., Short, A., Cooper, P., Jones, H., Manson, S., Buchwald, D., Eide, K., Gouldy, A., Kelly, E., . . . Womack, V. (2017). A new approach to mentoring for research careers: The National Research Mentoring Network. *BMC Proceedings, 11*, Article 22. https://doi.org/10.1186/s12919-017-0083-8

Tucker, J., & Vogtman, J. (2020). *When hard work is not enough: Women in low paid jobs*. National Women's Law Center.

Woods-Giscombé, C. L. (2010). Superwoman Schema: African American women's views on stress, strength, and health. *Qualitative Health Research, 20*(5), 668–683. https://doi.org/10.1177/1049732310361892

Yoder, J. D., Aniakudo, P., & Berendsen, L. (1996). Looking beyond gender: The effects of racial differences on tokenism perceptions of women. *Sex Roles, 35*(7–8), 389–400. https://doi.org/10.1007/BF01544128

Chapter 21

Multimedia
Changing the Narrative

CRYSTAL R. EMERY AND CARMEN CLARKIN

It is an act of deepest resistance to be unashamedly present in spaces of oppression. It requires tenacity, ingenuity, and the utmost resilience. For Black women, these qualities are not only vital, but seemingly intrinsic, as every moment and with every breath that a Black woman takes, her sheer existence pushes back against a world that seeks to silence. Despite residing squarely in the center of the -ism vortex between sexism and racism, Black women have prevailed in being the most remarkable contributors to their own liberation. They continue to adapt and overcome, finding new ways to reclaim space and subvert injustice, division, and cruelty to create a new, more inclusive paradigm. When their voices, stories, and perspectives are elevated, so are those of others who are marginalized, working against a multitude of oppressive systems deeply ingrained into American society. One of the many tools that Black women have utilized in their fight for justice and equality is multimedia. Leveraging the unique power of multimedia, Black women have been able to communicate their stories and experiences on a level that transcends barriers inherent to other forms of intervention.

For decades, Black women have used multimedia to amplify their voices and the voices of others. Through the true representation of Black women not only in voice, but also body and perspective, Black female artists and creators have been catalysts for change on pressing issues, ranging from racism and mental health to homophobia and sexism within and outside of the Black community. By harnessing this powerful tool, Black women have actively combated racism, one of the leading public-health crises in the United States, not only physically and psychologically, but politically and spiritually as well. Through dance, film, radio, and other forms of media expression, Black women have graced the airwaves, the screen, and the stage to proclaim that their lives matter; that they, too, are beautiful; and that they have a voice.

With the power to bring people together, shed light on issues in society, and bring healing and restoration to individuals and communities, multimedia offers a uniquely effective vehicle for intervention. Over the years, Black women in media have used their positions as musicians, dancers, artists, filmmakers, and poets to influence perceptions of Blackness, gender, and health. Through their respective crafts and the stories that their art conveys to audiences, Black female creatives have significantly contributed to important work that researchers would later find substantially impact an individual's overall well-being (Geronimus, 1992; Geronimus et al., 2006; Russell, 2016, p. 48; Stanton et al., 2017). Studies have shown that racism and bias have severe effects on both mental and physical health (Geronimus et al., 2006; D. E. Roberts, 2012; Seeman et al., 2001). Experiencing racism and bias on a constant basis takes a physical toll on the body on both a systematic and a cellular level. As many scholars across a range of disciplines have discussed, "long-term exposure to social and financial stress and prolonged active coping with stressful circumstances" (Russell, 2016, p. 48), such as those associated with racism, have been implicated in the high rates of hypertension, heart failure, diabetes, kidney disease, maternal mortality, low birth rates, and other health issues that disproportionately affect the Black population within the United States. Furthermore, "considerable energy . . . must be exerted on a daily basis to manage the psychological consequences generated by chronic exposure to stress" (Russell, 2016, p. 48; Geronimus, 1992; Geronimus et al., 2006). An individual's inability to return to homeostasis, the physiological state of equilibrium, due to persistent environmental stressors causes bodily distress on a cellular level (Adelman et al., 2014; C. Roberts, 2019; D. E. Roberts, 2012, p. 132; Seeman et al., 2001). High cortisol levels in the blood contribute to allostatic load and what scholar Arline T. Geronimus terms "weathering" (Geronimus, 1992; Geronimus et al., 2006). Nina Martin and Renee Montagne describe "weathering" as the way in which "continuous stress wears away at the body, caus[ing] health vulnerabilities and increases susceptibility to infection," as well as influences the "early onset of chronic diseases [and] accelerates aging at the cellular level" (Martin & Montagne, 2017b, para. 24). In light of the significant body of evidence linking systemic racism to negative health outcomes, it is clear that racism not only intersects with public health, but is, at its core, a pressing public health issue.

Knowledge about the multitude of ways that racism impacts an individual's health has long been understood by those who experience it. Black women in particular have historically taken on a significant share of the burden of dispelling stereotypes and fighting for equality. From their activism and the interventions that have arisen from their potent self-expression of identity and resilience, it is possible to learn ways to combat racism and prejudice. In spite of tropes and harmful stereotypes perpetuated by dominant culture, Black women have carved out space for themselves and, through the resilience and fortitude they have displayed in various art forms, crafted more accurate narratives to counter these harmful stereotypes. In this way, the role that Black women in media have played in promoting public health is undeniable. However, their work, and the gravity of their contributions, has largely been overlooked. From television, radio, and music to film and frontier science, there is a plethora of Black women whose stories tell a tale of overcoming obstacles, asserting their right to be represented, and contributing creative capital to mainstream and historic avenues impacting others in profoundly significant ways.

During the civil rights era, women with prominent presences in mainstream media, such as Nina Simone and Bernice Reagon, used their platforms and their art to elevate the voices of the marginalized. Simone's music held widespread appeal for audiences of many backgrounds, ethnicities, and musical tastes. Though she was trained classically, racist policies and practices prevented her from pursuing a career as a classical pianist. Nonetheless, Simone's skills and technical ability eventually made her a popular sensation. She became a voice that transcended genre and race. Black and White audiences alike loved her classic and poised musical style, providing her a unique platform.

While other vocalists might have lost their careers had they taken the risk of making a political pivot, Simone was able to take the style of the 1950s and 1960s and make it revolutionary. She derived power from her art by giving herself and others an authentic voice in her music, translating pain and struggle into something musical and utterly beautiful. According to Stokely Carmichael, Simone was the "true singer of the civil rights movement" (Kernodle, 2008). In this way, Simone became a voice for racial equality and justice, not just in the US but around the world, and a global icon of "protest music" whose anger and pathos carried hard-hitting critiques of injustice (Simone & Cleary, 1991). Unlike Simone's earlier work, songs like "Mississippi Goddam" that came to her in a "rush of fury, hatred and determination" as she "suddenly realized what it was to be Black in America in 1963" were political anthems and calls to action (Feldstein, 2005, p. 1349; Simone & Cleary, 1991, p. 89). Throughout her career, Simone was not only able to use her own pain to fuel her creativity and music, but she was able to tap into the pain of a nation and create art from the narratives arising out of the civil rights movement. Her resilience as an artist allowed her work to traverse decades and influence the fabric of American culture and civil rights.

In addition to promoting health for the Black community through her music and contributions to the civil rights movement, Simone also helped bring to light a historically taboo subject within the Black community: mental health. Nina Simone suffered from what is now known as bipolar disorder. For years, she did not receive help because even she did not know what she was experiencing. Later, however, after receiving a diagnosis, she would share her voice and experiences to bring mental illness to the forefront in the Black community (Simone & Cleary, 1991).

A contemporary of Simone's, and another influential musician during the civil rights movement who contributed to the improvement of Black health by advocating for social justice, was Bernice Johnson Reagon. Like Simone, Reagon is a songwriter and activist who helped to shape and document the "evolving political identity of young Black America" (Kernodle, 2008, p. 296), but has also made important contributions to the progression of Black health through other avenues. Not only a singer, Reagon is a professor, songwriter, poet, and social activist whose work has been an integral part of African American history and the women's movement in the United States. Reagon has worked as a music consultant, composer, and performer on a number of acclaimed films and videos. Her prolific catalog includes publications such as *We Who Believe in Freedom: Sweet Honey in the Rock—Still on the Journey*; *We'll Understand It Better By and By: Pioneering African American Gospel Composers*; and the anthology *Voices of the Civil Rights Movement: Black American Freedom Songs, 1960—1965* (About Dr. Reagon, n.d.).

During the 1960s, at the height of the civil rights movement, Reagon was a founding member of the Student Nonviolent Coordinating Committee Freedom Singers. From her hometown in Albany, Georgia, Reagon worked as a field secretary and Freedom Singer. In her work, she used the power of song to carry the message of the civil rights movement and the stories of activists to various locations around the United States (About Dr. Reagon, n.d.). At a pinnacle point during the movement, while holding hands and marching with Martin Luther King, Jr., she started singing "We Shall Overcome," the song that became the anthem of the civil rights movement, giving people hope and courage to keep fighting. In this way and others, Reagon's voice was integral in shaping the path to equal rights (Ruehl, 2018).

Throughout her life, Reagon has lifted her voice and inspired others to do the same, contributing to cultural and community work that promotes the betterment of the African American population. She began her most widely known work as the founder of the group Sweet Honey in the Rock in 1973 in Washington, DC, and performed with them until her retirement from the group in 2004. During her three decades with Sweet Honey in the Rock, Reagon solidified the group's place in American history as the musical oratory group of the civil rights movement (Ruehl, 2018).

Of course, Bernice Reagon did not do this important work in isolation. In collaboration with June Jordan, she was able to build a coalition with the LGBTQ+ community and push for social change on multiple fronts, exploring music and lyrics that integrated Black power, feminism, and other issues (Reagon, 1986). Together, Reagon and Jordan blended pressing cultural issues with new and old forms of music, always drawing from what Reagon refers to as the "core reservoir of Afro-American traditional song" (Reagon, 1987, p. 106). She believed that "selecting things from [their] culture, organizing them, and using them to bring back information, positions, and political stances to the community that had created the material in the first place" was her job as an artist engaging in cultural work (Reagon, 1986, p. 77). As MacPhail discusses, for "artists and listeners alike, the way to find . . . Blackness . . . is to look to each other" (MacPhail, 1999, p. 61). Over the course of their collaboration and throughout their respective careers, June Jordan and Bernice Reagon began a dialogue through poetry and music to voice social commentary in an extremely unique way. They used their respective skills, command of language, and emotion to craft a new narrative that was not only "in the service of social change" (Savonick, 2018, p.196), but also provided powerful new perspectives to audiences. Ralph Rinzler, assistant secretary of public service for the Smithsonian, said of Reagon and her work with Sweet Honey in the Rock:

> What Bernice has done with Sweet Honey is more innovative than what anyone has done to synthesize root and evolved forms into a new form. She's done it with vocal music, but in a sense she's done it with instrumental music, too, because she's taken the voice and used it as another kind of instrument. She has drawn on the richest wellspring of Black and in some cases, non-black, vocal tradition and created a brilliant new genre. It's the most important thing being done with traditional vocal styles and repertoire than anybody's done in this country. (Harrington, 1987, para. 43)

In a similar groundbreaking spirit, Jordan redefined preconceived notions about the role of Black intellectuals, subverting traditional assumptions about who Black intellectuals were, how they functioned, and who they wrote for (MacPhail, 1999). As a woman of many talents, Jordan's body of work, from her poetry and activism to her plays and novels, worked to change the images that Black people identified with, especially with regard to female roles, emphasizing the importance that "Black intellectuals not fall back on universal, idealizing images that ignore or devalue experience or difference" (MacPhail, 1999, p. 65). Across three decades, the unique, complex, and shifting positions that Jordan expressed in her writings pushed back against perceived boundaries between the roles of artist and intellectual. As a creative, Jordan synthesized the two, strategically shifting her approach to best reach her desired audiences. Using her craft to draw attention not only to racism and imperialism but also sexism and homophobia, June Jordan sought to address issues of inequity within the Black community itself and placed a large emphasis in her writing on intersectionality. Scholars acknowledge that Jordan's writing clearly indicates that she was "concerned with the ways that powerful male speakers presume to know what Black women would say and how this presumption silences any different perspective that women would bring to the dialogue (be it political social or personal)" (MacPhail, 1999, p. 66). For this reason, Jordan intentionally and unashamedly used her work to carve out space for herself and others, not only as a Black woman but as a queer Black woman operating in intellectual and artistic spaces.

Both Reagon's and Jordan's work exemplifies the spirit of resilience of Black Women, and the remarkable power to transmute fear, oppression, and negativity into creativity, positivity, hope, and inspiration. The spirit of Sweet Honey in the Rock and their interwoven commentary on the spiritual temperature of America and June Jordan's critical exploration of intersectional identity and need for ideological evolution are both evidence of the power of media to forge new understandings and empower marginalized voices. In their own ways, Reagon and Jordan were fighting the deleterious effects of racism on the health of their communities long before it was acknowledged as a public health issue.

Despite several prior attempts and an extensive amount of research to empirically support the claim, it was not until 2020, almost 60 years after the start of the civil rights era, that the American Medical Association and other entities officially declared racism as a public health issue (American Medical Association, 2020). Though such acknowledgment serves to propel research efforts and discussions about racism and health to the forefront of the academic realm, many researchers note that "interrupting the cycle will require multiple points of intervention to mitigate root causes and effects of implicit bias, institutional racism, community violence, excessive use of force in law enforcement and the long-term effects of violence-related trauma in [minority] communities" (Danis et al., 2016). Changing the status quo is never easy. Years of mistreatment and degradation of humanity cannot simply be erased from the consciousness of society overnight, especially when there is still denial of the severe repercussions that racism continues to have on Black lives. When racism and prejudice are so embedded in a culture, they seep into the fabric of the nation, becoming visible in every fiber and seemingly inextricable from the soiled cloth. Yet because of the versatility of multimedia, Black female artistic expression has been able to shed light on a multitude of ways to begin approaching the daunting work of dismantling institutionalized racism.

The first lesson to be taken from the long history of resilience among Black women in media is the importance of reclamation: the reclamation of space, the reclamation of narrative, and the reclamation of voice. From the beginning, the ability to regain a level of autonomy over the images and perceptions of Black women has worked to fight racism by countering pernicious stereotypes. For a long time, Black women had no control over their portrayal in the media. In fact, at one point in time, the uniquely effective tool of popular media was used primarily for subjugation and silencing by denying Black people a voice in shaping the mainstream narrative (West, 1995). When others were in charge of dictating what representations of Black women were seen in the media, depictions of Black females were either matronly or hypersexualized. There was an absence of true-to-life displays of Black female characters, and instead Black women were portrayed as one of two possible extremes: the homely cook "mammy" caricature or the depreciated, licentious sex object referred to as a Jezebel (West, 1995). Even more extreme than the Madonna-whore dichotomy that remains prevalent in the White patriarchal society of the US, this paradigm of Mammy and Jezebel offers no option of piousness or purity in relation to Black womanhood and sexuality (Monahan et al., 2005).

Bodies of literature, some dating as far back as the 1500s, served as the backbone of "empirical" and "objective" racial narratives that encoded harmful beliefs about the Black female body. In the travel narratives of European imperialists in Africa, Black individuals were typically seen and described as animals. Referencing African people as "beasts" and using evocative imagery to create an association between African people and the nonhuman, these works functioned to reaffirm the idea that the people in these new lands were merely something else to exploit along with the animals, plants, and other natural resources. By depicting Africans in this way, White explorers began the project of ascribing meanings of difference to Black bodies that would become pervasive in overarching lines of European thought, fueling oppressive colonial and imperialist action. As scholar Jennifer Morgan notes, "Abolitionists and anti-abolitionists alike accepted the connections between race, animality, [and] the legitimacy of slavery" (1997, p. 189). Any wonder at the cultures, customs, and appearances of Black individuals served only to underscore difference and amplify observed distance between Black people and their White counterparts. These narratives and patterns of depiction functioned to establish the separation between the educated White observer and the "other" that distinctly marks these writings and the ideologies that sprung from them. These travel narratives told solely from the point of view of White male explorers and imperialists inevitably painted Black women as the epitome of the "otherness" that they sought to depict. The unfamiliarity of Black women to these White men incited both fascination and fear in the imperialists that was representative of their sentiments toward the African population generally. In this way, Black women became cultural symbols of all that was deliberately portrayed as backward and uncivilized about African populations. These writings would directly compare African women to White women in order to help construct "stable categories of whiteness and blackness" (Morgan, 1997, p. 168). This dynamic is reflective of what is described by Morgan as the ongoing "inability to allow black women to embody 'proper' female space compos[ing] a focus for representations of racial difference" (p. 168). Furthermore, because women are mothers, and ultimately continue the bloodline of a people, juxtaposing Black women with their White counterparts, documenting their difference and proclaiming their inferiority, was an attempt to point to the "logical" conclusion of inhumanity among the entire race. In this respect, "the development of racist discourse was deeply implicated by gendered notions of difference and human hierarchy" (Morgan, 1997, p. 170). It is from this gendered comparison that the foundations of the stereotypes we often see in media were eventually derived (Morgan, 1997, p. 189; Monahan et al., 2005). These stereotypes worked to create and reinforce notions of Black inferiority that persist into the present, impacting everything from educational outcomes to life expectancy.

Limited voice and lack of narrative control meant that stereotypes and harmful portrayals of Black women went unchecked, significantly impacting the health and well-being of African Americans in the United States for centuries through the nexus of racism that they maintained. Due to the pervasiveness of negative stereotypes and racial stigma, there exists an acute and inescapable cultural awareness of their existence. Psychologists have found that even if an individual does not embrace these attitudes consciously, the awareness of and exposure to their existence can lead to what is known as implicit bias (Devine, 1989; Kirwan Institute for the Study of Race and Ethnicity, n.d.). As scholars Chapman, Kaatz, and Carnes discuss, "automatic activation of race, gender, ethnic, age and other stereotypes has been demonstrated to influence judgment of and behavior toward individuals from stereotyped groups" (Chapman et al., 2013, p. 1506).

This culturally entrenched implicit bias is particularly dangerous in the context of medicine and public health. Studies have shown that racism and ethnic discrimination are significant contributors to healthcare inequality, in addition to other factors like gender (Chapman et al., 2013; Paradies et al., 2015). For this reason, Black women, by virtue of their intersectional identities, are already facing what some refer to as a "double jeopardy" when entering the health-care system. In spite of what most health-care providers believe about their ability to conduct themselves in an unbiased manner, implicit bias functions on an unconscious level, creating an incongruence between intention and practice (Matthew,

2015). Health-care decisions are significantly shaped by implicit biases and present an extreme danger for individuals belonging to marginalized groups. Coupled with structural disadvantages rooted in stigma and reinforced by policies that have historically worked to disenfranchise people of color, stereotyping, even when unintentional, significantly impacts health, cost of care, and overall health quality to a significant degree, annually contributing to thousands of preventable patient deaths in the United States (Williams & Collins, 2004). Failure to appropriately counsel patients on diet, lifestyle changes, or possible medical interventions occurs more frequently to African American patients than their White counterparts, and this inferior preventative care leads to worse health outcomes (Matthew, 2015). For example, Black mothers are less likely to be properly classified as overweight or underweight in prenatal risk factor screenings performed by clinicians (Fuentes-Afflick et al., 1995). Studies have also indicated that Black individuals are less likely to receive more effective forms of treatment and are more likely to receive medically risky or harmful treatment (Matthew, 2015). Even with increased access to health care, Black women are two and a half times more likely to die due to childbirth-related complications than their White counterparts, and are significantly more likely to develop chronic health issues such as breast cancer, diabetes, and heart disease. In addition, Black women face an increased risk of sexual violence and harassment (Barlow, 2020; Martin & Montagne, 2017a; D. E. Roberts, 2012, p. 175). In 2011, African American women in the US were dying at faster rates from cancer, stroke, heart disease, and diabetes-related complications than any other group of women in the nation, and researchers believe that 70%–80% of these deaths were preventable (Gaston, 2011). In spite of, or perhaps in many ways *because* of, these harrowing realities, Black women have continued to climb. They have continued to persist, attaining positions of prominence and using their platforms to keep pushing for change.

From the strides taken toward equity during the civil rights era arose new opportunities and avenues for Black women to continue this fight, such as the formation of interdisciplinary coalitions and partnerships that would significantly shape the landscape of public health. In the 1970s and 1980s, within the Office of the Surgeon General and the Bureau of Primary Health Care, Black women like Drs. Joycelyn Elders and Marilyn Hughes Gaston became high ranking officials with considerable political influence, working at the intersection of race, public health, and multimedia in an unprecedented manner. Both of these women capitalized on opportunities in mainstream media to make revolutionary changes to the way public health was practiced in the United States, drawing attention to topics ranging from unexplored health issues that disproportionately impacted the African American community to sexual health, a topic that was seen as extremely taboo at the time.

In the early 1970s, sickle-cell anemia was an afterthought in the world of public health. Patients had a life expectancy of only eighteen years, and very little progress had been made in researching effective treatments. The fact that this disease appeared to disproportionately affect people of color was in part why it was not a public-health priority at the time. However, Dr. Doris Wethers, a researcher and the third Black female graduate of Yale School of Medicine, having worked extensively on the topic of sickle-cell anemia, received Hughes Gaston's approval (at the time, Gaston was deputy surgeon general) to do a large-scale study to explore possible treatments for the disease (S. Roberts, 2019). The resulting trial was so successful that it significantly changed the life expectancy of those born with the disease. It also led to a change in hospital protocols, requiring that infants be screened for sickle-cell anemia to allow for rapid treatment.

Around the same time, Sidney Poitier's film *A Warm December*, starring Esther Anderson, helped to draw significant attention to the issue of sickle-cell anemia. The film featured images that the public did not often see: a beautiful, educated, African woman struggling with sickle-cell anemia. *A Warm December* effectively brought this disease to the forefront of national consciousness, transcending racial boundaries and arousing both public and political support for increased research and intervention. Within the year, sickle-cell anemia was on the list of the top ten public-health issues that needed to be addressed, providing the opportunity for Wethers's research to get the attention it deserved. In an act of converging interest to spur the Black vote, President Richard Nixon declared sickle-cell anemia as one of the top diseases the United States needed to address.

Both on and off camera, other forms of art and expression have served to further the promotion of holistic Black health. In 1980, Debbie Allen brought a healthy and beautiful portrayal of Black women into mainstream media in the Broadway revival of *West Side Story*. In her breakout role as Anita, Allen provided a counternarrative to stereotypical portrayals, thus promoting self-esteem and combating internalized racism among Black women and girls. As Anita, Allen, who is known for her legacy of dance, choreography, and acting, portrayed a beautiful, fit,

Black woman in a popular production. *Representation matters*, and Allen's performance heralded a new era for celebrating Black beauty, talent, and diversity in media.

As of 2021, Allen's career has spanned over 30 years. Her achievements include three Emmys, one Golden Globe Award, ten NAACP Image Awards, and a Lifetime Achievement Award. She has produced over 17 shows for television and was appointed as a member of the Arts and Humanities Committee under President George W. Bush in 2001 (Debbie Allen Dance Academy, n.d.a). In the same year, Allen also opened the Debbie Allen Dance Academy, whose mission is to expand "the reach of dance and theater arts for young people in the greater Los Angeles area, and the world, enriching, inspiring and transforming their lives" (Debbie Allen Dance Academy, n.d.a). By focusing on empowerment, self-esteem, discipline, creativity, and self-confidence, this academy creates a space to foster success not just for those who want to pursue a professional career in dance or the arts, but any child (Debbie Allen Dance Academy, n.d.b).

Today, with a multitude of racial health disparities disproportionately affecting the African American population in the US, and racism and prejudice remaining paramount issues, many artists have also turned toward using their platforms to educate young people and to speak out directly against racism. Most notably, Alicia Keys has continually used her voice as an award-winning artist and well-known celebrity to promote racial equality. As a biracial woman who identifies as Black, Keys often uses her music and interview opportunities to discuss racial injustice (NOW Staff, 2021). In 2014, Keys released the song "We Are Here" that launched the We Are Here Movement, rallying fans to speak out against violence and injustice across the globe. As a part of the project, and in response to police brutality, Keys and others produced a short video entitled "23 Ways." This video takes a somber look at the reasons that Black people in the US have died as a result of police violence and calls on government officials to address the issue of police brutality. Three years later, in 2017, Keys was awarded the Ambassador of Conscience Award (Amnesty International's highest award) (Activism, n.d). In recent years, Keys has been involved with Colin Kaepernick's Million Dollar Pledge initiative, participated in paying tribute to Black women in Hollywood who broke barriers, and actively fought against racism in the industry. Furthermore, she hosted a children's program on Nickelodeon discussing race and racism, emphasizing that it is never too early to seek unity and equality.

In her song "Perfect Way to Die," Keys continues to address police violence, recalling the murders of Trayvon Martin, Michael Brown, and Sandra Bland (Mixon, 2020). The music and lyrics not only express the shared suffering and loss, but also the collective resilience of Black communities that continue to push for change in the wake of traumatic loss. As Sirry Alang et al. (2017) discuss, "The impact of police brutality is much broader than simply affecting the individuals who have experienced racialized violence. It is a constant reminder of the historic and current devaluing of Black lives. Understanding how police brutality affects health requires seeing it both as the action of individual police officers and as part of a system of structural racism that operates to sustain White supremacy" (p. 664). When communities witness or experience chronic police brutality and violence, there are significant psychological consequences, such as depression, anxiety, anger, and fear, which may lead individuals to engage in isolation or self-destructive behaviors (Rankine, 2015; Bryant-Davis et al., 2017). This has been one of the clearest ways that researchers and laypeople alike have been able to make the connection between racism and public health. Recognizing this impact, Keys has utilized other avenues to combat some of the consequences of living in a country plagued by racism and violence, and now COVID-19. Her brand Soul Care promotes holistic wellness of body, mind, and soul, offering products as well as free resources to encourage deep healing by "creat[ing] special moments everyday" to decompress from the chaos of the world (Underwood, 2020). In an interview for *Vogue* magazine, Keys is quoted saying:

> We keep calling Covid-19 a pandemic, but really, this injustice, this racism is the major pandemic. It's the pandemic we've been dealing with for hundreds of years. It's an all-out assault. For the first time, people of every color, background, and upbringing can bear witness to the assault and feel the pain of it. It's time to see as clearly as we possibly can to stop all of this. The more we uncover, the more you can see. It is really overwhelming. (Mixon, 2020, para. 16)

Keys says that in everything she does as an artist and an activist, from winning 15 Grammys to calling on newly inaugurated President Joe Biden to create a racial justice commission just a few days after taking office, her goal is to "empower Black America" (Barajas, 2021).

The women discussed here are not the only ones who have made strides toward change utilizing different forms of art and media, but their stories may serve as examples of those women who often go unacknowledged in the mainstream narrative surrounding public health in relation to racism and equity, though they were the very ones who were instrumental in changing it. As scholar Howard Brody states:

> There are times when we (usually unconsciously) choose not to see. At these times, we have a strong reason for wishing to see the world in a certain way and in not wanting to allow a divergent perspective to enter our consciousness. This is especially true when we are comfortable with a pattern of behavior, and when perceiving the world differently would cause us to seriously question the correctness of that entire pattern of longstanding, habitual behavior. In such a case, the act of seeing, finally, is life-changing. (2009, p. 106)

Multimedia helps us to see; to see accurate representations of Black women, their joy, sorrow, pain, anger, and triumph. To see *their* lived experiences, *their* lives. The lives and work of Black women creatives illustrate their resilience. They illustrate how Black women do not sit waiting for someone else to change their situation, but rather go out and make change themselves by sharing their stories and creating new understandings, whether it be through music, film, song, or poetry.

Black women play a central role in the realm of important cultural work (Reagon, 1986). For decades and through various multimedia platforms, Black women have acted courageously and lent their voices, bodies, and perspective to address systemic racism, perhaps the most significant and pervasive public health issue in the United States. By honing their craft and effectively using their platforms to fight for equity, Black women in media have continuously catalyzed social change. and the fruits of this creative labor are a clear manifestation of their resilience. Though Black women's contributions to the field of public health have often been overlooked, their efforts to eradicate negative stereotypes about Black women and take on the daunting work of dismantling racism in whatever forms it presents itself are undeniable. From artists like Nina Simone to Alicia Keys, Black women have used and continue to use multimedia to create accurate, nuanced representations of Black women in their full humanity for all to see.

Media is everywhere. Media is everything. It influences the psychology and behavior of its consumers, transforming their mindsets and belief systems. What people see depicted and discussed in media, whether it be on television, in music, or on stage, they internalize as true on some level. Repeated exposure to messages, images, and stories can serve to desecrate and destroy, or it can be used to build. Our resilience, the resilience of Black women, is deeply rooted in subverting tools of oppression and turning them into tools of liberation. Black women in media have used this resilience and their understanding of the power of multimedia to take control of the narratives surrounding their lives, for if they did not, we would be left with racist, oppressive, externally constructed representations of who we are. Poet, activist, and scholar Audre Lorde put it best when she said, "If I didn't define myself for myself, I would be crunched into other people's fantasies for me and eaten alive" (BlackPast, 2012).

Recommendations and Call for Action

There are opportunities all around us every single day to access the powerful intervention tool of multimedia and use it for liberation and justice. With the 2020 pandemic putting a spotlight on deep-seated social and racial inequities in the United States and increased political unrest, the nation is undergoing changes that will shape its future for generations to come. In this moment, we are presented with an opportunity to create a new paradigm, and multimedia will play an integral role. Public health is grounded in policy, data collection, and the scientific method, but also relies on creative means to capture and express the experiences of individuals in order to get through to people, for that is what brings the heart and soul into any project. When policy and creative narrative intermingle, that is when you begin to change the world.

Multimedia has the unique power to bring all people to the table from different disciplines and walks of life. The rapid development and use of new technologies, if used strategically, hold the potential to expand the scope and reach of what we are able to create, touching more individuals and inspiring exponential change. bell hooks said, "The function of art is to do more than tell it like it is—it's to imagine what is possible" (hooks, 2006, p. 281). For generations, Black female creators have been reaching, imagining, and creating better futures that they dreamed of being possible, and *we* must continue to do so now. By following the example of Black women before us, we have the power to bring the vision for a new, just, equitable, and healthy society into fruition. Audre Lorde writes, "Our feelings are our most genuine path to knowledge" (Lorde, 2004, p. 91). It is through the power of media and Black women's resilience that the endless possibilities of a new paradigm are revealed.

Resources

WEBSITES

Kirwan Institute for the Study of Race and Ethnicity. *Implicit bias module series.* http://kirwaninstitute.osu.edu/implicit-bias-training/

BOOKS

Bobo, J. (Ed.). *Black women film and video artists.* Psychology Press, 1998.
Turner, M. F. *Hidden in history: The untold story of female artists, musicians, and writers.* Atlantic, 2018.

SCHOLARLY ARTICLES

Brooks, D. A. (2008). "All that you can't leave behind": Black female soul singing and the politics of surrogation in the Age of Catastrophe. *Meridians, 8*(1), 180–204. https://doi.org/10.2979/MER.2008.8.1.180
Feldstein, R. (2012). "The world was on fire": Black women entertainers and transnational activism in the 1950s. *Organization of American Historians Magazine of History, 26*(4), 25–29.

References

About Dr. Reagon. (n.d.). Bernice Johnson Reagon [Website]. https://www.bernicejohnsonreagon.com/about/
Activism. (n.d.). Alicia Keys [Website]. https://aliciakeys.com/news/category/activism/
Adelman, L., Smith, L. M., & Herbes-Sommers, C. (Producers). (2014). *Unnatural causes, Episode 2, When the bough breaks: How racism impacts pregnancy outcomes* [Video file]. https://unnaturalcauses.org/video_clips_detail.php?res_id=70

Alang, S., McAlpine, D., McCreedy, E., & Hardeman, R. (2017). Police brutality and Black health: setting the agenda for public health scholars. *American Journal of Public Health*, *107*(5), 662–665. https://doi.org/10.2105/AJPH.2017.303691

American Medical Association. (2020, November 16). *New AMA policy recognizes racism as a public health threat* [Press release]. https://www.ama-assn.org/press-center/press-releases/new-ama-policy-recognizes-racism-public-health-threat

Barajas, J. (2021, January 19). Black musicians, led by Alicia Keys, ask Biden to create racial justice commission. *Los Angeles Times*. https://www.latimes.com/entertainment-arts/story/2021-01-19/black-musicians-call-on-biden-and-harris-to-take-on-racism-and-police-brutality

Barlow, J. N. (2020, February). Black women, the forgotten survivors of sexual assault. *In the Public Interest*. https://www.apa.org/pi/about/newsletter/2020/02/black-women-sexual-assault

BlackPast. (2012, August 12). (1982) Audre Lorde, "Learning from the 60s." https://www.blackpast.org/african-american-history/1982-audre-lorde-learning-60s/

Brody, H. (2009). *The future of bioethics*. Oxford University Press.

Bryant-Davis, T., Adams, T., Alejandre, A., & Gray, A. A. (2017). The trauma lens of police violence against racial and ethnic minorities. *Journal of Social Issues*, *73*(4), 852–871. https://doi.org/10.1111/josi.12251

Chapman, E. N., Kaatz, A., & Carnes, M. (2013). Physicians and implicit bias: How doctors may unwittingly perpetuate health care disparities. *Journal of General Internal Medicine*, *28*(11), 1504–1510. https://doi.org/10.1007/s11606-013-2441-1

Danis, M., Wilson, Y., & White, A. (2016). Bioethicists can and should contribute to addressing racism. *American Journal of Bioethics*, *16*(4), 3–12. https://doi.org/10.1080/15265161.2016.1145283

Debbie Allen Dance Academy. (n.d.a). Debbie Allen [Bio]. https://www.debbieallendanceacademy.com/debbie-allen

Debbie Allen Dance Academy. (n.d.b). Mission. https://www.debbieallendanceacademy.com/mission

Devine, P. G. (1989). Stereotypes and prejudice: Their automatic and controlled components. *Journal of Personality and Social Psychology*, *56*(1), 5–18. https://psycnet.apa.org/doi/10.1037/0022-3514.56.1.5

Feldstein, R. (2005). "I don't trust you anymore": Nina Simone, culture, and Black activism in the 1960s. *Journal of American History*, *91*(4), 1349–1379. https://doi.org/10.2307/3660176

Fuentes-Afflick, E., Korenbrot, C. C., & Greene, J. (1995). Ethnic disparity in the performance of prenatal nutrition risk assessment among Medicaid-eligible women. *Public Health Reports*, *110*(6), 764–773.

Gaston, M. H. (2011, July 8). Marilyn Gaston—Interview 1 [Personal interview for Black Women in Medicine].

Geronimus, A. T. (1992). The weathering hypothesis and the health of African-American women and infants: Evidence and speculations. *Ethnicity and Disease*, 2(3), 207–221.

Geronimus, A. T., Hicken, M., Keene, D., & Bound, J. (2006). "Weathering" and age patterns of allostatic load scores among Blacks and Whites in the United States. *American Journal of Public Health*, 96(5), 826–833. https://doi.org/10.2105/AJPH.2004.060749

Harrington, R. (1987, June 25). Singing the Freedom Song. *The Washington Post*. https://www.washingtonpost.com/archive/lifestyle/1987/06/25/singing-the-freedom-song/93cdb852-497f-48a9-9886-2221261474d7/

hooks, b. (2006). *Outlaw culture: Resisting representations*. Routledge.

Kernodle, T. L. (2008). "I wish I knew how it would feel to be free": Nina Simone and the redefining of the Freedom Song of the 1960s. *Journal of the Society for American Music*, 2(3), 295–317. https://doi.org/10.1017/S1752196308080097

Kirwan Institute for the Study of Race and Ethnicity. (n.d.). Understanding implicit bias. https://kirwaninstitute.osu.edu/research/understanding-implicit-bias

Lorde, A. (2004). *Conversations with Audre Lorde* (J. W. Hall, Ed.). University Press of Mississippi.

MacPhail, S. (1999). June Jordan and the new black intellectuals. *African American Review*, 33(1), 57–71. https://doi.org/10.2307/2901301

Martin, N., & Montagne, R. (2017a, May 12). U.S. has the worst rate of maternal deaths in the developed world. *NPR*.

Martin, N., & Montagne, R. (2017b, December 7). Nothing protects black women from dying in pregnancy and childbirth. ProPublica.

Matthew, D. B. (2015). *Just medicine: A cure for racial inequality in American health care*. New York University Press.

Mixon, I. (2020, June 20). Alicia Keys on her new song, "Perfect Way to Die," Blackness and fighting against racial Inequality: "Racism is the major pandemic." *Vogue*. https://www.vogue.com/article/alicia-keys-perfect-way-to-die-racism-breonna-taylor

Monahan, J. L., Shtrulis, I., & Givens, S. B. (2005). Priming welfare queens and other stereotypes: The transference of media images into interpersonal contexts. *Communication Research Reports*, 22(3), 199–205. https://doi.org/10.1080/00036810500207014

Morgan, J. L. (1997). "Some could suckle over their shoulder": Male travelers, female bodies, and the gendering of racial ideology, 1500–1770. *William and Mary Quarterly*, 54(1), 167–192. https://doi.org/10.2307/2953316

NOW Staff. (2021, January 24). Alicia Keys celebrates Black women fighting racism in Hollywood. *NOW*. https://nowtoronto.com/movies/alicia-keys-how-it-feels-to-be-free-exclusive-film-clip

Paradies, Y., Ben, J., Denson, N., Elias, A., Priest, N., Pieterse, A., Gupta, A., Kelaher, M., & Gee, G. (2015). Racism as a determinant of health: A systematic review and meta-analysis. *PLoS One, 10*(9), Article e0138511. https://doi.org/10.1371/journal.pone.0138511

Rankine, C. (2015, June 22). "The condition of Black life is one of mourning." *The New York Times Magazine.* https://www.nytimes.com/2015/06/22/magazine/the-condition-of-black-life-is-one-of-mourning.html

Reagon, B. J. (1986). African diaspora women: The making of cultural workers. *Feminist Studies, 12*(1), 77–90. https://doi.org/10.2307/3177984

Reagon, B. J. (1987). Let the Church sing "Freedom." *Black Music Research Journal, 7,* 105–118. https://doi.org/10.2307/779452

Roberts, C. (2019, Fall). Sickness and health in African American history. Lecture presented in Yale University.

Roberts, D. E. (2012). *Fatal invention: How science, politics, and big business re-create race in the twenty-first century.* New Press.

Roberts, S. (2019, February 7). Dr. Doris Wethers, 91, on front lines against sickle cell, dies. *The New York Times.* https://www.nytimes.com/2019/02/07/obituaries/dr-doris-wethers-on-front-lines-against-sickle-cell-dies-at-91.html

Ruehl, K. (2018, January 16). We who believe in freedom shall not rest: Sweet Honey in the Rock's four decades of music and freedom. *NPR.* https://www.npr.org/2018/01/16/577690049/we-who-believe-in-freedom-shall-not-rest

Russell, C. A. (2016). Questions of race in bioethics: Deceit, disregard, disparity, and the work of decentering. *Philosophy Compass, 11*(1), 43–55. https://doi.org/10.1111/phc3.12302

Savonick, D. B. (2018). *Insurgent knowledge: The poetics and pedagogy of Toni Cade Bambara, June Jordan, Audre Lorde, and Adrienne Rich in the era of open admissions* [Doctoral dissertation, City University of New York]. CUNY Academic Works. https://academicworks.cuny.edu/gc_etds/2604

Seeman, T. E., McEwen, B. S., Rowe, J. W., & Singer, B. H. (2001). Allostatic load as a marker of cumulative biological risk: MacArthur studies of successful aging. *Proceedings of the National Academy of Sciences, 98*(8), 4770–4775. https://doi.org/10.1073/pnas.081072698

Simone, N., & Cleary, S. (1991). *I put a spell on you: The autobiography of Nina Simone.* Ebury.

Stanton, A. G., Jerald, M. C., Ward, L. M., & Avery, L. R. (2017). Social media contributions to strong Black woman ideal endorsement and Black women's mental health. *Psychology of Women Quarterly, 41*(4), 465–478. https://doi.org/10.1177/0361684317732330

Underwood, B. (2020, December 3). Alicia Keys' new skincare brand urges us to rethink self-care. *Oprah Daily.* https://www.oprahdaily.com/beauty/skin-makeup/a34859953/alicia-keys-soulcare-interview/

West, C. M. (1995). Mammy, Sapphire, and Jezebel: Historical images of Black women and their implications for psychotherapy. *Psychotherapy*, *32*(3), 458–466. https://psycnet.apa.org/doi/10.1037/0033-3204.32.3.458

Williams, D. R., & Collins, C. (2004). Reparations: A viable strategy to address the enigma of African American health. *American Behavioral Scientist*, *47*(7), 977–1000. https://doi.org/10.1177/0002764203261074

Chapter 22

Anti-Racism Primer

Naming Racism and Moving to Action

CAMARA PHYLLIS JONES, CLARA Y. JONES, AND CAMILLE A. JONES

Racism is a system of structuring opportunity and assigning value based on the social interpretation of how one looks (which is what we call "race") (Jones, 2002a; Jones, Truman, Elam-Evans, et al., 2008). Furthermore, racism has three impacts: it unfairly disadvantages some individuals and communities, unfairly advantages other individuals and communities, and saps the strength of the whole society though the waste of human resources (Jones, 2002a; Jones, Truman, Elam-Evans, et al., 2008).

As president of the American Public Health Association (APHA) in 2016, Camara Phyllis Jones (one of the authors of this chapter, hereafter referred to as CPJ) used her platform to launch APHA and as many of its affiliates, partners, and communities as would join us on a National Campaign Against Racism (Jones, 2016a). She identified three sequential tasks for that campaign (Jones, 2018a): (1) Name racism. (2) Ask, "How is racism operating here?" (3) Organize and strategize to act.

Naming racism, saying the whole word, "race-ism," is essential because we must name a problem in order to get started on a solution. Naming racism is especially crucial in the United States' context because racism denial is so staunchly held by so many in this nation, and it is so seductive.

Racism denial is like a huge black hole in our national landscape, much like black holes in the universe. They are massive and powerful, sucking in everything that comes near. And they are also invisible because they even consume the light. The first step in anti-racism is to defy the black hole of racism denial by explicitly and unapologetically naming racism.

But as necessary as it is to name racism, it is necessary but insufficient. The disproportionate impact of COVID-19 on communities of color in the United States and the gruesome murder of Mr. George Floyd (a Black man) by Mr. Derek Chauvin (a White police officer whose job was to serve and protect Mr. Floyd and others) have led more people who are living as "White" in the United States to recognize that racism exists. However, we are at risk that those newly aware people will forget their new insights within a few months. If all they do is affirm that Black Lives Matter or utter the word "racism" out loud, or even put together the phrases "systemic racism" or "structural racism" on their social media, six months from now they may forget why they ever said those words and fall back into what we describe as the sleepiness, the somnolence of racism denial.

So we must all name racism and then move to action, because once we start acting we will *not* forget why we are acting. We must carry the question "How is racism operating here?" with us everywhere to unveil the myriad mechanisms of racism. After all, racism is not a cloud or a miasma that we can't get a handle on. It is a system of power with identifiable and addressable mechanisms that are in our structures, policies, practices, norms, and values. And when we understand that these structures, policies, practices, norms, and values are actually the elements of decision-making, dismantling them suddenly seems within our grasp. The question "How is racism operating here?" guides our identification of potential levers for intervention, fruitful targets for action.

Yet moving to action requires more than simply mapping out the terrain. It requires organizing and strategizing to act. It requires gathering a group of like-minded folks to focus on a single aspect of a structure, policy, practice, norm, or value using all the tools at their disposal, working from their centers of power, while also identifying and coordinating with other groups near and far who are working on the same, related, or vastly different targets. This coordinated effort is necessary because racism is so deeply entrenched in all facets of life and thought in the United States. A little tinkering here or there will be met with quick adjustment of the system of racism to the perturbance. We must abandon the perceived limits of power that seem to arise when we ask the question "What can

I do about racism?" and recognize that our power lies in the question "What can *we* do about racism?"

Collective action informs us, inspires us, motivates us, propels us, protects us, sustains us. And the collective is not just in the here and now. We all must invest in our children and mentor them and bring them up in the way of community consciousness and collective action. We must teach them the long histories of our struggles, struggles to be valued, protected, promoted, and nurtured in this society. We must let them see and learn about those strategies that have worked and those that have failed and how to be able to predict the differences in advance. They must know that they are not the first ones to recognize the injustices that characterize our deeply racist society. And as we equip our children with the tools and strategies from our own struggles, we need to lift up their tools and strategies that will carry them into times that we will never see.

We need to understand that this is a multigenerational struggle and that we have power, that action is power, and especially that collective action is power. And we must recognize that the fruit of our labors may not be fully realized in the time that we are on this earth. But that action and resistance have healing powers of their own. We must start imagining ways to place "back-up spikes" in the road after we have made progress, so that the efforts at backlash will be made more difficult. And we must be willing to plant acorns now so that our grandchildren will have shade.

The remainder of this chapter is structured as a "primer" with key lessons and talking points for eight different aspects of anti-racism that we have distilled over our careers in academia, clinical practice, and government service. We recognize that work on individual and community resilience, work on health issues that disproportionately impact women of color, work on elevating the voices of Black women in all areas of discourse, is work on naming, measuring, and addressing the impacts of racism on the health and well-being of our nation and the world.

Anti-Racism Primer: Review by the Numbers

The following summarizes eight elements that are of salience when addressing racism as a threat to the health and well-being of our nation and the world, and as the root cause of "racial"/ethnic disparities in health care and in health. The elements of our Anti-Racism Primer and their associated questions are:

1. **Launching a National Campaign Against Racism.** What is necessary to launch and sustain a National Campaign Against Racism? Are there examples already happening in the United States? Here we will review the three tasks of the National Campaign Against Racism mentioned above and share the current status of cities, counties, and states that have formally declared racism to be a public health crisis.

2. **Dimensions of health intervention.** Why should people who are interested in health interventions concern themselves with naming, measuring, or addressing racism? Here we will describe five levels of health intervention that can be displayed along the three dimensions of a cliff. Be clear that at whatever level you may be working, your success will be hampered if you do not recognize or address the impacts of racism (and other systems of structured inequity) that shape the conditions of our lives.

3. **Key messages when naming racism.** What are the four key messages when naming racism? What tools exist to help communicate those messages? Here we will identify four key messages and share links to some of CPJ's allegories that facilitate understanding those messages.

4. **Levels of racism.** How can we understand racism on three levels? How are the levels related to one another? How do these levels help us understand what we need to do to dismantle racism?

5. **Principles for achieving health equity.** What is health equity? How do we get there? How is health equity related to health disparities? Is there a core set of principles by which we need to abide to be sure that we are on the path toward achieving health equity?

6. **Barriers to achieving health equity** embedded in United States culture. We have some sense of the structural targets for action to dismantle racism, but are there also cultural or values-based targets for action that we need to consider? How do these operate to undergird the intergenerational transmission of racism denial? How do these operate to limit our societal efforts to achieve health equity?

7. **Actions we can take today** toward dismantling racism. Are there general principles or strategies that we can adopt to guide our anti-racism efforts today? And how do they relate to sustained strategies over the long term?

8. **Habits of mind for social justice warriors.** How do we sustain ourselves in this anti-racism struggle? And what guides to action do we instill in our children?

Launching a National Campaign Against Racism

There are *three essential tasks for a National Campaign Against Racism* (Jones, 2018a). A National Campaign Against Racism is necessary because racism is foundational in our nation's history, and yet many people are in staunch denial of its continued existence and its profoundly negative impacts on the health and well-being of our nation (and the world). The three tasks for a National Campaign Against Racism are:

1) Name racism (Jones, 2016h; Jones, 2018c). If you do not say the whole word "racism" in our national context of widespread and staunchly held racism denial, then you are complicit with that denial. As of February 10, 2023, there were 260 declarations by local jurisdictions (city councils, county commissions, state legislatures) across 41 U.S. states and the District of Columbia that "racism is a public health crisis" (American Public Health Association, 2023; see fig. 22.1).

2) Ask the question "How is racism operating here?" to identify levers for intervention and targets for action (Jones, 2018a). We must carry the question "How is racism operating here?" with us everywhere. How is racism operating in our children's daycare (or lack thereof) or their school? How is racism operating on our job (or lack thereof)? In our neighborhood? City? State? Nation? The world?

We ask this question to identify mechanisms of racism in our structures, policies, practices, norms, and values, which are the elements of decision-making.

Structures are the who, what, when, and where of decision-making, especially who is at the table and who is not, and what is on the agenda and what is not, as well as when and where decision-making processes can be accessed.

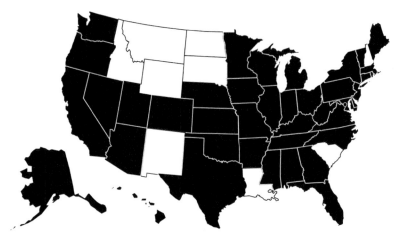

Figure 22.1. States with jurisdictions declaring "Racism is a public health crisis." Two hundred sixty cities, counties, regional bodies, or state-level entities across 41 states and the District of Columbia (shown in black) have declared that "Racism is a public health crisis" as of February 10, 2023. Figure based on data from the American Public Health Association, https://www.apha.org/topics-and-issues/health-equity/racism-and-health/racism-declarations.

Policies are the written how of decision-making, describing how we *should do* things, the written rules for how we claim and aim to act.

Practices are the unwritten how of decision-making in the short term—how we *actually do* things here and now, the ad hoc patterns of conduct.

Norms are the unwritten how of decision-making over the long haul—how we *have always done* things, the unwritten and deeply embedded rules of appropriate conduct.

Values are the why of decision-making—why we prioritize one group or action over another, the underlying judgments about who and what matters most.

As an example of how to examine these elements of decision-making, we have distilled four classes of policies that are core mechanisms of racism (Jones, 2002a): (1) policies allowing segregation of resources and risks, (2) policies creating inherited group disadvantage or its reciprocal inherited group advantage, (3) policies favoring the differential valuation of human life by "race," and (4) policies limiting self-determination.

Anti-Racism Primer | 371

3) Organize and strategize to act (Jones, 2016e). Collective action informs us, inspires us, motivates us, propels us, protects us, sustains us. As described in the introduction to this chapter, we need identify or create collectives where we are, decide on a focus of action, and then take turns leading the effort for our collective (distributed leadership) while also connecting with other anti-racism collectives in our local areas, across the nation, and around the world.

CPJ has articulated an Anti-Racism Collaborative with eight collective action teams, including guiding questions and early ideas for action, as one possible framework for anti-racism collaboration (Jones, 2018a).

Dimensions of Health Intervention

There are *three dimensions of health intervention* that can be understood and displayed using a Cliff Analogy (Jones, Jones, Perry, et al., 2009; Jones, 2018b). To care for people who have fallen off of the cliff of good health and to prevent others from falling after them, our health interventions must include all of the following:

1) Curative and preventive services (depicted as the ambulance, net, and fence) which can be placed on a vertical line along the edge of the cliff. The ambulance at the bottom of the cliff represents acute medical care as well as "tertiary" prevention, preventing complications from disease that is already manifest (for example, preventing amputations from diabetes).

The net or trampoline halfway up the cliff face represents our safety net programs (often in our social services) as well as "secondary" prevention, early detection (including screening programs in our communities and in health-care settings).

The fence at the top of the cliff represents "primary" prevention, keeping bad things from happening in the first place, which can also happen in both community and health-care settings. These include immunizations (including COVID-19), health promotion messages (for example, stay physically active, eat fresh fruits and vegetables, avoid tobacco products), anticipatory guidance (for example, what to expect in pregnancy or how to play with your child), self-help groups (for example, pregnancy circles, fatherhood support groups, Al-Anon family groups), and policies aimed at changing individual behaviors (for example, tobacco-21 policies to prevent easy access of young people to tobacco products).

2) Addressing the social determinants of health, including poverty and adverse neighborhood conditions, can be seen in a two-dimensional plane as moving the population away from the edge of the cliff. The social determinants of health are the determinants of health and illness that are outside of the individual. They are beyond our individual genes and beyond our individual behaviors. They are the contexts of our lives.

They include individual context, such as individual education, occupation, income, and wealth. They also include neighborhood context, such as the quality of housing, education, jobs, transportation, food choices, greenspace, physical safety, and the physical environment (air, water, cleanliness, noise) in an area. Addressing adverse social determinants of health at the place-based and group levels will result in larger, more sustained improvements in health outcome than interventions made one-on-one at the individual level.

3) Addressing the social determinants of equity, including racism, sexism, and other systems of structured inequity, involves acknowledging and addressing the three-dimensionality of the cliff and recognizing that intervention in only one of the dimensions will not be successful in improving health.

If the social determinants of health are the contexts of our lives, the social determinants of equity determine the range of contexts in our society as well as which groups are over- or underrepresented in each of the different contexts. For example, if the social determinants of health included the presence of bike paths in a neighborhood, the social determinants of equity would be about who was at the table deciding where the bike paths would go, or whether bike paths were really what a community wanted or needed.

The social determinants of equity are systems of power that differentially distribute resources and assign societal value. They operate at the most basic level through determining who is at the decision-making table and who is not, as well as what is on the agenda and what is not. They create a three-dimensional cliff, differentially distribute the resources along the cliff face, and push some populations closer to the edge of the cliff. In the United States, racism is the most foundational and pernicious social determinant of equity (see fig. 22.2).

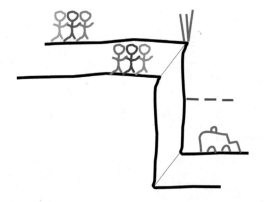

Figure 22.2. Levels of health and social intervention: A Cliff Analogy. The three dimensions of health and social intervention include provision of services (ambulance at the bottom of the cliff, net or trampoline half-way down, fence at the edge of the cliff); addressing the social determinants of health (including poverty and adverse neighborhood conditions) by moving the population away from the edge of the cliff; and addressing the social determinants of equity (including racism and other systems of structured inequity) by acknowledging and addressing the three-dimensionality of the cliff, the differential distribution of resources along the cliff face, and the differential distribution of populations in relation to the edge of the cliff. *Source*: Author.

Key Messages when Naming Racism

There are *four key messages that must be communicated when naming racism:*

1) Racism exists.

2) Racism is a system of power, not an individual character flaw or personal moral failing.

3) Racism saps the strength of the whole society through the waste of human resources.

4) We can act to dismantle racism.

Each of these key messages has been successfully communicated through allegories developed by CPJ (Jones, 2014a; Jones, 2019a; Jones, 2019b; see fig. 22.3).

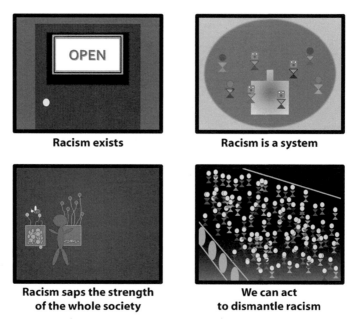

Figure 22.3. Allegories communicating four key messages about racism. Clockwise from the top left, the allegories from which these images are excerpted are "Dual Reality: A Restaurant Saga" (*Racism exists*); "Cement Dust in Our Lungs" (*Racism is a system*); "Levels of Racism: A Gardener's Tale" (*Racism saps the strength of the whole society*); and "Life on a Conveyor Belt: Moving to Action" (*We can act to dismantle racism*). The allegories and the artwork are original works of Camara Phyllis Jones.

"Dual Reality: A Restaurant Saga" (Jones, 2014a; Jones, 2016b) uses the image of an "Open"/"Closed" sign to communicate that racism structures dual realities. For those born inside a restaurant, sitting at the table of opportunity, eating, and looking up to see a sign posted on the door that proclaims "Open," it is difficult for them to recognize that there is there is a two-sided sign in operation. It is difficult for *any* of us to recognize a system of inequity that privileges us. But those on the outside of the restaurant are very well aware that there is a two-sided sign in operation, because the sign proclaims "Closed" to them, but they can look through the window and see people inside eating.

"Cement Dust in our Lungs" (Jones, 2020b) uses the image of a cement factory spewing cement dust in the air as a metaphor for racism.

The factory fills the air with so much dust that anyone near the factory for any amount of time will develop cement dust in their lungs. This cement dust in our lungs is problematic for all of us. Yes, it affects different ones of us differently, depending on our relationship to the factory. But yes, it affects all of us, even those who do not recognize that they have cement dust in their lungs.

The question arises, How should we address this problem of cement dust in our lungs? Should we focus on the individual, screening for the amount of cement dust each of us has in our lungs and creating temporary cleansing spas? Should we focus on the cloud of dust, donning gas masks one by one to start our individual anti-cement dust journeys? Or should we focus on the factory, naming it as the source of the dust and moving collectively to dismantle it? Only the structural intervention of dismantling the factory will position us to create a new system in which all of us can breathe free. Racism is a system, so we must address racism at the systems level.

"Levels of Racism: A Theoretic Framework and a Gardener's Tale" (Jones, 2000; Jones, 2002b; Jones, 2014a; Jones, 2016f) uses the image of a gardener who has two flower boxes, rich soil and poor soil, and flowers that differ only in the colors of their blossoms (red or pink), to illustrate three levels of racism: institutionalized (structural), personally mediated (interpersonal), and internalized. As shared in more detail in the section on "Levels of Racism" below, the Gardener's Tale allegory demonstrates that to set things right in the garden, we must at least address the structural racism, and when we do the other levels may take care of themselves.

"Life on a Conveyor Belt: Moving to Action" (Jones, 2014a; Jones, 2016i) starts with an image from Beverly Daniel Tatum's book *Why Are All the Black Kids Sitting Together in the Cafeteria? and Other Conversations about Race* (1997) that depicts the racism of many White people as a passive process, living their lives uncritically on a conveyor belt that is moving inexorably through and toward racism. CPJ expands on that image to illustrate how we become actively anti-racism.

First, we must acknowledge the signs of racism all around us. Then we must take action, turning around and walking backward on the conveyor belt. As we bump into people on the crowded belt, we must name racism and invite them to leave their comfort and join us in our walk against the grain. As we develop a critical mass, we will be able to walk faster than the conveyor belt is moving and make our way back to the motor that is running the system. There, we must ask, "How is racism operating here?" And as we identify the huge array of mechanisms, we must organize and strategize to act, coordinating our efforts to dismantle the system and put in its place a system in which all people can know and develop to their full potentials.

Levels of Racism

There are *three levels of racism* (Jones, 2000):

1) Institutionalized/structural racism: the constellation of structures, policies, practices, norms, and values that taken together result in differential access to the goods, services, and opportunities of society by "race." This is the kind of racism that does not require an identifiable perpetrator. Structural racism shows up as inherited disadvantage and its reciprocal inherited advantage. It can be seen in the differential distribution of material conditions and in the differential distribution of access to power.

When some would ask, "Why even talk about racism, doesn't everything boil down to social class?" we need to explain that in the United States (and in many parts of the world) the overrepresentation of people of color in poverty and of White people in wealth does not "just so happen." Each marginalized, stigmatized, oppressed group of color experienced some initial historical injustice. And each of those initial historical injustices is perpetuated by contemporary structural factors that are part and parcel of structural racism. Structural racism explains why we even see an association between social class and "race" in the United States—that is not just a happenstance or because some people are lazy or stupid.

Finally, structural racism occurs both through acts of commission ("acts of doing") and acts of omission ("acts of not doing"). In these times, structural racism very often shows up as indifference and inaction in the face of need.

2) Personally mediated racism: differential assumptions about the abilities, motives, and intents of others by "race," and differential actions based on those assumptions. This is what most people think of when they hear the word "racism"—someone has done something to someone else. It includes both prejudice (the differential assumptions) and discrimination (the differential actions).

Like structural racism, personally mediated racism can manifest both as acts of "doing" and acts of "not doing." Perhaps even more important is that this level of racism can be unintentional as well as intentional. A person does not have to intend to be racist to have had a racist impact.

3) Internalized racism: like the two levels of racism described above, internalized racism is differential by "race." For members of structurally disadvantaged, marginalized, stigmatized, oppressed "races," internalized racism shows up as acceptance of negative messages about our own abilities and intrinsic worth. Self-devaluation. The "White man's ice is colder" syndrome. Resignation, helplessness, and hopelessness.

For members of structurally advantaged "races," internalized racism manifests as a sense of entitlement. And this sense of entitlement undergirds the racism denial so deeply held by so many in the United States. If you are convinced that you are entitled to your status in life, how could there be an unfair system going on? Racism denial is a huge barrier to our anti-racism efforts in this country.

As briefly described above, CPJ has illustrated these three levels of racism with her "Gardener's Tale" allegory. For a full treatment of the story, please see Jones, "Levels of Racism: A Theoretic Framework and a Gardener's Tale" (2000) or view the 18-minute video produced by the Centers of Disease Control and Prevention where she describes the levels of racism and illustrates them with her "Gardener's Tale" allegory (Jones, 2002b).

Here is a quick version: A gardener has two flower boxes, one that she knows to have rich, fertile soil and the other that she knows to have poor, rocky soil. She has seed for the same kind of flowers, except some of the seed will produce pink blossoms and some of the seed will produce red blossoms. And the gardener prefers red over pink. So she puts the red seed in the rich, fertile soil and the pink seed in the poor, rocky soil.

In the rich, fertile soil, all of the red seed sprouts, with the strong red seed growing tall and vigorous but even the weak red seed making it to a middling height. But in the poor, rocky soil, the weak pink seed dies and even the strong pink seed needs to struggle to make it halfway up. And that first generation of flowers goes to seed. The next year, the same thing happens, and then those flowers go to seed. And year after year, the same thing happens. Finally, ten years later, the gardener looks at her flower boxes and says, "You know, I was *right* to prefer red over pink!"

Structural racism is manifest in the gardener's initial separation of the pink and red seed into the two types of soil, the differences in the heights and vigor of the pink and red flowers resulting from the differences in the quality of the soil, the flower boxes keeping the soil separate, and indifference and inaction in the face of need perpetuating the inequity. Personally mediated racism is reflected in the gardener's plucking of the pink flowers before they can even go to seed, or seeing a pink seed that has blown into the rich, fertile soil and plucking it out before it can establish itself. And internalized racism for the pink flowers is shown by a preference for pink pollen over red, while internalized racism for the red flowers is shown by a belief that they are entitled to the rich, fertile soil in which they find themselves (see fig. 22.4).

But perhaps the most important question is "Who is the gardener?" After all, the gardener is the one with the power to decide, the power to act, and control of resources (which are the elements of self-determination). Note that CPJ paints the gardener red, which is why she prefers red over pink. In the U.S. context, government is clearly a huge part of the gardener, but not the only part. Media, foundations, corporations, health-care sys-

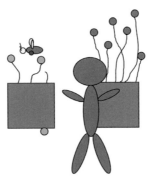

Figure 22.4. Summary image from the Gardener's Tale allegory "Levels of Racism: A Theoretic Framework and a Gardener's Tale" (Jones, 2000).
In this image, "red" appears dark gray and "pink" appears light gray.
Note the red gardener aligning herself with the red flowers. She has sown the red seed into the rich, fertile soil and the pink seed into the poor, rocky soil. The result is the difference in the numbers, heights, and vigor of the pink and red flowers. Note the pink blossom that has been plucked and thrown outside the flower box. Note the pink flowers shrinking away from the bee because they prefer red pollen over pink pollen. *Source:* Author.

tems, educational institutions, even communities (to the extent that they can achieve self-determination) can all be part of the gardener.

What are we to do about the gardener? Do we make the gardener striped, or polka-dotted, or fuschia? Do the pink flowers need to grow or recruit their own gardener? There are many questions that arise out of the "Gardener's Tale."

CPJ was asked the following question nearly two decades ago: "Why should the red flowers share their soil?" When she heard that question, she loved that question because it showed her the power of the "Gardener's Tale" to start conversations about racism that might otherwise be quite charged. Her answer to the question "Why should the red flowers share their soil?" was that actually, the rich, fertile soil does not belong to the red flowers. It belongs to the whole garden.

And here is a question that we leave with you, the reader: "What if the gardener that we are looking at is not the original gardener? What if that is the original gardener's great-great-great-great-grandchild?" Because here we are. And that great-great-great-great-grandchild has always seen the red flowers thriving and the pink flowers struggling. She may not even think there is a problem to be solved.

So what must we do? First, we must make the differences in the heights and vigor of the pink and red flowers a problem requiring urgent solution. We must put this on our urgent action agenda. Second, we need to make the flower boxes transparent so that we can see the differences in the quality of the soil and then address them. But third, as we make the flower boxes transparent, we must make sure that everybody understands that the pink seeds did not just launch themselves into the poor, rocky soil. So we must talk about history. And we must talk about how the gardener's initial (and ongoing) preference for red over pink set up and perpetuated (and continues to perpetuate) the situation. Some might call that initial (and ongoing) preference for red over pink "cultural racism." In the U.S. context, it is clearly White supremacist ideology.

We must directly address the gardener's preference for red over pink, because if we do not, even if we were able to compel the red gardener today to enrich the poor rocky soil today so that it was as rich as the rich fertile soil today, if she continues to prefer red over pink, she will continue to privilege red over pink going forward. Understanding that racism is a system that does two things, structures opportunity and assigns value, we must address both aspects of racism if we are to set things right in this nation and the world.

Principles for Achieving Health Equity

There are *three core principles that guide our actions toward achieving health equity* (Jones, 2014b; Jones, 2016d):

1) **Value all individuals and populations equally.** To operationalize this, generate and then apply a list of "valuing" verbs based on how we value our children unconditionally (nurture, celebrate, protect, invest, encourage, invite, respect, engage, listen, support, welcome, attend to, and so forth).

2) **Recognize and rectify historical injustices.** To operationalize this, learn the history of your own organizations and locales; learn the history of problems you aim to solve; take action to rectify historical injustices with both words and deeds, including sharing resources and power.

3) **Provide resources according to need.** To operationalize this, establish a metric of need upon which all stakeholders agree, and then have the political spine to distribute resources according to that metric of need without introducing other considerations of deservingness, readiness, or political expedience.

Barriers to Achieving Health Equity

There are *seven barriers to achieving health equity* that are embedded in United States culture and society (Jones, 2016c; Jones, 2020a; Jones, 2021). These can be usefully understood as seven "values" targets for anti-racism action. They include our:

1) **Narrow focus on the individual,** which makes systems and structures invisible or seemingly irrelevant.

2) **Ahistorical stance,** which pretends that the present is disconnected from the past and that the current distribution of advantage and disadvantage is just a happenstance.

3) Endorsement of the **myth of meritocracy** ("If you work hard, you will make it"), which denies the reality that there are many people working just as hard or harder than those who have made it, but who will never make

it because of an uneven playing field, a field structured and perpetuated by racism and other systems of structured inequity.

4) Endorsement of the **myth of a zero-sum game** ("If you gain, I lose"), which fosters competition over cooperation and masks the costs of inequity to the whole society.

5) Limited future orientation, which manifests as a disregard for the children and a usurious relationship with the planet.

6) Endorsement of the **myth of American exceptionalism** ("The United States is so different, so special, so ordained by God that the usual rules do not pertain to us"), which results in a sense of U.S. entitlement and limits our openness to learn from other countries.

7) Nation's foundational embrace of **White supremacist ideology** (the false idea of a hierarchy of human valuation by "race," with White people at the top as the ideal or norm), which results in a sense of White entitlement, dehumanization of people of color, and fear at the "browning" of America that underlies our current political divide.

Four of these societal attributes (narrow focus on the individual, ahistorical stance, myth of meritocracy, and White supremacist ideology) are the roots of racism denial. The remaining three (myth of zero-sum game, limited future orientation, and myth of American exceptionalism) further stymy our efforts to achieve health equity by dividing us one from the other, dividing us from our children and the planet, and dividing us from the knowledge and examples of success from other countries.

All of these "values" targets are in addition to the "structural" targets that are often more evident, including residential segregation (which invites and facilitates active disinvestment in communities of color), financing of public schools based on local property taxes, elements of the criminal-legal system that block police accountability, and the glib consignment of our communities to be environmental "sacrifice zones."

Actions We Can Take Today

The factors mentioned above help us distinguish *six actions toward dismantling racism* that we can begin taking today. These can be described using the image of a dual reality from the allegory "Dual Reality: A Restaurant Saga" described above (Jones, 2016b):

1) Actively look for evidence of two-sided signs (Jones, 2001): shine the bright light of inquiry to identify differences in outcomes *and* in opportunities by "race," language, immigration status, age, gender, rurality, religion, or any other potential axis of inequity.

2) Burst through our current bubbles of experience to experience our common humanity in different settings—this recognition of our common humanity in different settings is the basis for building common cause, critical mass, and collective action.

3) Be interested, believe, and join in the stories of others (Jones, 2016g): read widely, talk to strangers, accept the truths of others (for example, understand that some people are justifiably concerned about police violence without requiring them to provide cell phone video documentation), go across town and stay a while in an environment that is not your usual comfort zone.

4) Develop the ability to see "the absence of": Who is *not* at the table? What is *not* on the agenda? What policies are *not* in place that could have a pro-justice, anti-racism impact?

5) Reveal inaction in the face of need (Jones, 2016k): lack of action in the face of demonstrable need is how structural racism often manifests these days.

6) Recognize that collective action is power: collective action informs, inspires, propels, and protects us—we each can bring our gifts and tools and contribute to the greater effort from our centers of strength.

Habits of Mind for Social Justice Warriors

There are *four charges to individuals committed to social justice* (Jones & Corbie, 2020a; Jones & Corbie, 2020b). These "4 BCs" are habits of mind for social justice warriors as we aim to positively impact our world:

1) Be courageous: speak your truth; embrace challenge; be unafraid of controversy; recognize that the edge of your comfort is your growing edge.

2) Be curious: ask "Why?" and then "Why?" and then "Why?" again—these serial "Why?"s will lead you from accepting superficial explanations to understanding root causes; read widely/read history; stay "woke" to current events; learn more than one language; travel as much as you can, both across town and around the world; walk in wonderment at what others have to teach you.

3) Be collective: care about the whole; share your ideas, time, energy, and material possessions with others; recognize yourself as a global citizen; organize and strategize to act, because collective action is power.

4) Build community: be interested, believe, and join in the stories of others; talk to strangers; create "bubble-bursting" opportunities for yourself and others—these are opportunities to experience our common humanity, to recognize that there are people who are just as kind, funny, generous, hard-working, and smart as you are who are living in very different circumstances; speak up and take action on behalf of others; go across town and stay a while, investing your presence and time to turn strangers into friends.

Naming Racism and Moving to Action

Anti-racism is an essential strategy for resilience, for Black women, and for public health. At the level of individual resilience, recognizing our power and engaging in action, especially collective action, gives us purpose and reveals to us our strengths. But we must also acknowledge that our ultimate goal is not simply to strengthen individual people to persist and thrive in the face of adversity. The ultimate goal is to eliminate the adversity.

Anti-racism is a process with three sequential tasks: name racism, ask "How is racism operating here?", and organize and strategize to act (Jones, 2016e). But once you have gone through that process once, are you done? Oh no! Anti-racism is also iterative. We must continue to name racism because some will insist that racism is only a thing of the past. We must continue to ask "How is racism operating here?" because our reach may now be longer or some of our earlier progress may have become undone. And we must continue to organize and strategize to act, because racism is a shape-shifting system that seeks to beguile us into complacency.

Which highlights the need for us to understand that anti-racism is a sequential and iterative process that will likely span generations. We are planting and nurturing acorns today so that our grandchildren can have shade. And we must involve the young people in the work, being intentional about mentoring them and making space for them to inform our efforts today. If we are focused, persistent, resilient, we will dismantle the system of racism and put in its place a system in which all people can know and develop to their full potentials. And that is for the good of all.

Recommendations and Call for Action

The Black woman's imperative is to continue to be critical thinkers, investigators, instigators, and advocates, then to braid that genius, insight, and power into a *mighty collective* across sectors, across regions, across generations. Some ideas to build a critical mass and catalyze collective action:

- Add anti-racism to the agendas of collectives to which you already belong, including neighborhood organizations, religious institutions, sororities and other social groups, parent groups, and book clubs.
- Familiarize yourself with the meeting times and places of local decision-making bodies (school boards, city councils, county commissions), stay abreast of their agendas, attend their meetings, and introduce anti-racism as an agenda item for their consideration (including passage of a resolution that "racism is a public health crisis").
- Learn the histories of your neighborhood, city, workplace, and local institutions, and then share that knowledge with others.
- Learn national and world history and then share that knowledge with others.
- Identify the public elementary, middle, and high schools in your neighborhood, and then contribute your time and other

resources to at least one of them. This is whether or not you have children, or your children are currently school-age, or your children ever did or ever will attend the public schools. In the end, there is no such thing as "my children" versus "your children" (Jones, 2016j)—*all* children are *our* children and an investment in our children is an investment in our collective future.

Resources

All-In Cincinnati Coalition—Greater Cincinnati Foundation. gcfdn.org

American Psychological Association. *Racism in America*. First in a video series on *Facing the divide*, 2018. https://vimeo.com/282358544/7d1a26949d

American Public Health Association. *Research and intervention on racism as a fundamental cause of ethnic disparities in health* (APHA policy no. 20017). American Public Health Association, 2001. http://www.apha.org/advocacy/policy/policysearch/default.htm?id=246

Berney, B. (Producer). *Power to heal*. BLB Film Productions, 2018.

Boyd, R. W., Krieger, N., Jones, C. P. In the 2020 US election, we can choose a just future. *Lancet*, 396, no. 10260 (2020):1377–1380. https://doi.org/10.1016/S0140-6736(20)32140-1

Crowder, James A. *All-In Cincinnati: Equity is the path to inclusive prosperity*. https://nationalequityatlas.org/sites/default/files/All-In_Cincinnati_10-17-18e.pdf

Jones, C. P. Coronavirus disease discriminates, our health care doesn't have to. *Newsweek*, April 7, 2020. https://www.newsweek.com/2020/04/24/coronavirus-disease-discriminates-our-health-care-doesnt-have-opinion-1496405.html

Jones, C. P. Foreword. In C. L. Ford, D. M. Griffith, M. A. Bruce, & K. L. Gilbert (Eds.), *Racism: Science and tools for the public health professional*. APHA Press, 2019.

Jones, C. P. *Maori-Pakeha health disparities: Can treaty settlements reverse the impacts of racism?* (1999 Ian Axford Fellowship Report). New Zealand-United States Educational Foundation, 1999.

Jones, C. P., Caunca, M., & Hung, E. Confronting racism denial, Part 1, Racism exists in medicine. *The takeaway: A leadership podcast for residents and fellows*, University of California, San Francisco School of Medicine, August 25, 2022. https://podcasts.apple.com/us/podcast/confronting-racism-denial-part-1-racism-exists-in-medicine/id1641336985?i=1000577329726

Jones, C. P., Gilbert, K. L., & Castle, A. Exploring Antiracism with Dr. Camara Jones and Dr. Keon Gilbert. *The HPP podcast, health promotion practice*, Season 3, Episode 1, January 2, 2023. https://anchor.fm/health-promotion-practice/

episodes/S3-Ep--1-Exploring-Antiracism-with-Dr--Camara-Jones-and-Dr--Keon-Gilbert-e1svs94

Jones, C. P, Hatch, A., & Troutman, A. Fostering a social justice approach to health: Health equity, human rights, and an antiracism agenda. In R. L. Braithwaite, S. E. Taylor, H. Treadwell (Eds.), *Health issues in the Black community* (3rd ed.). Jossey-Bass, 2009.

Jones, C. P., Kishnani, S., & Hung, E. Confronting Racism Denial, Part 2, Racism is a system. *The takeaway: A leadership podcast for residents and fellows*, University of California, San Francisco School of Medicine, August 25, 2022. https://podcasts.apple.com/us/podcast/confronting-racism-denial-part-2-racism-is-a-system/id1641336985?i=1000577329703

Jones, C. P., LaVeist, T. A., & Lillie-Blanton, M. "Race" in the epidemiologic literature: An examination of the *American Journal of Epidemiology*, 1921–1990. *American Journal of Epidemiology,* 134, no. 10 (1991):1079–1084. https://doi.org/10.1093/oxfordjournals.aje.a116011

Jones, C. P., Powell, D., & Hung. E. Confronting racism denial, Part 4, We can act to dismantle racism. *The takeaway: A leadership podcast for residents and fellows*, University of California, San Francisco School of Medicine, August 25, 2022. https://podcasts.apple.com/us/podcast/confronting-racism-denial-part-4-we-can-act-to-dismantle/id1641336985?i=1000577329777

Jones, C. P., Sudler, A., & Hung, E. Confronting racism denial, Part 3, Racism saps the strength of the whole society. *The takeaway: A leadership podcast for residents and fellows,* University of California, San Francisco School of Medicine, August 25, 2022. https://podcasts.apple.com/us/podcast/confronting-racism-denial-part-3-racism-saps-the/id1641336985?i=1000577329727

Lee, T. L. (Producer). *Crisis in the crib: Saving our nation's babies* [Documentary film]. US Department of Health and Human Services, Office of Minority Health, 2009.

LaVeist, T., Cheers, I., & LaVeist, W. (Producers). *The skin you're in: Racial health injustice—Overcoming an American crisis* [Documentary film]. Tulane School of Public Health and Tropical Medicine. https://www.tsyi.org/the-film

National Academies of Sciences, Engineering, and Medicine. Advancing Antiracism, Diversity, and Equity Inclusion in STEMM Organizations: Beyond Broadening Participation. Washington, DC: National Academies Press, 2023. https://doi.org/10.17226/26803.

Racism in America. Part of video series *Facing the divide*. American Psychological Association, 2018. https://vimeo.com/282358544/7d1a26949d

Unnatural causes: Is inequality making us sick? Episode 2, *When the bough breaks*. California Newsreel, 2008.

Wallis, C. Why racism, not race, is a risk factor for dying of COVID-19 [Interview of C. P. Jones]. *Scientific American*, June 12, 2020. https://www.scientificamerican.com/article/why-racism-not-race-is-a-risk-factor-for-dying-of-covid-191/

References

American Public Health Association. (2023). Racism is a public health crisis. https://www.apha.org/Topics-and-Issues/Health-Equity/Racism-and-health/Racism-Declarations

Jones, C. P. (2000). Levels of racism: A theoretic framework and a gardener's tale. *American Journal of Public Health, 90*(8), 1212–1215.

Jones, C. P. (2001). "Race," racism, and the practice of epidemiology. *American Journal of Epidemiology, 154*(4), 299–304.

Jones, C. P. (2002a). Confronting institutionalized racism. *Phylon, 50*(1–2), 7–22.

Jones, C. P. (2002b). *A discussion with Camara P. Jones*. National Center for Chronic Disease Prevention and Health Promotion. https://www.youtube.com/watch?v=1QFCcChCSMU

Jones, C. P. (2014a). Telling stories: Allegories on "race" and racism. YouTube video. TEDxEmory. https://www.youtube.com/watch?v=GNhcY6fTyBM

Jones, C. P. (2014b). Systems of power, axes of inequity: Parallels, intersections, braiding the strands. *Medical Care, 52*(10, suppl. 3), S71–S75.

Jones, C. P. (2016a). Launching an APHA presidential initiative on racism and health. *The Nation's Health, 45*(10), 3.

Jones, C. P. (2016b). How understanding of racism can move public health to action: Allegory highlights dual reality of privilege. *The Nation's Health, 46*(1), 3.

Jones, C. P. (2016c). Achieving health equity: The crisis in Flint, and what should be done next. *The Nation's Health, 46*(2), 3.

Jones, C. P. (2016d). Creating the healthiest nation: Equity barriers pose obstacles to progress. *The Nation's Health, 46*(3), 3.

Jones, C. P. (2016e). Becoming actively anti-racist: The need to organize and act. *The Nation's Health, 46*(4), 3.

Jones, C. P. (2016f). Strength and beauty everywhere: Extensions of the Gardener's Tale. *The Nation's Health, 46*(5), 3.

Jones, C. P. (2016g). A whole world of stories: Be interested, believe, join in. *The Nation's Health, 46*(6), 3.

Jones, C. P. (2016h). The urgency of naming racism: Adding clarity in time of conflict. *The Nation's Health, 46*(7), 3.

Jones, C. P. (2016i). Life on a conveyor belt: Making a choice to take action on racism. *The Nation's Health, 46*(8), 3.

Jones, C. P. (2016j). Pondering the meaning of life: "And how are the children?" *The Nation's Health, 46*(9), 3.

Jones, C. P. (2016k). Overcoming helplessness, overcoming fear, overcoming inaction in the face of need. *American Journal of Public Health, 106*(10), 1717.

Jones, C. P. (2018a). Toward the science and practice of anti-racism: Launching a national campaign against racism. *Ethnicity and Disease, 28*(Suppl. 1), 231–234. https://doi.org/10.18865/ed.28.S1.231

Jones, C. P. (2018b). Dr. Camara Jones explains the Cliff of Good Health. *Urban Institute*. https://www.youtube.com/watch?v=to7Yrl50iHI

Jones, C. P. (2018c). #MeToo against racism. *Journal of Human Lactation, 34*(2), 232.

Jones, C. P. (2019a). Action and allegories. In C. L. Ford, D. M. Griffith, M. A. Bruce, & K. L. Gilbert (Eds.), *Racism: Science and tools for the public health professional*. Washington, DC: APHA Press.

Jones, C. P. (2019b). Allegories on "race," racism, and anti-racism. 2019–2020 Fellows' Presentation Series, Radcliffe Institute for Advanced Studies, Harvard University. https://www.radcliffe.harvard.edu/event/telling-stories-allegories-on-race-racism-and-anti-racism

Jones, C. P. (2020a). Seeing the water: Seven values targets for anti-racism action. *Harvard Primary Care Blog*. http://info.primarycare.hms.harvard.edu/blog/seven-values-targets-anti-racism-action

Jones, C. P. (2020b). Cement dust in our lungs. Acceptance speech, Executive Director Citation Award, *American Public Health Association*. https://www.youtube.com/watch?v=BGmIXV859YQ&t=26s

Jones, C. P. (2021). Addressing violence against children through anti-racism action. *Pediatric Clinics, 68*(2), 449–453.

Jones, C. P., & Corbie, G. (2020a). "Be courageous, be curious, . . ."—Interviewing Dr. Camara Jones. *A different kind of leader*, Season 2 opener, Part 1 [Podcast]. https://www.differentkindofleader.com/episodes/episode/4bb6851e/be-courageous-be-curious-interviewing-dr-camara-jones-part-i

Jones, C. P., & Corbie, G. (2020b). "Be a citizen, and build community"—Interviewing Dr. Camara Jones. *A different kind of leader*, Season 2 opener, Part 2. https://www.differentkindofleader.com/episodes/episode/4a606685/be-a-citizen-and-build-a-community-interviewing-dr-camara-jones-part-ii

Jones, C. P., Jones, C. Y., Perry, G. S., Barclay, G., & Jones, C. A. (2009). Addressing the social determinants of children's health: A cliff analogy. *Journal of Health Care for the Poor and Underserved, 20*(4 Suppl.), 1–12. https://doi.org/10.1353/hpu.0.0228

Jones, C. P., Truman, B. I., Elam-Evans, L. D., Jones, C. A., Jones, C. Y., Jiles, R., Rumisha, S. F., & Perry, G. S. (2008). Using "socially-assigned race" to probe White advantages in health status. *Ethnicity and Disease, 18*(4), 496–504.

Tatum, B. D. (1997). *Why are all the Black kids sitting together in the cafeteria? And other conversations about race*. New York: Basic Books.

Commentary

Looking Back to Move Forward

Camara Phyllis Jones, Byllye Y. Avery,
Linda Rae Murray, and Kisha Braithwaite Holden

This dialogue of significance is based on a wide-ranging conversation on February 2, 2022, between four powerful Black women. We met as sisters across decades of life experience to reflect on the importance of looking back to move forward. As our community understands the power of collective action, we also need to understand the importance of the elders connecting with the younger generations, both teaching and learning from them. We need to embrace the practice of mentoring, of passing our batons of knowledge and experience to those who follow.

We need to fashion barrels of batons and then pass them on. This tapestry of life with its joys and struggles is not just for our times. Our communities bridge both space and time. Our wisdom and collective action need to do the same.

The following record of our conversation is broken down into 16 short themes. Feel free to read through these sequentially or to hop around as you please:

- One Word on Black Women
- On Resilience
- On Black Women Saving Democracy and the Roles of White Women

- On Listening to Young People
- On Knowing Our Power
- On Breaking Our Silence
- On Racism and Capitalism and Structural Factors—Multiple Pandemics
- On Maternal Mortality
- On Hope
- On Our Sick Care System
- On Habits of Mind for Social Justice Warriors
- On Knowing Yourself
- On Trauma
- On Values Targets for Anti-racism Action
- On Principles for Achieving Health Equity
- Pearls of Wisdom

One Word on Black Women

Kisha Holden [as a discussion prompt]: What one word would you use to describe Black women, and why?

Byllye Avery: Political. One word that describes Black women to me is "political." And I sort of hadn't thought of it that way until I can remember back in the 1980s and we were all up in Dahlonega in that big room up in Forest Hills, and a woman was there from Amsterdam. She was called "Black" you know, and she was like Korean, she was Asian. And she said, "It's a political term. It's about our politics." And so I sort of thought, hmm, that is interesting. If you think about what happens when a Black woman enters the room, you know, her politics come in with her.

I got a call from Tijuana Malone yesterday or the day before saying that she'd gotten a call at 7:00 a.m. that morning to not come to work cause they'd gotten a bomb threat and all. She works at Albany State, an HBCU in Georgia. She said, "Yeah, the idea of a Black woman being on the Supreme Court makes these White people totally crazy." Here goes our politics again. So I'm pretty much sticking with "political" as my answer.

Linda Rae Muray: Resistance. To build on that, to me, the key thing about Black women is resistance. That's our politics. We are being oppressed and misused, not the only people in the world, but clearly on the bottom of so many piles, of so many hierarchies, and in order for us to survive, in order us to get up the next morning, it's an act of resistance against our oppression. It's an insistence that we in fact are really human.

I think the role of Black women has historically been that. In fact, you know, we have to remind ourselves "Black" women were created by this oppression, by this system of slavery. Before that, we were many different things in many different parts of the continent. But today we've been forged into a new identity.

And we've been added to, so not only do we have Black women that come from the continental United States in our system of slavery, we have our cousins that were enslaved in the rest of the hemisphere, and more recently we have the rest of the diaspora joining us. I was reading an article recently and saw that 25% of the Black population in the United States today—this may be higher because this was on a 2010 census—are immigrants or first-generation immigrants. And so I think that Black women represent for the world one wonderful example of resistance.

Camara Phyllis Jones: Power. Power is the word that keeps coming to me. But it's little power and big power. It's political power, resistance power, but power to protect our kids as we try to bring them to adulthood. It's creative power, power to inspire, and multidimensional power. I'm thinking like the sun. At first, I was thinking like one of those disco balls, but not reflecting. I'm thinking multifaceted, like a disco ball, but not reflecting but instead emanating like that. Sometimes they try to constrain our power, to wrap it up in something, but we still find that ray of light that comes through in some way.

Different ones of us in our different positions are still expressing our power in at least one kind of way. Some people have more latitude—they haven't been tied up so much. So they're able to express their power more fully. But all of us have that power.

On Resilience

Jones: And so, the expression of power is to recognize the onslaught and try to dismantle that, as opposed to try to equip our sisters and brothers or the next generation to be resilient.

Murray: A lot of the normal jargon we use to talk about resilience is missing those three words: power, political, and resistance.

Resilience is an academic paradigm that's trying to describe something that oppressed people have known for centuries. It's not that the concept of resilience is unimportant, but what we have to do as Black women is decolonize that word and decolonize that concept.

I don't think individuals—I don't want to overstate this—I think it's a mistake, and I think the book is so correct for expanding on this, I think it's absurd to talk about individuals being resilient. To me that just means figuring out how to adapt to getting your ass whipped. Community resilience, on the other hand, means being able to fight back. That's why I chose the word resistance. The critical thing for Black women historically has been, "How has our oppression changed." What new shit have they added to our oppression, and how can we organize and build power politically, which inherently means making allies and having solidarity with Native American women.

You know, today we're really challenged with that. None of this is brand new, but today they're back to banning books. They don't even want you to talk about basic Black history. Last night on Steven Colbert, in his little monologue he was talking about this attack on Black History Month. The band took Marvin Gaye's "What's Going On" and they changed the lyrics. You know, "Mother, mother, ..." They changed the lyrics so it was stripped of any cultural context, any resistance, any anything, and the refrain was, "Nothing's going on." He said, "You know, this is what they're trying to take, Marvin Gaye, and change Marvin Gaye into saying that nothing's going on and you don't have to worry about it."

We're really challenged today to not just know history, but the issue is to continue the fight against the suppression, which is getting worse, unfortunately.

Avery: And it has to get worse before it can get better. The thing that is happening now is that we are in the fight. We are beginning to be in the fight. Before, it was sort of away because folks were hiding who they really were. We *knew* who they were, but they thought we couldn't see them, because they thought we were blind. But the one thing I can say about Black women as a whole is that we have our eyes pretty open.

And kind of collectively, this question about our status in today's world, I am so proud of the way we as a community of Black women are conducting ourselves. We are about the business. It's like we know that civilization came out of us. We birthed it. We are the mothers. Everything on this earth came from a Black woman, and we are claiming that, and that is a part of what our legacy is. And, of course, we're resilient, because that's what it takes to withstand all of this bullshit that people are tossing around in their angst and their craziness.

Part of the problem is that the White supremacists know how mean and nasty they are. And they just can't imagine that we wouldn't be as mean and nasty as they are.

On Black Women Saving Democracy and the Roles of White Women

Avery and Holden: Absolutely. Yeah, we saved this country. I mean let's just put it on out there like it is. We saved the democracy for at least for these four damn years. Who knows what's going to happen? What they're going to have cooked up by the next time, because the White women aren't doing their part? They're sitting back, being all up in it, wearing those jeweled hats and carrying on like fools and acting like they're not a part of this.

I say to the White women activists all the time, y'all need to go to White women. You aren't talking to White women. And why are you so afraid to go and talk to your sisters? Why don't you have these hard conversations? They are and they have to be acknowledged as a part of the problem.

On Listening to Young People

Murray: My son always challenges me. He says, "I'm not sure your gen"—now, I think he distorts what our generation did, but—"I'm not sure your generation did the right thing." And so this is my concern and question. Certainly, as Brother Clyburn went with Biden, I was unhappy. You know, we're not a monolith. Are we afraid as Black women to really say what we need? I think this is something Byllye has really added to our struggle and our concept of health. Are we afraid to say that we really did need universal medical care? We really do need child support payments? We really do need free college tuition?

Are we functioning like we were in 1940 in terms of what we demand? Is it appropriate today? Is that adequate for my child, who's 50, or for his children who are in their early twenties? I'm not sure it is.

I think that part of what Black women should be doing, and I think this has happened historically, is to recognize that it's a two-way street. We have to listen to the younger generations in addition to transferring the knowledge that we've learned and that of our ancestors. I am really concerned—I feel like we're faced with fascism. We have climate change. There are so many huge things going on. I don't care whether you talk about the fact that there are fewer Black men in medical school today than when I was in medical school. That is stressful enough. But then when you realize that these people are organizing for good old-fashioned fascism. They haven't even changed it that much. It's not even more sophisticated.

Avery: I think for a long time, a lot of us didn't know what we needed. We didn't allow ourselves to think or come up with that. We just didn't know. But you know, we broke that silence 40 years ago now, and people are talking and claiming and moving and progressing. While we got all this retro activeness—just reactive shit going on with these White people who are just totally crazy and a few Black men who are all tied up in that, there's still a whole bunch of us who are still working really hard and making advances and making things happen. We have some who don't know, but I think there's a lot of voice out there to what we need. And I think that we we've got to give ourselves a little time to press.

Jones: The young people have clearer eyes about what's going on here, but maybe they aren't positioned yet. Or maybe they are, if they come together in collectives, perfectly positioned to call it out and to move things.

On Knowing Our Power

Jones: Byllye, I want to pick from when you were talking about talking, moving, claiming, progressing, about the fact that Black women do know our power. I agree with you and Linda Rae on the importance of collective action, which starts with talking to one another. It starts with joining in collectives. So, I want you to just say a little bit about the National Black Women's Health Project and how you got people just talking about health, sitting around kitchen tables. About how that work 40 years ago started people understanding their power, because we can walk around atomized, and maybe have a sense we have some power, but it's not until we connect with one another that we start recognizing, oh, Sis, you're strong. You got this. And here's the little piece I can put in this too. And that's that the talking, moving, claiming, progressing isn't automatic. Some communities do that better than others. We used to do it when we lived more in compounds and families could give you a sense of power. But we are so atomized sometimes in some parts of the country and so mobile. So I want you to maybe hit upon that and the importance of us being in dialogue and forming collectives.

On Breaking Our Silence

Avery: Well, the most important thing that we started doing was breaking the conspiracy of silence. We had lived with our stories inside of us. And when we started telling our stories and talking out loud about the things that happened to us, including what was good and what was bad, we found out that we had institutions within our families. bell hooks says some of the most oppressive things that can happen to you happen within our families. We found out how we are passing things on, generation to generation, whether it be sexual abuse, physical abuse, psychological abuse. But the mere fact of putting those words out in the air and others hearing them meant that we learned that it wasn't just our business. "Oh, oh so you got this. This one got this." So no longer anything you need to be protective of or feeling bad about or feeling ashamed of. That was an important thing.

And one thing I'm proud to say is that we were doing that in the eighties, before Oprah was doing it on her show at four o'clock in the afternoon. She came more in the nineties. And even now, when I hear these folks on these talk shows saying, "Oh, but I don't love myself, I have to love myself," we were doing that in the eighties when women had to learn how to love themselves. How to love your arms, how to love your hands, how to love your feet, how to love your hair. Even though people were telling us that the way our hair grows out of our head, that there's something wrong with that. And to love our skin, to love our color, to love all of that. So that basic work had a kind of ripple effect, and people got the word that we could look at all of this stuff that has happened to us. We could look at it. We can heal. We can learn from it. We can move on.

And the most important thing is to stop that cycle, that intergenerational conspiracy cycle that was going on, especially around sexual abuse and domestic violence. We all had to own up. We all had to talk about it. Talk out loud about it so that we could look at it and then handle it.

Then you can start thinking about the family unit and you can start thinking about health, because how in the heck can you think about going and getting a pap smear if somebody might be ready to beat you because you walked out of the door and went to the doctor? Think about the psychological abuse and all of what goes on and how that affects how we seek health care.

On Racism and Capitalism and Structural Factors— Multiple Pandemics

Avery: Now, we're in a different whole place with looking at it, when you ask, what are the significant health concerns Black women face. It's a lot of racism in health-care delivery—racism among the providers. Provider biases they call it. I call it plain old racist attitude, you know, just making decisions about me, on my life. And I mean when you get a person like Beyonce, who was in the top echelon up there in the Cadillac of the suites of the hospitals, you know, the ones they have on the top, top floors where all the ultra-wealthy go, and she couldn't get care? Serena Williams, and she couldn't get care? She's up there. She wasn't on the ward. You know what I mean? She's up there paying high dollar, top dollar, and they are not listening to her? What are you going to think about Miss Sally, who's down here on the ward saying something? So I'm just saying, it's plain overt racism that is at the core.

Not having access to health care and the racism of health-care providers, not just physician bias but all of the health-care provider bias that goes on, is one of the biggest threats to our health today. *The* biggest threat to our health today. And if you think about the politics of what's happening in the country, that gets spread around. You aren't going to tell me that some of those people working there aren't Trumpets.

Murray: Right. I remember a few years ago I was talking to some Latinx brother from South America. He's an epidemiologist. And I asked, because I had read somewhere that the life expectancy for White women in the South was falling. It was a little snippet, maybe *MMWR*, one of these little government pieces. And I asked him, "Because I'm not an epidemiologist, help me understand this. Now I know this is a crude measure, but when you have life expectancy for anybody falling, but especially for White women falling, isn't this like a fire alarm?" And he, being an epidemiologist, laid it out for me. He said, "You know, it's not only that. It's the healthy. It's not White babies that are dying or White old women." He said, "It's the healthy working population," and then he made some discussion about how they calculate these measures.

So what I'm saying is, when we see plants blooming a month early, okay, flowers in your garden blooming, and these so-called unusual weather events that are supposed to occur once in a hundred years happening every other year, we are not paying enough attention to these structural factors that are causing these issues.

When you're getting beaten every day, when you've got a whip on your back every day, it's easy to miss when the rhythm changes, it's easy to miss when the whip changes. But it's critical that we not miss that, because otherwise we will not survive. We really have to understand these changes in the structure. And we really have to challenge ourselves and future generations on how to address this. We really have to reach out and have a better understanding of what's going on in the world.

Avery: Right. We've got to connect all of these pandemics together. Cause we are living in several of them at one time, you know.

Murray: We have to refashion the social relations around the world to promote health. It's not just a question of resisting forces that are trying to kill us. We have to do that, obviously, but we also have to understand deeply what we need to do to repair, or I would prefer to say, recraft the conditions that we need to be healthy. That's the difference between being able to put pressure on a wound that's bleeding to try to stop the bleeding, and being able to surgically go in and do the repairs necessary to make sure that that person is able to function in a healthy way in the future.

I have one comment, and it's the same comment I always make, Camara, but I'll ask it as a question. Is it possible to eliminate racism without eliminating capitalism?

Jones: There are other systems, economic systems, where racism also exists.

Murray: That's true.

Jones: They're intertwined, but I don't put one above the other.

Murray: I try not to do that either. But it's just, when you look at that list of barriers to achieving health equity, is it possible to achieve health equity when we allow for the notion that a tiny fraction of the world's population can have all the wealth? That's my crude definition of capitalism for the time being. If we don't address the structural cause of the world's inequities on so many levels, which are growing around the world, then that's the one thing I feel is missing from that list [of barriers to achieving health equity].

Jones: It's a both/and. When I'm doing talks and I'm talking about structural racism and people ask me, "Camara, don't you care about poor White people?" I say, "Even if we were to eliminate poverty or go beyond that and eliminate income inequality today, even if we did that, if we did that without addressing the background structures, policies, practices, norms, and values that are the mechanisms of racism, then in one generation we would start to see a stratification by 'race' in terms of income again." So it is not an either/or, anti-poverty or anti-racism, it is a both/and. I say "anti-poverty." I don't say "anti-capitalism," which would be what you would want me to say. The other—

Murray: No, hold on. No, you know, especially when I'm in a small town in West Virginia, I don't be talking about capitalism. I talk just the way you do.

Jones: But this is the thing that I say: "Eliminating capitalism will not eliminate racism."

Murray: Right? That's correct.

Jones: "Eliminating racism will not eliminate capitalism."

Murray: Yes.

Jones: You asked me the question, "Can we eliminate racism without eliminating capitalism?" In this country, no. In other countries we might have to eliminate a feudal system or something, so the economics—because the racism manifests in economics and it manifests in some people seeing and clinging to their positionality as "White," not serf, not sharecropper, or something like that. So in this country, racism and capitalism are intertwined. They are both foundational in our nation's history.

Murray: Well, you know, we're only doctors. We're out of our league here. You know, this is all economics, and they argue about this still. And I'm going to mention Cuba, so this may help you with some of your talks. There's no doubt in my mind, Cuba tried to eliminate capitalism. One can argue if they were really successful or if that's possible. It's a small island in this world. But one thing I'm clear about is that they haven't eliminated racism. So, I encourage us to think that it's not like you're drawing a picture. This is a complicated thing.

You can't expect to eliminate racism, and I think Fidel Castro pointed this out in a speech he gave in New York City where he said, "We thought if we eliminated capitalism, if we had a socialist state, we would solve the problem of racism." And he said, "That was a mistake. That's not enough. It didn't happen." Some of this has to do with timing, if we had a[n anti-capitalism] change tomorrow, it'd be two or three, four generations for the reasons Kisha talked about—historical trauma—before all of these problems or these barriers [to achieving health equity] that you're listing would go away. It's not like you can suddenly change the material reality and think that human beings aren't still carrying burdens.

But in terms of these barriers, there is an economist who has a whole website now about inequality in the world. And obviously it's not just economic inequality, but he argues that the widening of inequalities in the world starting with economics—he's an economist—is a major threat. This continual growth of inequality in wealth and resources in the world is a major problem that's dragging us down. Maybe just calling it that, "the continual growth of inequality of wealth and resources." I am not sure that just getting people to *say* the word "capitalism" is enough.

On Maternal Mortality

Avery: That's why the maternal health crisis has just blown up. I started talking about this in the early nineties. I had a whole thing saying, "You don't hear this term 'she died in childbirth.'" During my mother's time, I said, "Well, what about my cousin?" "Oh, she died in childbirth." So and so died in childbirth. Now, we've got people dying in childbirth. We've got young Black women—I heard a young Black women say, "I'm scared to get pregnant cause I think I might die."

Pregnancy is a healthy condition. This is when you're excited. You're bringing creative life into the world. It should be the opposite experience. And you've got Black women walking around fearful that they might die because some fool over here won't listen to them or take good care of them.

Murray: I'm glad Byllye brought up the maternal mortality issue, which we don't completely fully understand. Again, this is something that public health people, none of us on this call, are surprised with the fact that the maternal mortality is going up for Black women. This is what I find frightening, as you begin to look into it, and this is what I think we have a special obligation to deal with. The maternal mortality rate is going up for *all* women in this country, including White women. Not as bad—not as high as us. So then you say to yourself, what are we coming to where these fools will let their own women die in childbirth? So, again, if we look at the structural problems, then it's like the bridges that are falling. It's our societal infrastructure that's crumbling.

On Hope

Murray: So, I have hope. I want to be clear about that. I don't think this is a pessimistic notion. But I feel like you have to see the things coming down the track in order for you to derail the train or get out the way or whatever you have to do.

On Our Sick Care System

Avery [in a discussion about COVID-19 and the disproportionate impact on communities of color]: "Tasha" won't even get a ventilator. That's why I said, before the shot came out, "I'm 82 years old." I was 82 then. I said, "I'm keeping my butt home cause if I go down there to Cape Cod Hospital, they are not going to give me a ventilator." You know what I'm saying? In this kind of political system that we have today, it has affected our health care, and it's going to affect it for many, many years. When we get past COVID, when we go through our Greek alphabet and then double back around and find another alphabet, we're going to find out that our sick care system is even going to be sicker than it was. I'll stop there.

On Habits of Mind for Social Justice Warriors

Jones [as a discussion prompt]: I have what I call my "Four BCs" that I describe as habits of mind for social justice warriors. They are Be Courageous, Be Curious, Be Collective, and Build Community.

The first one, "Be Courageous," is to speak your truth, to embrace challenge, to be unafraid of controversy, and to know that the edge of your comfort is your growing edge. So it's basically "be out there." And I should say "recognize your power," because a lot of people who get in positions, a lot of Black women who are in positions and could be doing more than what they're doing, don't recognize the power that they have. Or they're trying to hold back, so they can get up to that next rung. They say, "Then I'll act." But if you practice not acting, if you practice not using your power where you are, you will never use your power.

The second one, "Be Curious," starts with asking "Why?" when you see something or when somebody tells you something, and then asking "Why?" again, and "Why?" again, asking serial "Why?"s so that we don't get complacent or accept superficial explanations of things. That we dig to root causes, which is a lot of our analysis in this room here. "Be Curious" is also to speak more than one language, to travel widely, across town or around the world, to be in other people's experiences. Reading widely and reading history. Don't be threatening Black institutions in Black History Month, right.

The third one is "Be Collective," which is to care about the whole. I used to frame it as "Be a Citizen," but "citizen" is so narrowly constrained as national citizenship, not global citizenship. So be collective to share your ideas, your energy, your time, and your stuff with others. But especially to organize, because collective action is power. So I was really appreciating what you were saying, Byllye, the whole thing about talking, moving, claiming, progressing, that collective piece.

And the fourth one is "Build Community." I talk about being interested in the stories of others, then believing the stories of others, and then joining in the stories of others. Talk to strangers. I think about bursting through bubbles to experience our common humanity, because all of us are in some kind of bubble. I even started thinking about how some people's small bubbles with thick Plexiglas boundaries are being hardened by fear. But whatever kind of bubble we are in, most of us do not really, really know that there are people who are just as kind, funny, generous, hardworking, and smart as we are just across town who are living in very different circumstances from ours.

Byllye, you were describing some of the work of bubble bursting that people were doing with the National Black Women's Health Project (now the Black Women's Health Imperative) and before. It helps Black women bubble burst with each other to know that the thing that I was hiding inside me is a collective experience. We need to burst through our bubbles and then we can start planning and acting. Really, it's about going across town and staying a while.

So, be courageous, be curious, be collective, build community. Do you like those? Would you want to add to them? Would you want to take some out? Is there one that speaks to you most loudly? Should I have a T-shirt with the "Four BCs"?

Avery: Well, first of all, I like them. The only piece that was missing for me is that a lot of times people don't know who they are. They haven't done any work on themselves, you know? And they can be so reflective of a narrow way of looking at life. I like the part about go across town, go sit at somebody else's table, go see how other people live their lives, look at it. But a lot of us haven't looked at our own lives. So if somewhere that comes under being curious, be curious about who you are. Do you know yourself? Sometimes you can say something, and you think, "Where did that come from?" or "Whose voice was that? What am I listening to?"

People carry a lot of these voices with them everywhere they go. And they sometimes forget to unplug those negative tapes. So maybe it'll come in be courageous and interrupt that tape that's going on in your head. Don't always play the same thing, cause you're going to get the same answers and you're not going to be moving forward. So that was my thought, that a lot of people don't know themselves. They're afraid to know themselves. They're afraid to go and clean out the cobwebs of their minds.

They have a lot of them. That's one of my favorite sayings, that you need to go clean out the cobwebs of your mind. That's what you can do on your walks every day. Don't be afraid to go in there and examine. You can come out, you know? A lot of people won't open those doors. They keep them sealed off.

Murray: When you first went through these four, I got stuck on the first one, be courageous. And then after Byllye's comment, I have an actual suggestion. Don't put it first, because when you start off "Be Courageous" as the first thing, any rational person will be, "I don't want to do that!" I mean what idiot would just say, "Oh, I'm going to just go out here and be courageous and get lynched." No rational human being would do that. But if you put it last—you go through these other scenes first, then you come to what Byllye is saying. If you're going to be true to yourself, okay, then you will end up being courageous. If you really understand yourself, if you love yourself, if you do all—and I think curious is great to start off because first you gotta figure out what the hell's going on here. So I think starting with curious; put "Be Courageous" at the end, because your courage is not a personality trait. It's based on your curiosity, the collective, the community. You can't be courageous outside of that. So that would be my one suggestion. And then I think you can weave the individual aspect of these things into the collective and community aspects. That would be my only suggestion.

On Knowing Yourself

Jones: How do you do it, Byllye? Maybe we don't know how to know ourselves.

Avery: Well, you do it by thinking, first of all, why won't you do it? What do you have in your mind that you don't want to deal with? Was it that this person said something at work today that made you have a weird feeling, but you don't know where that came from? That you had an overreaction? Do some sort of self-examination and ask, "Why is this bothering me so? What about this is restimulating?"

Or you see a person who's having a really bad time and you can't help them. I remember once when I was there out in Atlanta. A young woman came. She was an intern over at CDC and she needed a place to stay. And they called me at the last minute, and I said, yeah, she could stay with me, a little White woman. I didn't know her, but you know, anyway, whatever.

I got sick in the night and was throwing up, and this woman stood in the door and just looked at me. She didn't go get a bucket. She didn't say, "Do you need something?" She didn't say nothing. And so I was kind of bothered. I'm giving this woman my house, a bed to sleep in, and she can't even go get a darn bucket or towel or anything.

Jones: Oh, Byllye.

Avery: No, I found out that she was anorexic. She was bulimic. And my vomiting—

Jones: Okay. But still—

Avery: I know. Hey, I'm with that too, but you know things like that can paralyze people and they don't know why they are paralyzed. Maybe later on she went back—I hope she went back and examined that situation—and said, "I couldn't help Byllye because it reminded me too much of myself." But people can get stopped by—they can get frozen by—unresolved things that have happened to them.

Holden: In that same situation, had it been a Black woman, the initial reaction would've instinctually been to get a bucket or something.

Avery: I want to think so. I don't think race had anything to do with it to tell you the truth, Kisha. I would like to think that, but I have seen many, many sisters that, you know you can get frozen and not understand why you didn't help that person. What was going on? You know what I'm saying. Or why are you in a group and someone is picking on somebody and clearly they're wrong and you don't speak up on behalf of the person being picked on? It's hard to say. I like to think a Black woman would've helped me, but I can no longer think that because I've just seen too many dysfunctional Black women that probably would've been as messed up as this woman was in her head

Jones: Because of the trauma.

Avery: Yeah, the trauma, and the trauma is something else.

On Trauma

Avery: There was one of the studies that really stayed with me. They did a study down at Emory University on mice, and they would hit the male mouse with a cattle prod. And they would present it with a smell of a chemical that was something like almonds. When they mated that male mouse and pups were born, when they put the chemical in front of the pups, they had a traumatic response just from the chemical, not the cattle prod.

I think about slavery and the trauma of slavery and how—can trauma be passed down through our DNA, through our genes?

Holden: I didn't know about that study, but I'm a psychologist, and I do some work on PTSD with Black women. And the generational trauma piece is real. And so it's nature and nurture. It's a part of the picture.

On Values Targets for Anti-Racism Action

Jones [as a discussion prompt]: I talk about racism as a system of doing two things, structuring opportunity and assigning value. And I think we know a lot of the structural stuff, how we fund public schools based on local property taxes, or environmental racism, or the child welfare system and how it participates in the school to prison pipeline, and all of those things. These are structural things, and we have some idea. We've mapped out that at least these are some targets for action.

But the values pieces of racism as a system that does those two things, structures opportunity and assigns value, have been largely invisible, because they're part of our capitalist society. They're part of the Western canon. Pull yourself up by your bootstraps—it's all of that.

I first talked about seven societal or cultural barriers to achieving health equity. I now describe them as the seven values targets for anti-racism action. They are: narrow focus on the individual; ahistorical stance; myth of meritocracy; myth of a zero-sum game; limited future orientation; myth of American exceptionalism; and White supremacist ideology. You can find these in my Harvard Primary Care Blog from August 2020.

Murray: You know the students insisted at the school of public health on a course on racism, which I taught now twice. But I use these principles in lots of the talks I give. In the racism class, this is what we think of it. I make a distinction in the class and when I have more time, the whole semester. Some of these things are inherent in the Western scientific method, and that's why the global south is arguing for decolonization of knowledge. And then some of this stuff is just American pathology, you know, like American exceptionalism.

Jones: There is this list of seven barriers to achieving health equity. But I describe a subset of four of them as the roots of racism denial. These four are:

1. The narrow focus on the individual, which makes systems and structures invisible or seemingly irrelevant.

2. The ahistorical stance, which acts as if the present were disconnected from the past and as if the current distribution of advantage and disadvantage were just a happenstance.

3. The myth of meritocracy, the story that goes like this, if you work hard, you will make it, which misses the point that, yes, most people who've made it have worked hard (but not even everybody who's made it has worked hard—we've got Trump and all of them). Yes, we acknowledge that most people who have made it have worked hard. But there are many other people working just as hard or harder who will never make it because of an uneven playing field. And when we deny racism and these other systems of structured inequity that have created and are perpetuating the uneven playing field, we blame those who haven't made it for being lazy or stupid.

4. White supremacist ideology, which I put last in my list so people can listen to the others before they go crazy.

Actually, when you talk about racism as a system that structures opportunity and assigns value, the foundational "values" piece is White supremacist ideology. It should be number one on my lists, but I always put it last because I am being strategic.

On Principles for Achieving Health Equity

Jones [as a discussion prompt]: When I talk about health equity, there are many things that we need to be doing, many principles for achieving health equity. I've distilled at least these three: valuing all individuals and populations equally, recognizing and rectifying historical injustices, and *especially* providing resources according to need.

Murray: If you look at all of that stuff, I ask myself, "Okay, so if we did that, would that be enough?" And my answer would be no. And you might have to think of a more appropriate way to say this, but the only way that that's going to happen is if you take some stuff from these folks that stole it. I mean you can't do that.

Jones: You're going hard. That's going high.

Murray: Well, you know, think about climate change. What's going to happen quickly? Millions of people are not going to be able to live where they live now. So it's not enough to say providing resources according to need. You know, they don't think providing resources means giving up their stuff, so you have got to clearly say that. It's a tiny group of people.

Jones: Redistribution.

Murray: That is critical to what's going on.

Pearls of Wisdom

Jones [as a discussion prompt]: What else do Black women and the whole world need to know from you now? What pearls of wisdom do you want to share?

Avery: Keep your eyes open. This is not the time to fall asleep. Stay on it. I wanted to say, "Keep your eyes on the prize," except I don't quite know what the prize is.

Holden: And the young people say, "Stay woke."

Avery: Yes. Stay woke! And we really do have to keep paying attention. We cannot afford to become complacent. We have to stay on this.

But on the other side, I have to say I am just so pleased that so much attention is being given to Black women's health. You know, things are happening. Books are coming out. Sisters are getting into it. People are doing things to help make sure that we look at all parts of Black women's health, and the way Black women are taking charge of this maternal stuff with midwives and doulas and looking at what we need. I just say, I am so pleased. I am so pleased.

And I don't want to toot my horn, but maybe I will. I'm just so damn proud of the Black Women's Health Imperative and Linda Goler Blount, she has taken it way beyond anything that I could have ever dreamed of. You know? And the only hope I had in those long dark days of 40 years, there were some dark ones, was that there would be some Black women who would come along, take this thing, and make it happen.

Murray: Oh, they're standing on your shoulders, Byllye. Standing on your shoulders.

Avery: And I'm happy to provide them for them. You know, I am so glad. You know, it's just wonderful. So, I'm pleased. I'm very pleased.

Murray: I think we have to have our eyes on the international problems. We're in an existential crisis here. We have to remember what's unique about this historical period. And what's unique about this historical period is that we really are in an existential crisis, not only just with climate change, but you know, movements of people around the world because of war and corruption and all of those kind of things.

Avery: Yeah. It's a small world, you know?

Murray: Yeah.

Jones: And we're all on it, and people don't want to recognize our neighbors, you know. That we are all in this together.

Holden: Most definitely

Avery: Absolutely. Absolutely.

Conversations with Thought Leaders: Beacons of Light

MELISSA HARRIS-PERRY, CHRISTINE BEATTY, AND SANDRA HARRIS-HOOKER

Question: What one word describes Black women to you? Why? What does that word mean to you?

SELECTED EXCERPTED RESPONSES

- Versatile. Whether Black women are in the professional world/high-level career or not, it really doesn't matter, we [Black women] have to be versatile. Black women have the mindset to pivot at a moment's notice/anytime. She has to be educator, mother, wife, sister, friend, motivator, culinary artist, family financier, etc. It is not just one path that we are on.

- Humanistic. We [Black women] can be vulnerable but must disentangle expectations of who we are.

- Powerful. We [Black women] have an innate ability to go "inside of ourselves" for whatever we need—and it is a true gift from God. Our perseverance is unmatched—we perform well in so many different roles including problem solver, mom, wife, partner, sister, aunt, friend, teacher, doctor, employee, etc.

Question: Can you describe how you see Black women as a critical part in establishing cultural norms and/or trends in our society?

SELECTED EXCEPTED RESPONSES

- Young Black people create popular culture. This is done creatively through music, tv, social media. Nevertheless, Black women are the ones that encourage collaboration, community, and charity—we give regardless of our income.

- Black women have always set the norm re: fashion, hairstyles, etc., yet the credit goes unrecognized; and Black people established in music—jazz, R & B, hip-hop, spoken word, etc.

- Black women are now being recognized. Thanks to strong women such as Michelle Obama. We [Black women] always knew we were fabulous; and now the world is finally seeing us for the remarkable women that we are. But the fight is not over—the pay disparity between men and women still exists.

- We [Black women] set the cultural norms for many things from fashion to work ethic. We are the "hidden figures"—and established what it means to be an overachiever. Many people emulate our styles and ways of being.

Question: What are some of the challenges that you believe Black women must overcome in navigating through our society? How do you think we demonstrate resilience?

SELECTED EXCEPTED RESPONSES

Challenges

- We [Black women] have the challenge of "always being seen, but not heard." Also, we have experienced extreme "mansplaining" regardless of education and/or experiences. Black women must work twice as hard for less recognition.

- Among the most critical work is the need for of Black women to put ourselves at the top of the nation's political and social agenda. We need structure in our society and to care for each other regardless of descent—Caribbean, African, Indigenous. We are all Black women.

- Handling multiple identities and being undervalued simultaneously in a society fraught with deleterious systemic issues. We [Black women] have unfairly been at the "bottom of the totem pole" for many things.

Resilience

- We [Black women] demonstrate resilience by aiming to balance multiple roles and responsibilities, which typically results in stellar outcomes. We must fully establish our rightful place and engender power.

- Resilience is demonstrated by how we [Black women] live and thrive daily by overcoming the plethora of challenges. And, we do it while looking fashionably amazing. Our power is unmatched.

Question: What do you believe are the most significant health concerns facing Black women and families today?

SELECTED EXCERPTED RESPONSES

- Currently it is the COVID-19 pandemic. Not only risk for the coronavirus itself, but the other health issues, such as exacerbating co-occurring health problems that impact families. Our Black women and men are negatively affected; and the full impact of the disease is not known.

- Among all of the health disparities, Black women are on the list and very negatively impacted.

- Heart disease/cardiovascular health problems. For many years, attention was only placed on men as at risk. We [Black women] need to participate in more clinical trials which will help with better diagnoses for women.

- Cancer. Especially breast cancer. It is less diagnosed among Black women regardless of SES.
- The fact that there are limited doctors that look like us [Black women] and some providers that simply do not believe us relative to many issues (i.e., pain). This limitation contributes to the health disparities that exists—especially when it comes to Black maternal health; and it is related to poor access to affordable healthcare.

Contributors

Tabia Henry Akintobi, PhD, MPH, is Professor and Chairperson of the Department of Community Health and Preventive Medicine and Associate Dean of Community Engagement at Morehouse School of Medicine in Atlanta, Georgia.

Ndidiamaka N. Amutah-Onukaga, PhD, MPH, CHES, Associate Professor, Department of Public Health and Community Medicine, Assistant Dean of Diversity and Inclusion, Tufts University School of Medicine, Founder and Principal Investigator, Maternal Outcomes for Translational Health Equity Research (MOTHER) lab.

Yoann Sophie Antoine, MPH, CHES, Research Assistant, Maternal Outcomes for Translational Health Equity Research (MOTHER) lab, Research Associate, Amaka Consulting and Evaluation Services.

Ifeyinwa V. Asiodu, PhD, RN, is on faculty in the Department of Family Health Care Nursing at University of California, San Francisco School of Nursing.

Byllye Y. Avery, MEd, founder of the Black Women's Health Imperative, formerly the National Black Women's Health Project, has been a healthcare activist for over 40 years, focusing on the specific needs of women.

Christine Beatty, MSW, is a Woman on a Mission. In 2002, Christine became the youngest Chief of Staff in the City of Detroit's history, where she managed two winning mayoral campaigns. She was named one of Michigan's Most Influential Women by Crain's Detroit Business in 2004 and her drive and talent produced solid results for Detroit, where she was born and raised.

Allyson S. Belton, MPH, is Director of Education and Training for the Satcher Health Leadership Institute (SHLI) at Morehouse School of Medicine. In this role, she is responsible for the design, delivery, and evaluation of SHLI's health equity–based leadership training programs for diverse learners.

Linda Goler Blount, MPH, President, CEO, Black Women's Health Imperative (BWHI). As president and CEO, Linda oversees the strategic direction for the Imperative and is responsible for moving the organization forward in its mission to achieve health equity, as well as reproductive justice for Black women.

Katrina M. Brantley, DrPH, MPH, Community Relations Manager, Georgia Department of Public Health, serves as the Community Relations Manager in the Maternal and Child Health Section of the Georgia Department of Public Health. Dr. Brantley has two decades of experience in the areas of public health research, program management, and evaluation.

Donna L. Brazile is a veteran democratic political strategist. She is an adjunct professor, author, syndicated columnist, television political commentator, Vice Chair of Voter Registration and Participation at the Democratic National Committee, and former interim National Chair of the Democratic National Committee, as well as the former chair of the DNC's Voting Rights Institute.

Addie Briggs, MD, FAAP, is board certified in pediatrics. She received her bachelor of science with honors from Howard University in Washington, DC. She then went on to earn her medical degree from the Virginia Commonwealth University School of Medicine (formerly Medical College of Virginia) in Richmond, Virginia. Dr. Briggs completed a primary care pediatric residency at Cincinnati Children's Hospital in Cincinnati, Ohio.

Raquel Brown, JD, is an experienced attorney, mother, and proactive community servant. She has a BBA from Howard University and a JD from Southern Methodist University. Raquel has two sons, Blake and Joshua, who provide lasting experiences of resilience for her. As a single mother and professional, Raquel has faced difficulties with maintaining balance.

Kimarie Bugg, DNP, MPH, is President and CEO of Reaching Our Sisters Everywhere (ROSE). Dr. Bugg, a career perinatal and neonatal nurse professional, recognized her calling alongside her grandmother, a lay midwife in rural Arkansas, at the age of 12.

Yvette C. Cozier, ScD, is an epidemiologist at the Slone Epidemiology Center and Associate Professor and Assistant Dean for Diversity and Inclusion in the Boston University School of Public Health. Dr. Cozier has also worked on the Black Women's Health Study since its inception.

Joia Crear-Perry, MD, is a physician, policy expert, thought leader, and advocate for transformational justice. As the founder and president of the National Birth Equity Collaborative (NBEC), she identifies and challenges racism as a root cause of health inequities.

Cedrice Davis, MD, Family Medicine, Urban Family Practice Associates, Adjunct Clinical Assistant Professor, Department of Community Health and Preventive Medicine, Morehouse School of Medicine. Dr. Davis was born in Cleveland, Ohio, and grew up in New Orleans, Louisiana. She completed her undergraduate degree at Howard University in Washington, DC, and received her MD from Case Western Reserve University in Cleveland, Ohio.

Shubhecchha Dhaurali is a first-generation student originally from Kathmandu, Nepal. She is double majoring in community health and sociology at Tufts University.

LeConté J. Dill, DrPH, MPH, is a scholar, educator, and a poet originally from South Central Los Angeles. Her work focuses on safety, resilience, resistance, and wellness, particularly for urban Black girls and other youth of color. Dr. Dill earned her BA degree in sociology and creative writing from Spelman College, her MPH degree in community health sciences from the University of California, Los Angeles, and her DrPH degree from the University of California, Berkeley, and she was a Health

Policy Post-doctoral Fellow in the Satcher Health Leadership Institute at Morehouse School of Medicine.

Jemea Dorsey, MS, is the President and CEO, Center for Black Women's Wellness. She is responsible for the overall management and operations of a community-based, nonprofit organization that provides low-cost health-care services, microbusiness training, prenatal case management, and youth development programming to over 2,000 families annually.

Crystal R. Emery, MA, is known for producing narratives aimed at creating a more equitable society. She is the Founder and CEO of URU The Right to Be, a nonprofit content production company that addresses issues at the intersection of humanities, arts, and sciences.

Paige E. Feyock is a Research Assistant for the Maternal Outcomes for Translational Health Equity Research (MOTHER) lab. She is a junior at Wellesley College, double majoring in sociology and Africana studies on the pre-medicine track.

Adrienne Chevelle Glymph Foster, MPH, earned a Bachelor of Science at Howard University and her master's in public health from the George Washington School of Medicine and Health Sciences. Her research interests are in infectious disease and surveillance. Foster currently works as the Senior Director of Programs at the National Association of County and City Health Officials (NAACHO).

Helene D. Gayle, MD, MPH, is President and CEO of the Chicago Community Trust, one of the nation's oldest and largest community foundations, since October 2017. Under her leadership, the Trust has adopted a new strategic focus on closing the racial and ethnic wealth gap in the Chicago region.

Malika B. Gooden, DC, MPH, CMT, is Principal Doctor, Chiropractic and Physical Therapy Specialty for Premier Spine Center (PSC), Silver Spring, Maryland. Dr. Gooden's areas of special clinical interest include integrative medicine, public health, women's health issues, family health, and patient education.

Lisa Grace-Leitch, EdD, MPH, MA, currently serves as Associate Professor and Deputy Chair of the Health Education department at City

University of New York-Borough of Manhattan Community College. She teaches courses in women's health, gerontology, spirituality, community health education, public health, health communication, and the social and behavioral determinants of health.

Lesley Green-Rennis, EdD, MPH, has over 18 years' experience in public health research and evaluation. She currently serves as Associate Professor and Chair of the Health Education department at City University of New York-Borough of Manhattan Community College.

Sandra Harris-Hooker, PhD, is Vice President, Executive Vice Dean, and Professor of Pathology and Anatomy at Morehouse School of Medicine. Her research interests are cardiovascular biology and delineating ways to enhance the integration of basic, clinical, and population-based research in order to address disparities in health.

Melissa Harris-Perry, PhD, is the Maya Angelou Presidential Chair in the Department of Politics and International Affairs, the Department of Women and Gender Studies, and the Program in Environment and Sustainability at Wake Forest University. For nearly two decades, Harris-Perry has contributed to American public life through her distinct combination of scholarly analysis and grounded wisdom applied to analysis of race, gender, politics, and power.

Rhonda C. Holliday, PhD, is an Associate Professor in the Department of Community Health and Preventive Medicine at Morehouse School of Medicine. Dr. Holliday conducts HIV and substance use prevention, minority health issues, and community-based participatory research.

Elizabeth O. Ige, MSW, has research interests in youth violence, juvenile justice, and inequities within the education system, particularly the school-to-prison pipeline and the invisibility of Black girls and other girls of color in these spaces. She thrives as a social worker and as an independent scholar.

Brenda Ingram, EdD, LCSW, is a licensed clinical social worker and an educator who has over 30 years working in the trauma, mental health, and education fields. She directs Relationship and Sexual Violence Prevention and Services for USC Student Health; and she is Associate Director, USC Counseling and Mental Health Division and Clinical Assistant Professor, Psychiatry and Behavioral Sciences, USC Keck School of Medicine.

Bridg'ette Israel, PhD, currently serves Florida Agricultural and Mechanical University as assistant professor in pharmaceutics. Dr. Israel's passion for teaching is deeply rooted in her love for empowering others with knowledge.

Camille A. Jones, MD, MPH, is a physician, board-certified in both internal medicine and preventive medicine, with a Master of Public Health degree focused on health policy and management and epidemiology. She is passionate about public health! She has worked at many levels of government, including as an Epidemiology Program Director at the National Institutes of Health (1991–2001), as Medical Director for the Arkansas Minority Health Commission (2003–2007), and most recently as Assistant Health Commissioner for the City of Cincinnati Health Department (2007–2019).

Clara Y. Jones, MD, MPH, is an internal medicine physician with a lifelong commitment to fostering and providing excellent primary care in underserved communities. She is currently an internal medicine physician with the Cambridge Health Alliance at the Windsor Street Clinic in Cambridge, Massachusetts.

Kristian T. Jones, MD, is currently pursuing residency at Morehouse School of Medicine, Department of Psychiatry and Behavioral Sciences, where she is Chief Resident.

Jennifer F. Kelly, PhD, ABPP, Director, the Atlanta Center for Behavioral Medicine, Atlanta, Georgia, was the 2021 President of the American Psychological Association. She is board-certified in Clinical Health Psychology and is the Director of the Atlanta Center for Behavioral Medicine in Atlanta, Georgia.

Ricardo D. LaGrange, PhD, MPH, is Vice President, US Health for ideas42 and Adjunct Professor at Howard University. He is a licensed psychologist, applied research scientist, and public health specialist. Dr. LaGrange brings over 25 years' experience advancing public health, educational, and youth development initiatives.

Blessing Chidiuto Lawrence, MPH, is the Epidemiology Data Coordinator, Partners in Health, Research Assistant, and Writing Cochair for Maternal Outcomes for Translational Health Equity Research (MOTHER) lab. She is a Research Associate for Amaka Consulting and Evaluation.

Cynthia Major Lewis, MD, maintains a limited part-time private practice, providing independent medical examinations and fitness for duty evaluations for injured and at-risk workers. Dr. Lewis was recently named Cochair of the Baltimore City Suicide Prevention Legislative Workgroup, along with Councilmember Danielle McCray, by Baltimore City Council President, Nick Mosby. She is a member of the legislative committee for the Maryland Psychiatric Society and the Johns Hopkins Medicine Behavioral Safety Steering Committee.

Sydney Love, BA, is a fourth-year health-care management undergraduate student at Clayton State University. Her current line of work focuses on medical billing and health insurance claims. Ms. Love intends on pursuing a master's in public health.

Imani Ma'at, EdD, MEd, MCP, is an award-winning author, wellness coach, speaker, and CEO of Focused Health and Healthy Haiku Productions. She is a goal-oriented, public health manager and trainer, researcher and evaluator; and she has expertise in youth, women, and incarceration health education, and in focus group facilitation. Previously, she was employed at the Dekalb County Sheriff's Office in Georgia, where she was responsible for inmate services and educational programs.

Tamia A. McEwen, PhD, is a State Certified Recovery Peer Specialist (CRPS), mental health and wellness advocate; E-RYT 200, YAEP author of *Mind as Well*; Founder of Be Well, Friends, LLC, and Treasure Coast Peer Network; qigong instructor; Board Member of Peer Support Coalition of Florida (PSCFL); and Digital Facilitator Orlando Peer Support Space.

Brian McGregor, PhD, is Adjunct Clinical Assistant Professor, Department of Psychiatry and Behavioral Sciences, Staff Psychologist, Cardiovascular Research Institute, Morehouse School of Medicine, and Owner, McGregor Research and Consulting. Dr. Brian McGregor is a community psychologist with over 15 years of experience in needs assessment, program evaluation, and clinical and community-based research.

Tonyka McKinney, DrPH, is currently completing a postdoctoral fellowship at the Morehouse School of Medicine leading public health projects focused on the political determinants of health.

Ashley Kennedy Mitchell, DrPH, MSPH, is passionate about creating and retaining a diverse and competent health workforce. She currently serves as Director of Learning Communities and Assistant Director of the Office of Academic and Community Innovation at Morehouse School of Medicine.

Nia Mitchell, MPH, is a Birth Equity Research Scholar with the National Birth Equity Collaborative. As an evaluator and researcher, she is committed to centering on Black women and birthing people's lived experiences, models of care, scholarship, and activism in her work.

Nicole Taylor Morris, MTS, is a womanist scholar-activist, doula, and aspiring movement chaplain and healer. She recently graduated from Harvard Divinity School with a Master of Theological Studies focused on the intersections of Black women and community's health, community-centered healing, and the role of spirituality in wellness.

Regina Davis Moss, PhD, MPH, MCHES, is the Associate Executive Director of the American Public Health Association. She oversees a broad portfolio of programs addressing the social determinants of health and has nearly 20 years of experience managing national health promotion initiatives addressing women's health, health equity, and public health system capacity building.

Bahiyyah M. Muhammad, PhD, is an Associate Professor of Criminology in the Department of Sociology at Howard University (HU) in the District of Columbia (DC). She is an expert on mass incarceration and the collateral consequences on families, specifically focused on resilience among children of incarcerated parents.

Linda Rae Murray, MD, MPH, has spent her career serving the medically underserved. Currently, she serves as the Chief Medical Officer for the Cook County Department of Public Health of the Cook County Health and Hospital System. She practices as a general internist at Woodlawn Health Center, is an attending physician in the Division of Occupational and Environmental Medicine at Cook County Hospital, and is an adjunct Assistant Professor at the University of Illinois at Chicago School of Public Health (Occupational and Environmental Health and the Health Policy and Administration Departments).

Julie R. Palmer, ScD, is Director of the Slone Epidemiology Center at Boston University and Karen Grunebaum Professor in the Boston University School of Medicine. Dr. Palmer is one of the Principal Investigators and Founders of the Black Women's Health Study.

Kimberly A. Parker, PhD, MPH, MCHES, is Founder and Principal Investigator, Parker Owens Research Group, Independent Consultant. She conducts research on the intersection of social injustice and minority health issues.

Anana Johari Harris Parris is Founder of the SisterCARE Alliance, which promotes and educates populations at risk on Strategic Self Care Programming and social justice advocacy and the Self Care Agency. Currently, Ms. Parris is the Women of Color Initiative Strategic Self Care Curriculum Design Consultant and Leadership Program Developer.

Annelle B. Primm, MD, MPH, is a community psychiatrist and the Senior Medical Director of the Steve Fund, a nonprofit focused on the mental health of young people of color. She chairs the All Healers Mental Health Alliance, a group of mental health professionals, faith leaders, first responders, and public health advocates that facilitates culturally aligned responses to the mental health needs of marginalized communities affected by natural and human-caused disasters.

Sharon A. Rachel, MA, MPH, is an Associate Project Director in the Satcher Health Leadership Institute at Morehouse School of Medicine in Atlanta, Georgia, where she directs an NIH-funded research study aiming to promote culturally centered, trauma-informed mental health care and wellness for African American/Black women with Post-Traumatic Stress Disorder (PTSD).

Rhonda Reid, MD, is Chief Resident Physician in the Department of Psychiatry and Behavioral Sciences at Morehouse School of Medicine.

Valerie Montgomery Rice, MD, is the sixth president of Morehouse School of Medicine (MSM) and the first woman to lead the freestanding medical institution; Montgomery Rice serves as both the president and CEO. A renowned infertility specialist and researcher, she most recently served as dean and executive vice president of MSM, where she has served since 2011.

Bianca D. Rivera, DrPH (c), MPH holds an MPH degree from SUNY Downstate School of Public Health, where she is also currently pursuing a DrPH degree in epidemiology. Through her applied research, she focuses on examining violence as an infectious disease from a social and environmental perspective, and its subsequent relationship to urban adolescent educational experiences and trauma-related health outcomes.

Alyssa G. Robillard, PhD, MCHES, is an Associate Professor in Community Health in the Edson College of Nursing and Health Innovation at Arizona State University. She is also an Affiliate Faculty with the Voices/Voces Project in the Institute for Families in Society at the University of South Carolina.

Amorie Robinson, PhD, is a licensed clinical psychologist serving as the Behavioral Health Lead Therapist at the Ruth Ellis Center in Highland Park, Michigan. She previously worked at the Third Circuit Court (juvenile/family) Clinic for Child Study in Detroit for 15 years, providing psychotherapy and psychological assessments.

Jennifer Rooke, MD, MPH, is a Clinical Assistant Professor in the Department of Community Health and Preventive Medicine at Morehouse School of Medicine. She is certified in lifestyle medicine and founded the Optimal Health and Wellness Clinic at Morehouse Healthcare. Dr. Rooke envisions a world free of preventable diseases, where all people may enjoy the physical, emotional, and social health necessary to reach their full potential.

Lynn Rosenberg, ScD, is an epidemiologist at the Slone Epidemiology Center at Boston University and Professor of Epidemiology in the Boston University School of Public Health. Dr. Rosenberg is one of the Principal Investigators and Founders of the Black Women's Health Study.

Andrea Serano, BS, holds a Bachelor of Science in Maternal Child Health with an emphasis in human lactation from Union Institute and University. Her work in breastfeeding advocacy stems from her passion for addressing maternal and infant health issues, especially among communities of color.

Calah Singleton, MSc, is a writer, editor, and mental health advocate. She is a graduate of Yale University and the London School of Economics and Political Science. Originally from Atlanta, Georgia, she now lives in London, United Kingdom, where she is an editor at Profile Books and Souvenir Press. She is also the cofounder of Mendü, a start-up focused on the mental well-being of women of color.

Vivian C. Smith, PhD, is the Chair and Associate Professor in the Department of Sociology and Criminology at Cabrini University. Her research focuses on understanding the collateral consequences of mass incarceration, factors related to substance abuse, drug policy, gender, and crime.

Maisha Standifer, PhD, MPH, is the Director of Health Policy in the Satcher Health Leadership Institute at Morehouse School of Medicine. In her role, Dr. Standifer conducts studies and administers evidence-based prevention initiatives that effectively employ targeted strategies to reduce negative health outcomes throughout underresourced, racially and ethnically vulnerable populations. She brings her wealth of experience, including health program administration, evaluation and research expertise, health policy development and analysis, mixed methods research, and examining social and political determinants of health.

Shavaun S. Sutton is a doctoral student in the Department of Sociology at Northeastern University. She holds a Master of Public Health degree in community health sciences from SUNY Downstate School of Public Health. She strives to promote equity via the analysis of nuanced narratives and lived experience.

Cheryl Taylor, PhD, MN, RN, FAAN, is an Associate Professor, Southern University College School of Nursing.

Shenique Thomas-Davis, PhD, is an Assistant Professor in the Criminal Justice Program at the City University of New York-Borough of Manhattan Community College. Her research sits within a criminology and human development framework and examines the social consequences of mass imprisonment efforts on individuals, family systems, and communities, race-related stress, and public policy.

Anika Thrower, PhD, MPH, served in Women, Infants, and Children's (WIC) programs around the United States for over 16 years. Because of her background, service, and research, she has expertise in utilizing the transtheoretical behavioral health model in underrepresented populations. She serves as an Assistant Professor within the Health Education department at City University of New York-Borough of Manhattan Community College.

Henrie M. Treadwell, PhD, is Founding Director of Community Voices: HealthCare for the Underserved and is Research Professor, Department of Community Health and Preventive Medicine. Prior to joining the Morehouse School of Medicine, she served for 17 years as Program Director, Health, at the Kellogg Foundation and was responsible for grantmaking in the United States, Central and Latin America, southern Africa and China.

Beverly Udegbe is a sophomore at Tufts University. She is on the premedicine track with a major in community health and minor in Spanish. Also, she is Research Assistant for Somerville Homeless Coalition and the Maternal Outcomes for Translational Health Equity Research (MOTHER) lab.

Rachel Villanueva, MD, is a Clinical Assistant Professor of Obstetrics/Gynecology at the NYU Grossman School of Medicine. Dr. Villanueva is a women's health expert and advocate who is committed to reproductive justice, health equity, workforce diversity, and disease prevention. She was recently elected President of the National Medical Association.

Christopher Villongco, MD, a psychiatrist, is faculty at Morehouse School of Medicine, Department of Psychiatry and Behavioral Sciences. His current research focuses on addiction medicine and collaborative care in the Philippines.

Chidi Wamuo, MD, is a graduate of the residency program of the Department of Psychiatry and Behavioral Sciences at Morehouse School of Medicine. His interests include child/adolescent mental health, mental health advocacy, and increasing diversity within health care.

Mildred Watson-Baylor, PsyD, is the Founder and Director of Clinical Services at Ferris Healthcare Group. Dr. Mildred Watson is a licensed professional counselor (LPC) who specializes in reproductive and maternal mental health providing empathic, quality care to women experiencing infertility, reproductive loss, and birth trauma.

Taylor A. Wimbly, MPH, is passionate about working to improve minority health within her community. She currently serves as a Program Manager at Morehouse School of Medicine, managing a research project to increase COVID-19 testing among minorities at risk for or living with diabetes.

Asha S. Winfield, PhD, is an assistant professor at LSU's Manship School of Mass Communication. Winfield is a critical/cultural media scholar with a focus on the stories (creation, rituals, and practices) of Black individuals and groups occurring in the media, culture, and society. As a researcher and filmmaker, she aims to use intersectionality, counternarratives, and Black feminist thought to frame and center the experiences of Black people as they relate to audience reception.

Glenda Wrenn Gordon, MD, MSHP, is the Chief Medical Officer, 180 Health Partners, Associate Professor, Department of Psychiatry and Behavioral Science, Morehouse School of Medicine, and Adjunct Associate Professor at Emory University in the Department of Psychiatry. She is a nationally recognized expert in mental health policy, trauma and resilience, and mental health equity. A board-certified psychiatrist, her professional mission is to create and foster environments where people impacted by mental health challenges and adversity can build a good life and recover.

Gail E. Wyatt, PhD, has been awarded the Dena Bat Yaacov Endowed Chair in Psychiatry. A clinical psychologist and licensed sex therapist, Dr. Wyatt is a Distinguished Professor of Psychiatry and Bio Behavioral Sciences at the Semel Institute of Neuroscience and Behavior at the David Geffen School of Medicine and the first African American Psychologist at DGSOM to be so awarded.

About the Coeditors

Kisha Braithwaite Holden, PhD, MSCR, is a psychologist, the Poussaint-Satcher Endowed Chair in Mental Health, and Associate Director of the Satcher Health Leadership Institute at Morehouse School of Medicine (MSM), located in Atlanta, Georgia. Also at MSM, Dr. Holden is Professor and Director of Research and Scholarship for the Department of Psychiatry and Behavioral Sciences; and Professor in the Department of Community Health and Preventive Medicine. Dr. Holden is an Adjunct Professor at Emory University School of Medicine, Department of Psychiatry and Behavioral Sciences.

Camara Phyllis Jones, MD, MPH, PhD, is a family physician and epidemiologist who is currently a Leverhulme Visiting Professor in Global Health and Social Medicine in the School of Global Affairs at King's College London. As President of the American Public Health Association (2016), she launched the association on a National Campaign Against Racism with three tasks: name racism; ask, "How is racism operating here?"; and organize and strategize to act. Her presidential initiative catalyzed the first of what are now 260 declarations by local jurisdictions (city councils, county commissions, state legislatures) across 41 states and the District of Columbia that "racism is a public health crisis."

Index

abortion, 199–200, 201–4
Abrams, Stacey, 50, 318, 320, 323–24, 325, 328
activism: communicating experiences and, 397–98; demands for maternity care and breastfeeding support, 175; need for organized resistance, 297–301; and political office, 210; and recovery from trauma, 240; for reproductive justice, 199–204; and well-being, 232; White women and, 395. *See also* anti-racism primer; Black feminism; Black Mamas Matter Alliance (BMMA); multimedia; political power; Reaching Our Sisters Everywhere (ROSE); resistance; violence
adaptability, 22–26, 213
adinkra symbols, 11–12, 85–86, 213–14, 307, 308
Adverse Childhood Experiences Study, 236
Affordable Care Act (ACA), 79
African American Breastfeeding Blueprint, 178
African Americans: experience of stress by, 143, 150–51; media consumption of, 41; and mental illness, 157, 162; microaggressions experienced by, 186; religiosity of, 285. *See also* Black children; Black women
African Baobab tree, 17
Agricultural Research Service (ARS), 103
AIDS service organizations, 135. *See also* HIV
Alang, Sirry, et al., 357
Alghanee, Njere Akosua Aminah, 325
Ali, Qairo "Shevevyah," 294
Allen, Debbie, 355–56
alopecia, 147–48
Ameena Matthews, 325
American exceptionalism, myth of, 382–83, 407
American Medical Association (AMA), 102, 351
American Psychiatric Association, 164
American Psychological Association, 4–5, 164
American Public Health Association (APHA), 365
Anderson, Esther, 355
Anderson, J. R., and W. L. Turner, 270
Angelou, Maya, 17, 65, 231
anti-racism primer: barriers to equity, 368, 382–83, 407; collective action, 366–67, 371, 384, 385–86; eight

anti-racism primer *(continued)*
    elements in, 367–69; essential tasks in a national campaign, 369–73; habits of mind for social justice warriors, 368, 384–85, 402–4; key messages in naming racism, 368, 374–76, *376*; levels of racism, 368, 375, 381; naming racism and moving to action, 365–67, 369, 385–86; principles for equity, 368, 381; recommendation and call for action, 386–87; resources, 387–88; strategies to dismantle racism, 368, 383–84; values targets, 406–8
anxiety disorders, 159, *159*
Aretha Franklin, 291
Arts and Humanities Committee, 356
assisted reproductive technologies (ART), 189, 190
Association of Black Psychologists, 165
atherosclerosis, 110–11
Atlanta Reproductive Justice Commission, 328
Aunt Jemima, 32–33
autoimmune disorders: Black women and, 145, 152; case study, 147–50; diagnosis, causes, and treatment of, 144, 145, 149–50; incidence of, 144; list of, *145*; progression of illness, 151–52; recommendation and call for action, 152–53; and stress, 143, 146, 150–51; symptoms, 147
Avery, Byllye Yvonne, 290, 327, 392, 394–99, 401, 402, 404–6, 408, 409
Avery Institute for Social Change, 290

Baby-Friendly Hospital Initiative (BFUSA), 176, 179
Bailey, A., 24
Bailey, Moya, 322
Baker, Ella, 320, 325

Baldwin, James, 297
Bandura, A., 71
Banks-Wallace, J. A., 69
bariatric surgery, 109
Barnhill, Sandra, 324, 325
Bartmann, Sarah (Saartjie) (aka Hottentot Venus), 39
Bass, Charlotta, 325
Baumfree, Isabella. *See* Truth, Sojourner
beauty, 11, 35
Benjamin, Lila, 18
Bessie Smith, 291
Beyonce, 73, 398
Biles, Simone, 163
biocultural citizenship, 258
bioethics: and death, 265–67; and end-of-life care in Black communities, 266–68; equity-oriented perspectives in, 271–73; and impacts on Black women, 270–71; need for change, 273; resources, 274; violent deaths, 269
Black children: foundation of resiliency in, 16; incarceration of parents and trauma for, 219–20; media stereotypes and, 40; programs to reduce infant mortality, 178. *See also* Black girls
Black consciousness, 24–25
Black female artists, 346, 347–48
Black feminism, 67, 73
"Black Girl Magic," 2, 21, 73, 129–30, 138
Black girls: advocacy and support for developing and pregnant, 326–27; risks experienced by, 233–34, 235
Black Girls Rock! (BGR!), 2, 41
Black intellectuals, 350
Black Lives Matter movement, 271
Black Mamas Matter Alliance (BMMA), 26, 181, 326

Black Maternal Health Week, 326
Black motherhood: adaptability in, 23–26; advancement of, 26–28, 27–28; coordinated interventions to assist mothers, 326; and infertility, 188, 193; Lucy as the original Black mother, 15–16; matriarchs' stories of resilience, 17–21; and mindfulness, 21, 22; mother-child bond, 16–17, 172; and professional opportunities, 57; resilience in, 15, 16, 26; seeking professional help, 25; and sexual stereotypes, 32; and social activism, 210; and weight, 354; and work-life balance, 21–23, 23
Black Power movement, 321
Black womanhood: and collective consciousness, 7; core issues in, 2; and strength, 72. See also Black feminism
Black women: as caregivers, 270; dehumanization of, 31; and drive to prove worthiness, 47–48; experiments using, 39; looking to the past to build strength, 334–35, 391; Malcolm X on, 15; morbidity and mortality statistics regarding, 52–53, 119, 121, 172, 186, 187; multiplicity of roles played by, 122, 319; need for social support, 335; and objectification, 132; as political, 392–93; and politics of respectability and silence, 36–37; powerlessness, responsibility, and survival, 217–18; and the quilt of experiences, 73–74; quotes about, 65–66; shaming of, 108, 133; stress experienced by, 21; terms used to refer to, 279; use of the term *African American*, 2; vulnerability of, 322; and wealth, 51–52. See also

African Americans; Black female artists; Black girls; health and well-being; intersectionality; political power; resilience; stress; thought leaders
Black Women's Health Imperative (BWHI, formerly NBWHP), 61, 327, 409
Black Women's Health Study (BWHS): description of, 90; findings, 91–94; recommendation and call for action, 94–95; willingness to participate in, 90–91
Black Women Vote (BWHI), 327
Bland, Sandra, 288, 357
Blount, Linda Goler, 409
BLWH, 134, 137
Bond, Beverly, 41
Boosie, Lil', 66
Boston Medical Center, 177
Bottoms, Keisha Lance, 324
Braun, Carol Moseley, 318
Brave Heart, Maria Yellow Horse, 299
bravery and strength, 307
breast cancer, 89, 92, 94, 287, 318
breastfeeding: benefits of, 172; decolonization and promotion of, 180–81; historical perspective on, 172–75; men's roles in, 178; mentoring and lactation support, 179–80; rates of, 171–72, 174, 178; recommendations and call for action, 181–82; ROSE and lactation support, 175–78, 179, 180
Breastfeeding and Equity Summits, 176
Brewer, Rosalind, 50
Brinson, Esther, 19
Brody, Howard, 358
Brown, Linda, 20
Brown, Michael, 357
Browne, Adele, 20; "Face Your PACE," 87–88

Bruner, Jerome, *Making Stories,* 69
Bryant, Ma'Khia, 312–13
Bureau of Primary Health Care, 354
Burke, Yvonne Braithwaite, 17
Burton, L. M., and K. E. Whitfield, 151
Buttigieg, Pete, 79
BWHI. *See* Black Women's Health Imperative
BWHS. *See* Black Women's Health Study (BWHS)

Cahill, Lisa, 266
California's anti-discrimination laws, 36
cancers: CDC fact sheet, *206–7*; as continuing concern, 414; mortality rates, 354. *See also* specific types
capitalism and public health, 6
cardiovascular disease (CVD): Black women's incidence of, 89, 101, 105; as continuing concern, 413; COVID-19 and, 94; hypertension, 109, 110, 152, 172, 186, 211, 224, 270, 346; meat consumption and, 104, 105; morbidity and mortality from, 53, 109–10, 152, 354; and PCOS, 190; and rheumatoid arthritis, 152; and trauma, 161
caregivers for children of incarcerated parents: Black women's burden as, 219; devotion in caregiving, 221; extent of need, 219; health of caregivers and children, *224*; methods for studying lived experience of, 220–21; recommendations and call for action, 227; and resilient faith, 225–26; resources for, 228; surrender-resilience, 221–23, 226–27
Carlton, Carl, 66
Carmichael, Stokely, 348

Carnes, M., 353
CATO Institute, 312
CDC. *See* Centers for Disease Control and Prevention (CDC)
Center for Reproductive Rights, 326
Center for Social Inclusion, 181
Centers for Disease Control and Prevention (CDC): Black researchers at, 293; cancer fact sheet, *206–7*; Hear Her Campaign fact sheet, *205*; HIV prevention, 131; information on CVD, 110; lupus reports, 144; and risks to youth, 248, 249
CHAMPS. *See* Communities and Hospitals Advancing Maternal Practices (CHAMPS)
Chapman, E. N., 353
charisma, adinkra symbol for, 85
Charleston Code, 321
Chávez, V., 257
Chisolm, Shirley, 318, 320, 324–25
Christensen, Donna, 341
chronic disease, 55, 60, 89, 104–5, 186, 354. *See also* autoimmune disorders; cardiovascular disease (CVD); diabetes; stress
cisgender women, 240n2
civil rights movement, 175, 185, 320, 321, 347–49, 354
Clance, Pauline Rose, 336
Clarke, John Henrik, *Black/White Alliances,* 320
Clayton, Dominque, 313
Clemetson, L., 21–22
Cliff Analogy for levels of health intervention, 371–73, *373*
Clifton, Lucille, "won't you celebrate with me," 273–74
Colbert, Steven, 394
Collaborative Group on Hormonal Factors in Breast Cancer, 89

collective action: Black women's history of, 7; building, 384, 386; importance of, 2, 4, 367, 371, 396; power of, 384, 385, 391, 403
colorectal cancer, 94
Coltrane, Alice, 291
commentaries: on abortion as a reproductive justice issue, 199–204; on achieving health equity, 408; on activism and activists, 397–98, 402–3; on anti-racism action and values, 406–8; on Black women, 392–93, 395, 396–97; on community resilience, 393–94; on the health care system, 398, 402; on hope, 402; on listening to young people, 395–96; on maternal mortality, 401–2; need for organized resistance, 297–301; pearls of wisdom, 408–9; on racism and capitalism, 398–401; on resilience in sexual and gender difference, 77–80; on self-knowledge, 405–6; on trauma, 406
Communities and Hospitals Advancing Maternal Practices (CHAMPS), 177, 179
community: and breastfeeding in Black communities, 175; as foundation of health and wellness, 7; improving health and, 95. *See also* collective action
community resilience, 5
complementary and alternative medicine (CAM), 25
complex trauma, 160–61, 162, 235
cooperation and interdependence, 12
courage, 85
COVID-19 pandemic: Angela Geter's work during, 324; and bioethics, 272; Black women as frontline workers during, 66–67, 120–22; and Black women's mental health, 118–19, 120, 121; and carceral facilities, 218–19; and the caregiver burden, 122–23; as continuing concern, 413; and CVD, 94; and health equity, 402; impact on communities of color, 118, 366; Keys on, 357; and maternal health, 119–20; recommendation and call for action, 123–24; and spotlight on social inequities, 359
Creary, M. S., 258
Crenshaw, Kimberlé Williams, 41, 117, 123; "Mapping the Margins," 232
Crown Act, 36, 284, 325–29
Crumpler, Rebecca Lee, 17
culture: Black women's contributions to, 304; cultural norms, 412. *See also* beauty; Black motherhood; education; hair; mass media; quilters; stereotypes of Black Women; storytelling; Superwoman Schema (SWS)
culture of dissemblance, 257
CVD. *See* cardiovascular disease (CVD)

Danis, M., et al., 267
Danner, Deborah, 315
death and dying: bioethical approaches to, 265–67; death anxiety, 269, 270; end-of-life care in Black communities, 267–69; equity perspectives in public policy and end-of-life care, 271–73; and impacts on Black women, 270–71
Debbie Allen Dance Academy, 356
decolonization, 179, 180–81, 394, 407
Defense of Marriage Act (DOMA), 79
Degenholtz, H. B., et al., 268
Department of Health and Human Services (DHHS), *Healthy People*, 103, 171

depression, 159, 161
dermatitis, 148–49
Destiny's Child, 66
diabetes, 89, 92, 109, 354
Diabetes Care in General Practice study, 109
diet and nutrition: and CVD, 109–11; fasting, 287–88; food consumption by ethnicity, *105*; guidelines for, 101, 102–4, 111; human milk in, 172; infant formula, 174; meat consumption patterns, 104, *106*, 110; recommendation and call for action, 111
Dietary Goals for the United States, 102–3
Dietary Guidelines for Americans, 101, 103, 104, 111
dignity and self-respect, 37
discrimination: anti-discrimination laws, 36; and the CROWN Act, 36; and White medical workers' assumptions, 38
Dixon Diallo, Dazon, 290
Dobard, R. G., 320
Dobbs v. Jackson Women's Health Organization, 200
domestic violence, 234, 257, 312, 397
Drucker, Ernest, 218
DuBois, W. E. B., 37, 298
Durvasula, R., 130

Economic Research Service (ERS), 103
education: and Black history, 194; learning from the past, 308; marginalization of girls within the educational system, 234; mission of Black education, 299–300
Elbert, Donnie, 65
elders, connecting with, 391
Elders, Joycelyn, 354–55

emotion and feelings, expressing, 24
end-of-life care. *See* death and dying
endurance, 214
eugenics, 200
European Prospective Investigation into Cancer and Nutrition-Physical Activity, Nutrition, Alcohol, Cessation of Smoking, Eating Out of Home and Obesity (EPIC-PANACEA), 108

faith and religion: Black women as leaders in, 285; and caregiving for children with incarcerated parents, 225–26; in end-of-life care, 268; faith community and sexual and gender minorities, 78, 79; meaning of faith, 280; and mental health, 53–54, 56, 133, 137, 163; religious institutions and HIV stigma, 133; resilience and, 237; and womanist theological bioethics, 271–72. *See also* spirituality
families, survival and socialization through, 218
fatigue, debilitating, 147–48
Fauset, Crystal Bird, 318
"Feel some type of way," 248, 258
Ferebee, Dorothy Boulding, 341
Fitzgerald, Ella, 291
Floyd, George, 366
Foley, Lelia, 318
food industry, 102, 103, 173, 174
Forbes Fortune 500, 50
Ford, Hester, 17
Foreverfamily, 324
fortitude, 213, 308
Fossil Hominid Sites of South Africa, 15
Foxx, Jamie, 66
Frank, Arthur, 70–71
Franklin, Aretha, 73

French, B. H., 257
Full Frame Initiative, 232

Gaston, Marilyn Hughes, 341, 354–55
Gaye, Marvin, 394
gender and gender equity, 132, 161, 248, 321
Georgia, political power in, 323–24
Georgia election of 2020, 50
Geronimus, Arline T., 23–24, 346
Geter, Angelica, 324
Giddings, P., 290
Global Gag Rule, 201
grandmothers as caregivers, 219, 220, 222–23, 224, 226
Gray, Freddie, 322
Gregory, Lillian E., 18
griottes, 68
Gurusami, S., 220

hair: alopecia, 147–48; discrimination related to, 284, 328; hirsutism, 190; pride in, 304; self-image, and opportunity, 35–36
Hammer, Fannie Lou, 320, 325
Harris, Kamala, 17, 50, 317, 318, 320, 322, 323, 325
Harris v. McRae, 201
Hatshepsut, 320
Hayden, Dolores, 251
HBCU. *See* Historically Black Colleges and Universities
health and well-being: adaptability and, 22–26; as communal processes, 2; community as foundation of, 7; curative and preventive services for, 372; discrimination, microaggressions, and, 186; epidemiologic snapshot of Black women, 89–95; factors in achieving, 232, 237; frontline workers, 120–21; incarceration and, 122, 131, 220; journaling and, 22; promotion of, 3; racism as detriment to, 346–47; and risks facing girls, 233–34; social determinants of health, 372; socioeconomic status and, 6, 79, 187; spirituality and faith in, 280, 285; stereotype threat and, 38; structural inequities and disparities affecting, 174–75. *See also* activism; AIDS; autoimmune disorders; bioethics; Black girls; breastfeeding; cancers; cardiovascular disease (CVD); caregivers for children of incarcerated parents; COVID-19 pandemic; death and dying; diabetes; infertility; intersectionality; maternal health; mental health; public health; reproductive justice; spirituality; stress; violence
healthcare practitioners: diversity and professionalization of, 181, 193; frontline workers, 120–21; and naming racism, 368; public health professionals, 280, 284
health equity: achieving, 1, 328, 398–400; community resilience in, 5; examples of inequity, 186–87; and infertility, 193; principles of and barriers to, 381–83; social determinants of, 373
Health Security Act, 202
Healthy People, 103, 171
Henry, John, 48
Herman, Judith, 236
heroism, 85
Hill Collins, Patricia, 41, 42–43, 185, 220
Historically Black Colleges and Universities (HBCUs), 180, 181
HIV: experience of living with, 129, 135–37; rates of infection

HIV *(continued)*
    and interventions, 130–31, 132; recommendation and call for action, 138; and resilience, 133–35, 138; risk for, 131–33; self-efficacy and social support, 135, 136, 137
HIV National Strategic Plan, 2021–2025, 131
Holiday, Billie, 291
hooks, bell, 359, 397
Houston, Whitney, "I Didn't Know My Own Strength," 129
humility, 213
Hurston, Zora Neal, 289
Hyde Amendment, 201
hysterectomies, 93, 186

Ibarra, H., et al., 340
IBCLC. *See* International Board-Certified Lactation Consultants
identity: and caregivers of children of incarcerated parents, 222; commentary on resilience in difference, 77–80; defining, 67; gender, justice, and equality in, 37; intersectionality and, 231, 233; the quilt as a metaphor for, 74; resilience in, 71–73. *See also* intersectionality
IDP. *See* individual development plans
Imes, Suzanna, 336
immune system, functioning of, 144
imperialists and Black women, 352–53
implicit bias, 353–54
imposter syndrome, 335–37
incarceration: and Black communities, 218–19; of Black girls and women, 234–35; and child visiting centers, 324; mass incarceration and the Black community, 218–19, 225, 226–27; study of caregivers for children affected by, 220–27
individual development plans (IDP), 341, 342
infertility: assisted reproductive technologies (ART), 189, 190; Black women's higher rates of, 188–89, 318; causes of, 189–90; cultural factors and, 192–93, 194; and intersectionality, 185, 194; need for research on, 192, 194; as public health issue, 188–89; recommendation and call for action, 194–95; support for Black women experiencing, 191–92
In Our Own Voice, 202
intelligence and ingenuity, 12
International Association of Women (IAW), 61
International Board-Certified Lactation Consultants (IBCLCs), 177, 180, 181
intersectional complex trauma: Black women's risk of, 231, 239; definition of, 231; description of, 235–36; psychological effects of, 238; recommendation and call for action, 240; recovery from, 236–37, 239
intersectionality: axes of power and division in, 185; coinage and meanings of, 117–18; and COVID-19, 123; experience of, 77, 232–33; and health, 118, 119, 138; Jordan's work on, 351; and mental illness, 157–59; and public health policy, 293; of racism and sexism, 31, 123, 160, 231–33, 270, 336, 338, 353; and risk factors for HIV, 132–33; of spirituality and health, 280, *281–83*. *See also* COVID-19 pandemic

in vitro fertilization (IVF), 189, 190–91, 193
IVF. *See* in vitro fertilization (IVF)

Jackson, B., 24
Jackson, Ketanji Brown, 21
Jackson, Mary, 17
James, Etta, 291
James, Rick, 66
Jarrett, R. L., 248
Jefferson, Atatiana, 313
Jenkins, Aleah, 314
Jezebel stereotype, 31–32, 37, 49, 352
John Henryism (JH) framework, 48
Johnson, Katherine, 17
Johnson & Johnson, 328
Jones, Camara Phyllis (CPJ), 365, 371–76, *376*, 378–80, *379*
Jones, Leslie Salmon, 287
Jones, L. M., et al., 270
Jordan, Barbara, 318, 325
Jordan, June, 349, 350–51
Judy M. Braithwaite Family Foundation, Inc. (JMBF Foundation), 26

Kaatz, A., 353
Kaepernick, Colin, Million Dollar Pledge initiative, 356
KAVI. *See* Women's Program of the Kings against Violence Initiative (KAVI)
Keys, Alicia, 356–57, 358
kidney health, 110
Kiehl, E. M., 24
King, Barbara, 285
King, Coretta Scott, 335
Krieger, Nancy, 300
Kryst, Cheslie, 163

Lacks, Henrietta, 186

leadership: adinkra symbol for, 85; building a support network, 338–40, 342; challenges faced in positions of, 320; definition and characteristics of, 333–34; growing pains in achieving success, 334–35; imposter syndrome and tokenism, 335–37; and life/work balance, 50–51; overcoming stereotypes, 337–38; recommendation and call for action, 342; resources for, 342; seeking and maintaining positions of, 50–51; and self-management, 60, 61; servant leadership approaches, 4; strategies for growth and resilience, 340–41, 342; and stress, 57
lesbian women: and complex trauma, 231; dating violence, 253–54; incarceration of, 234–35; and liberation psychology, 238–39; and sexual abuse, 234; use of *cisgender* for, 240n2
Levin, P. D., and C. L. Sprung, 267–68
Levine, Rachel, 79
LGBTQ+ people: and community coalitions, 349; and conversion therapies, 240; and dating violence, 253–54, 258; definition of, 240n1. *See also* lesbian women; transgenders
liberation psychology, 238–39
life expectancy, 94, 158
LookAHEAD trial, 109
Lorde, Audre, 42, 279, 359, 360
Lucy (Dinknesh), 15–16
Lupus Foundation of America, 145
Luth, E. A., and H. G. Prigerson, 269
Lyles, Charleena, 314
Lynch, Loretta, 325

Ma'at, Imani, "Sandra Bland," 308–9
MacPhail, S., 349
Mahoney, Mary Eliza, 341
Malcolm X, 15, 49, 66
Malcolm X weekend (Harvard University), 42
Mammy stereotype, 32–33, 49, 352
Marsh, E. E., et al., 327
Martin, Mimi, 19
Martin, Nina, 347
Martin, Trayvon, 357
mass media: Black biopics, 69; portrayals of Black women in, 40–41, 42. See also multimedia
maternal health: adequate care for Black women, 95; and breastfeeding, 171, 172; Hear Her Campaign fact sheet (CDC), 205; impact of COVID-19 on, 120; maternal mortality, 119, 271, 300, 318, 326, 354, 401–2; and mental illness, 120; political advocacy for, 326–27; structural inequities and disparities affecting, 174–75. See also infertility; pregnancy and childbirth
maternal mortality: and chronic stress, 38, 346; as critical health issue, 270, 271, 326, 354, 401–2; increase in, 119–20, 121, 174, 187, 203, 300, 401; societal inequities and, 318
Matriarch stereotype, 34
McBride, Jasmine, 314
McCurn, A. S., 256
McDaniel, Ozella, 321
McEwen, Tamia A., "Corona Reflections," 215–16
medical establishment: Black doctors in, 414; invisibility of Black women in, 24; mistreatment of Black women by, 186; rates of misdiagnosis by, 192; training and education needed in, 42
Mental Health (Surgeon General), 158
Mental Health America, 165
"Mental health and COVID-19," 66–67
mental health therapists, cultural competence of, 162, 164
mental illness: anxiety disorders, 159; definition of, 158; depression, 159, 161; incidence of, 157, 158, 159; and infertility, 190; post-traumatic stress disorder (PTSD), 160–61; promoting resilience and recovery, 162–64; racism and, 346–47; recommendation and call for action, 164; stigma from, 161–62; support resources, 162, 164–65; types of stressors, 161
mentors and coaches, 339–40
meritocracy, myth of, 382–83, 407
mindfulness, practicing, 163, 164
miscegenation, 33
misogynoir, 322
Montagne, Renee, 347
morbidity and mortality for Black women: all-cause, 52–53, 108, 109–10, 270; cancers, 53, 92, 254; COVID-19, 121–22; CVD, 53, 109–10, 152, 354; obesity, 94, 108–9; stress, 52, 186, 346. See also maternal mortality
Morgan, Jennifer, 352–53
Morrison, Toni, *Beloved,* 289
Mosby, Marilyn, 322
mother, definition and role of, 16. See also Black motherhood
Mother Ozen, 65
motherwork, 220
Moynihan, Daniel Patrick, 34
mulatto stereotype, 33
Mullings, Leith, 48

multimedia: art and what is possible, 359; artists and the promotion of holistic Black health, 351, 355–57; Black women's activism and influence through, 345–47, 358; depiction of Black women in, 351–53, 355–56; and implicit bias, 353–54; musical artists' influence in social justice and health, 347–51, 356–57; racial narratives in literature, 352; recommendation and call for action, 359–60; resources, 360; and seeing accurate representations of Black women, 358–59; and sickle-cell anemia, 355; as tool of liberation, 345, 359
Murray, Linda Rae, 393, 394, 395–96, 398–402, 404, 407, 408, 409
Musgrave, C. F., et al., 279
My Brothers' Keeper, 234

National Association for the Advancement of Colored People (NAACP), 37, 61–62
National Association of Colored Women, 37
National Black Women's Health Initiative, 289–90
National Black Women's Health Project (NBWHP, now BWHI), 290, 327, 384–85, 396–97
National Black Women's Justice Institute (NBWJI), 26
National Campaign Against Racism, 365, 368, 369–71
National Cancer Institute, 90
National Center for Health Statistics, 326
National Coalition of 100 Black Women (NCBW), 62
National Council of Negro Women (NCNW), 62

National Health and Nutrition Examination Survey (NHANES), 103
National Institute of Allergies and Infectious Disease, 144
National Institute of Mental Health, 159
National Institutes of Health (NIH), 110, 293
Naylor, Audrey, 180
NBWHP. *See* National Black Women's Health Project
The Negro Family: The Case for National Action, 34
New Jersey anti-discrimination laws, 36
New York State anti-discrimination laws, 36
Nixon administration, 218
Nonviolent Coordinating Committee Freedom Singers, 349
Note: Illustrations and tables are indicated by italicized page numbers.
nurturing and discipline, 12

Obama, Michelle, 17, 95, 188, 322
Obergefell v. Hodges, 79
obesity: and bariatric surgery, 109; Black women's rates of, 101, 105, 106, 107; chronic disease and, 108; definition and measurement of, 105–6; European study on, 108; factors in, 92, 93, *104*; federal dietary goals to address, 102; genetic factors in, 107; meat consumption and, 104, 107–8
Office of the Surgeon General, 354
Office of Women Health Helpline, 145
organizational resources: for antiracism, 387–88; for bioethics,

organizational resources *(continued)* 274; for caregivers for children of incarcerated parents, 228; for families affected by incarceration, *228*; for infertility, *191,* 195; for leadership, 342; for mental illness, 164–65; for multimedia narratives, 360; for political power, 329; for Sojourner Syndrome, 61–62; for spirituality, 294; for teens experiencing relationship violence, 259; for those with complex trauma, 240–41
Osaka, Naomi, 163
othermothers, 220
Overstreet, Mikkaka, 336
oxysterols, 110–11

Panel Study of Income Dynamics (PSID), 52
Patton, Lydia, 19
Payne, Charles, 321
peace and harmony, 86
Pedler, M., 337
perseverance, 307
Phillips, Abby, 21
physical activity, 25
poetry: "Corona Reflections" (McEwen), 215–16; "Face Your Pace" (Browne), 87–88; "Jubilation" (Singleton), 13–14; "Sandra Bland" (Ma'at), 308–9; in workshops to study experience, 250–51
Poitier, Sidney, *A Warm December,* 355
police violence, 270–71, 311–15, 356, 357
political power of Black women: to achieve public health goals, 325–29; categories of support in developing, 323–24, 329; development of resilience and, 319–25; and health and safety, 317–19, 324–25; leveraging of, 318; recommendation and call for action, 329; and resistance, 393; resources for resilience in, 329; through collective action, 366–67, 394, 395
politics, goal of, 321
polycystic ovarian syndrome (PCOS), 190
Porter, T., et al., "Bioethical Issues Concerning Death," 266, 267
post-traumatic stress disorder (PTSD), 160–61, 162
power: adinkra symbol for, 86; Black women as embodiment of, 393, 394–95, 396–97, 411
pregnancy and childbirth: adequate care for Black women, 95; forced, 201; Hear Her Campaign fact sheet (CDC), *205;* maternal mortality rate, 300, 326, 401–2; stress and negative outcomes, 38. *See also* infertility; maternal health
Pregnancy Risk Assessment Monitoring System (PRAMS), 178
Price, Leontyne, 291
Prograis, L., and E. D. Pellegrino, *African American Bioethics,* 267
Progressive Era reforms, 36–37
psychosocial stress, 93
PTSD. *See* post-traumatic stress disorder (PTSD)
public health: bioethics and, 273; Black women's presence in, 280, 284; Black women trailblazers in, 341, 354–55; creative narratives in, 359; cultural factors affecting Black Americans' relationship with, 193; curative and preventive services, 372; definition and scope of, 5–7; equity in, 41, 273, 324; Latin Americans and public health

theory, 300; Legionnaire's disease, 314; national policy agenda for Black women, 327; policies and practices, 101, 380; and political power, 317–19, 325–29; racism as crisis in, 346, 351, 357, 358, *370*; recommendations regarding spirituality and health, 292–93; social determinants of health, 372; stereotypes in health awareness campaigns, 38–39; women's success as leaders in, 334
public policy and Black Woman stereotypes, 41

Quaker Oats, 33
Queen Afua, 286, 287, 288
quilters, 74, 320–21

racism: allegories about, 374–76, *376*, 378–80, *379*; and Black history in education, 194; and capitalism, 399–401; and continued oppression, 173, 194–95; and COVID-19, 122; definition, 365; denial of, 378; harmful health effects of, 93, 106, 138, 186; and health care inequities, 186–87, 398–400; imperialism and, 352–53; implicit bias, 353; intersection with sexism, 231, 233; levels of, 377–79; mechanisms of racism in policies and practices, 370–71, 376; and mental illness therapy, 162; naming racism and moving to action, 365–66; oppressive nature of, 233; partnering to dismantle, 179; spiritual and faith practices and, 284; strength as protection from, 334; and texturism, 35–36; trauma and stress from, 160–61
Rao, D., et al., 134, 135, 136, 137

Reaching Our Brothers Everywhere (ROBE), 178
Reaching Our Sisters Everywhere (ROSE): African American Breastfeeding Blueprint, 178, 181; founding of, 175–76; and lactation support partnerships, 179; mission and strategies of, 176; ROSE Community Transformers, 176–77, 180; train the trainers initiative, 177–78
Reagon, Bernice Johnson, 348–51
recommendations and calls for action: and anti-racism, 386–87; for autoimmune disorders, 152–53; for Black motherhood, 26–28; for breastfeeding, 181–82; and BWHS, 94–95; for caregiving related to incarceration, 227; for diet and nutrition, 111; for dismantling stereotypes, 41–43; for HIV, 138; for infertility, 194–95; for intersectional complex trauma, 240; for leadership, 342; lessons from the elders, 74; for mental illness, 164; and multimedia narratives, 359–60; for political power, 329; and questions regarding COVID-19, 123–24; for reproductive justice, 199–204; Sojourner Syndrome best practices, 59–61; for spirituality and health, 292–93; for violence prevention, 258
renin-angiotensin-aldosterone system (RAAS), 110
Representation matters, 356
reproductive justice, 199–204, 328
resilience: Black mothers and survival, 22, 23; in Black women's history, 129–30, 319–20; and the decision to be resilient, 297–98; definition and conceptualization of, 4–5,

133–34, 236–37; factors related to, 134; importance of reclamation in, 351–52; and infertility, 190–91, *191*; and liberation psychology, 238–39; as nuanced in the Black community, 66–67; and political power, 317–19; protective factors in, 237; and recovery, 124; research on, 247–48; spiritual dimensions in, *291*. *See also* activism; antiracism primer; Black women; commentaries; culture; health and well-being; power; slavery; stereotypes of Black Women
resistance, 251–56, *255,* 297–301, 393, 394
respectability, politics of, 36–37
rheumatoid arthritis, 147, 150, 152
Rinzler, Ralph, 350
Roe v. Wade, 200, 201, 203
ROSE. *See* Reaching Our Sisters Everywhere (ROSE)
Ross, Loretta J., 41, 200, 202

Sacks, Alexandra, 24
Sanchez, Sonia, 289
San Diego lactation program (WellStart), 179, 180
Sapphire stereotype, 33–34, 188
SARS-CoV-2. *See* COVID-19 pandemic
Satcher, David, 176, 333
#SayHerName, 271, 311–15
Scott, K. Y., 222
self-care: and mental health, 163, 164; public health policies for, 329; scheduling, 58–59; and Sojourner Syndrome, 54–55, 59–60
Self Care Matters (Parris), 329
self-efficacy, 136
self-esteem, 137
self-love, 397

self-worth, 24
Senate Select Committee on Nutrition and Human Need, 102–3
Sentencing Project, 234
sexism: and Black women's lives, 231, 233; and equity and access, 79; heterosexism and public health, 6; and limited access to resources, 320; misogynoir, 322; and public health, 6; trauma and stress from, 160
sexuality: and health challenges for minorities, 78–80; repression of, 37; stereotyping and, 38–40. *See also* Jezebel stereotype; LGBTQ+ people
sexually transmitted diseases (STDs), 192
sexual misconduct by police officers, 311–12
sexual violence and abuse, 234, 397–98
Shabazz, Betty, 335
shaming, 108, 133, 257, 327
sickle-cell anemia, 355
Simone, Nina, 291, 347–48, 358
Simpson, Monica, 202, 329
Sims, J. Marion, 39
Singleton, Calah, "Jubilation," 13–14
SisterCARE Alliance, 329
sister circles, 289–91
Sister Love, Inc, 290
Sister Song, 329
SisterSong Women of Color Reproductive Justice Collective, 202
Slater, Priscilla, 313
slavery: forced reproductive labor during, 31, 173, 201; "health care" under, 186; interracial rape during, 33; and stereotypes of Black Women, 32, 33, 132; and uninvited vulnerability, 49
social determinants of health, 118, 119, 171

Index | 443

social justice warriors, 368, 384–85, 402–4

social learning theory, 71

social support networks, 163–64, 335, 338–39, 342

Sojourner Syndrome (SS): description of, 48–49; and life/work balance, 50–51, 56, 57; managing, 57–59; organizational resources, 61–62; and psychological, spiritual, physical, and emotional health, 52–56; recommendation and call for action, 59–61; and the responsibility of wealth, 51–52

Song, H., et al., 146

Sorkness, C. A., et al., 339

Soul Care, 357

Southern Prisoners' Defense Committee, 324

Special Supplemental Nutrition Program for Women, Infants, and Children (WIC), 174

Spencer, M. B., 248

spirituality: in Black women's resilience, *291*, 292; as core value in Black culture, 279–80; fasting, 287–88; meaning of, 279–80; meditation, 286–87; music, 291–92; recommendation and call for action, 292–93; resources regarding, 294; review of literature on, *281–83*; sister circles, 289–91; worship and prayer, 285–86; yoga, 287. *See also* faith and religion

Standifer, Maisha, 4

stereotypes of Black Women: actions to examine and change, 41–43; and adverse health outcomes, 187–88, 354; common stories about, 298; discarding negative images, 304; impact on health and sexuality, 38–39; and imposter syndrome, 336; in the media, 352–53; media influence on, 40–41; overcoming, 337–38, 347; politics of respectability and silence, 36–37; prevailing types, 31–35, 69; and risk for HIV, 133; stress caused by, 49; texturism, 35–36

Stokes, Dorothy, 19

storytelling: African oral traditions of, 68; as continued tradition, 72; and identity, 68–69; in media's Black biopics, 69; modern artists' stories, 73; structuring reality through, 70–71

stress: anxiety disorders and stressors, 159, *159*; black women, 157; the body's response to, 143; breastfeeding and, 172; and chronic conditions, 270; physiology of, 146–48; on public health professionals, 284; and returning to state of equilibrium, 346–47; types of stressors, 161. *See also* trauma

Strong Black Woman (SBW) stereotype: *Berkeley News* on, 334; description of, 34–35; and the hard work of resilience, 73; and imposter syndrome, 336–37; and loss, 71–72; and the mystification of strength, 70; as a survival technique, 69–70; and themes in stories regarding, 72. *See also* Superwoman Schema (SWS); Truth, Sojourner

structural racism, 377, 379, 380–81, 406

Substance Abuse and Mental Health Services Administration (SAMHSA), 237–38

Superwoman Schema (SWS), 49, 55, 122, 123, 188, 334, 336

Surgeon General's Call to Action to Support Breastfeeding, 176

surveys: experience and management of stress, 55–56; National Health and Nutrition Examination Survey (NHANES), 103; University of Michigan Health and Retirement Survey, 187
survival habits, 217–18
Sweet Honey in the Rock, 349, 350, 351
syndemics, 120
Systematic Lupus Erythematosus (SLE), 144–45, 147–50

The Talented Tenth, 37
Tatum, Beverly Daniel, *Why Are All the Black Kids Sitting Together in the Cafeteria?*, 375
Taylor, Breonna, 313, 322
Teigen, Chrissy, 188
tenacity, 85
Thomas, "Able" Mable, 325, 328
Thompson, CaShawn, 21
thought leaders: on Black women and their resilience, 81–82, 209–11, 303–5, 411, 413; on Black women's health concerns, 82–83, 211, 305, 413–14; challenges to overcome, 413–14; on contributions to society, 412; interviews with, 4
Tobin, J., 320
tokenism, 336
Townes, Emilie, 272
transgenders, 234–35
trauma: adverse health effects from, 236; Black women's risk for, 231; complex, 160–61, 162, 235; and DNA, 406; experienced by Black women with political power, 322; lived experience and historical trauma, 299; police violence and, 357; trauma-informed care, 237–38, 239. *See also* intersectional complex trauma
trust and empowerment, 136, 137, 238, 239
Truth, Sojourner, 47–49, 65, 325, 334; "Ain't I a Woman?," 47, 48, 284–85
Tubman, Harriett, 17, 48, 286, 320, 325, 334
Tucker, R. T., 269
Turner, Pamela, 314
"23 Ways," 356
Tyson, Cicely, 294

Ufot, Nsé, 323–24
Underground Railroad, 320, 321
unemployment rates for Black women, 123
Ungar, M., 134
United States Department of Agriculture (USDA), 101, 103
United States v. Windsor, 79
unity, 86
Urban League, 37
U.S. Supreme Court, 21, 79, 200, 201, 392
uterine fibroids, 93, 189–90

Vaughn, Dorothy, 17
Veatch, Robert, 266
violence: coping strategies, 257–58; domestic violence, 257; psychological and emotional abuse, 254, 257; sexual violence, 252–53, 255, 256–57; street harassment, 251–52, 256; teen dating violence, 248–49. *See also* death and dying
violence prevention for Black girls: Black girls' experiences, 251–54, 256–58; coping strategies, 254–55, 257–58; data and analysis in studying KAVI, 250–51; KAVI

program, 249; prevalence of dating violence, 248–49; recommendation and call for action, 258; resources for, 259; spaces of Black girl resilience and resistance, 251–56, 255
voter registration, 321

Waite, R., and P. Killian, 161
Walker, Alice, 272, 289
Walker-Barnes, C., *Too Heavy a Yoke*, 35
Ward, E. C., and colleagues, 161
Washington, Booker T., 37
We Are Here Movement, 356
weathering, 52–53
Webster v. Reproductive Health Services, 200
Welfare Mother stereotype, 34, 40, 49, 188
Wells, Ida B., 325
We Remember: African American Women for Reproductive Freedom, 199, 200
"We Shall Overcome," 349
West African oral traditions, 68
West Side Story, 355
Wethers, Doris, 355
White House Office of Sexual and Reproductive Health and Well-Being, 202, 203
White supremacist ideology, 69, 181, 265, 273, 298, 357, 380, 383, 407–8

White supremicists, 395
WIC, 177
William Lloyd Garrison Ally Award, 180
Williams, Serena, 398
Wilson, Wylin, 272
Winfrey, Oprah, 397
wisdom, traditional, 11–12
wisdom and patience, 214
W. K. Kellogg Foundation grants, 176
Wojtasiewicz, M. E., 267
Wolf, Susan, 266
womanist frameworks, 280
womanist theological bioethics, 271–74
Women of African Descent for Reproductive Justice, 202
Women's Program of the Kings against Violence Initiative (KAVI), 249–51, 254–55, 257–58
Woods, Alteria, 314–15
Woods-Giscombe, Cheryl, 49, 53
work cultures and imposter syndrome, 337
World Health Organization, 159

Youth Risk Behavior Surveillance System (YRBS), 248

Zaw, K., et al., 51
Zeitlin, Jide, 50
zero-sum game, myth of, 382–83, 407